Current Developments in
Stem Cell Transplantation

Current Developments in Stem Cell Transplantation

Edited by **Rex Turner**

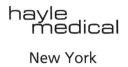

New York

Published by Hayle Medical,
30 West, 37th Street, Suite 612,
New York, NY 10018, USA
www.haylemedical.com

Current Developments in Stem Cell Transplantation
Edited by Rex Turner

© 2015 Hayle Medical

International Standard Book Number: 978-1-63241-102-0 (Hardback)

Printed in the United States of America.

Contents

             Permissions

             List of Contributors

Preface

Every book is a source of knowledge and this one is no exception. The idea that led to the conceptualization of this book was the fact that the world is advancing rapidly; which makes it crucial to document the progress in every field. I am aware that a lot of data is already available, yet, there is a lot more to learn. Hence, I accepted the responsibility of editing this book and contributing my knowledge to the community.

This book presents a number of basic applications, outlook for the future and research related to stem cell. It encompasses a broad spectrum of matters in regenerative medicine and cell-based therapy, and consists of information on preclinical basis contributed by renowned authors associated with this field. It elucidates the basics of stem cell physiology, hematopoietic stem cells, mesenchymal cells, tissue typing, dendritic cells, neuroscience, endovascular cells and other tissues. Evidently, the continued use of biomedical engineering will rely greatly on stem cells, and this book is well designed to educate the readers by providing elaborative coverage of these advancements.

While editing this book, I had multiple visions for it. Then I finally narrowed down to make every chapter a sole standing text explaining a particular topic, so that they can be used independently. However, the umbrella subject sinews them into a common theme. This makes the book a unique platform of knowledge.

I would like to give the major credit of this book to the experts from every corner of the world, who took the time to share their expertise with us. Also, I owe the completion of this book to the never-ending support of my family, who supported me throughout the project.

Editor

Basic Aspects of Stem Cell Transplantation

Generation of Patient Specific Stem Cells: A Human Model System

Stina Simonsson, Cecilia Borestrom and Julia Asp
Department of Clinical Chemistry and Transfusion Medicine,
Institute of Biomedicine, University of Gothenburg, Gothenburg
Sweden

1. Introduction

In 2006, Shinya Yamanaka and colleagues reported that only four transcription factors were needed to reprogram mouse fibroblasts back in development into cells similar to embryonic stem cells (ESCs). These reprogrammed cells were called induced pluripotent stem cells (iPSCs). The year after, iPSCs were successfully produced from human fibroblasts and in 2008 reprogramming cells were chosen as the breakthrough of the year by Science magazine. In particular, this was due to the establishment of patient-specific cell lines from patients with various diseases using the induced pluripotent stem cell (iPSC) technique. IPSCs can be patient specific and therefore may prove useful in several applications, such as; screens for potential drugs, regenerative medicine, models for specific human diseases and in models for patient specific diseases. When using iPSCs in academics, drug development, and industry, it is important to determine whether the derived cells faithfully capture biological processes and relevant disease phenotypes. This chapter provides a summary of cell types of human origin that have been transformed into iPSCs and of different iPSC procedures that exist. Furthermore we discuss advantages and disadvantages of procedures, potential medical applications and implications that may arise in the iPSC field.

1.1 Preface

For the last three decades investigation of embryonic stem (ES) cells has resulted in better understanding of the molecular mechanisms involved in the differentiation process of ES cells to somatic cells. Under specific *in vitro* culture conditions, ES cells can proliferate indefinitely and are able to differentiate into almost all tissue specific cell lineages, if the appropriate extrinsic and intrinsic stimuli are provided. These properties make ES cells an attractive source for cell replacement therapy in the treatment of neurodegenerative diseases, blood disorders and diabetes. Before proceeding to a clinical setting, some problems still need to be overcome, like tumour formation and immunological rejection of the transplanted cells. To avoid the latter problem, the generation of induced pluripotent stem (iPS) cells have exposed the possibility to create patient specific ES-like cells whose differentiated progeny could be used in an autologous manner. An adult differentiated cell has been considered very stable, this concept has however been proven wrong experimentally, during the past decades. One ultimate experimental proof has been cloning

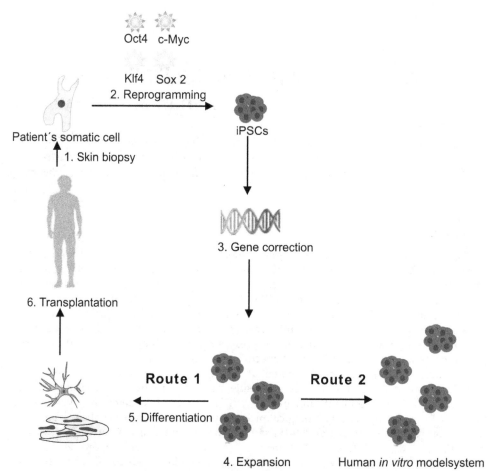

Fig. 1. Schematic picture of establishment of patient-specific induced pluripotent stem cells (iPSCs), from which two prospective routes emerge1) *in vivo* transplantation 2) *in vitro* human model system. Patient-specific induced pluripotent stem cells that are similar to embryonic stem cells (ESCs) are produced by first 1) collecting adult somatic cells from the patient, for example skin fibroblasts by a skin biopsy, 2) and reprogramming by retroviral transduction of defined transcription factors (Oct4, c-Myc, Klf4 and Sox 2 or other combinations) in those somatic fibroblast cells. Reprogrammed cells are selected by the detection of endogenous expression of a reprogramming marker, for example Oct4. 3) Generated patient-specific iPSCs can be genetically corrected of a known mutation that causes the disease. 4) Expansion of genetically corrected patient-specific iPSCs theoretically in eternity. First prospective route (Route 1): 5) upon external signals (or internal) iPSCs can theoretically be stimulated to differentiate into any cell type in the body. 6) In this way patient-specific dopamine producing nerve cells or skin cells can be generated and transplanted into individuals suffering from Parkinson´s disease or Melanoma respectively. Second route (Route 2): Generated disease-specific iPSCs can be used as a human *in vitro* system to study degenerative disorders or any disease, cause of disease, screening for drugs or recapitulate development.

animals using somatic cell nuclear transfer (SCNT) to eggs. Such experiments can result in a new individual from one differentiated somatic cell. The much more recent method to reprogram cells was the fascinating finding that mouse embryonic fibroblasts (MEFs) can be converted into induced pluripotent stem cells (iPSCs) by retroviral expression of four transcription factors: Oct4, c-Myc, Sox2 and Klf4. iPSCs are a type of pluripotent stem cell derived from a differentiated somatic cell by overexpression of a set of proteins. Nowadays, several ways of generating iPSCs have been developed and includes 1) overexpression of different combinations of transcription factors most efficiently in combination with retroviruses (step 2 in Figure 1), 2) exposure to chemical compounds in combination with the transcription factors Oct4, Klf4 and retroviruses, 3) retroviruses alone, 4) recombinant proteins or 5) mRNA. The iPSCs are named pluripotent because of their ability to differentiate into all different differentiation pathways. Generation of patient-specific iPSC lines capable of giving rise to any desired cell type provides great opportunities to treat many disorders either as therapeutic treatment or discovery of patient specific medicines in human iPSC model systems (Figure 1). Here, some of this field's fast progress and results mostly concerning human cells are summarized.

2. Reprogramming-Induced Pluripotent Stem Cells (iPSCs)

Reprogramming is the process by which induced pluripotent stem cells (iPSCs) are generated and is the conversion of adult differentiated somatic cells to an embryonic-like state. Takahashi and Yamanaka demonstrated that retrovirus-mediated delivery of Oct4, Sox2, c-Myc and Klf4 is capable of inducing pluripotency in mouse fibroblasts (Takahashi and Yamanaka, 2006) and one year later was reported the successful reprogramming of human somatic fibroblast cells into iPSCs using the same transcription factors (Takahashi et al., 2007). Takahashi and Yamanaka came up with those four reprogramming proteins after a search for regulators of pluripotency among 24 cherry picked pluripotency-associated genes. These initial mouse iPSC lines differed from ESCs in that they had a diverse global gene expression pattern compared to ESCs and failed to produce adult chimeric mice. Later iPSCs were shown to have the ability to form live chimeric mice and were transmitted through the germ line to offspring when using Oct4 or Nanog as selection marker for reprogramming instead of Fbx15, which was used in the initial experiments (Meissner et al., 2007; Okita et al., 2007; Wernig et al., 2007). Various combinations of the genes listed in table 1 have been used to obtain the induced pluripotent state in human somatic cells. The first human iPSC lines were successfully generated by Oct4 and Sox2 combined with either, Klf4 and c-Myc, as used earlier in the mouse model, or Nanog and Lin28 (Lowry et al., 2008; Nakagawa et al., 2008; Park et al., 2008b; Takahashi et al., 2007; Yu et al., 2007). Subsequent reports have demonstrated that Sox2 can be replaced by Sox1, Klf4 by Klf2 and c-Myc by N-myc or L-myc indicating that they are not fundamentally required for generation of iPSCs (Yamanaka, 2009). Oct4 has not yet been successfully replaced by another member of the Oct family to generate iPSCs which is logical due to the necessity of Oct4 in early development. However, Blx-01294 an inhibitor of G9a histone methyl transferase, which is involved in switching off Oct4 during differentiation, enables neural progenitor cells to be reprogrammed without exogenous Oct4, although transduction of Klf4, c-Myc and Sox2 together with endogenous Oct4 was required (Shi et al., 2008). Recently, Oct4 has been replaced with steroidogenic factor 1, which controls Oct4 expression in ESCs by binding the

Oct4 proximal promoter, and iPSCs were produced without exogenous Oct4 (Heng et al., 2010). Remarkably, exogenous expression of E-cadherin was reported to be able to replace the requirement for Oct4 during reprogramming in the mouse system (Redmer et al., 2011). iPSCs are similar to embryonic stem cells (ESCs) in morphology, proliferation and ability to form teratomas. In mice, pluripotency of iPSCs has been proven by tetraploid complementation (Zhao et al., 2009). Both ESCs and iPSCs can be used as the pluripotent starting cells for the generation of differentiated cells or tissues in regenerative medicine. However, the ethical dilemma associated with ESCs is avoided when using iPSCs since no embryos are destroyed when iPSCs are obtained. Moreover, iPSCs can be patient-specific and as such patient-specific drugs can be screened and in personalized regenerative medicine therapies immune rejection could be circumvented. However the question surrounding the potential immunogenicity remains unclear due to recent reports that iPSCs do not form teratomas probably because iPSCs are rejected by the immune system (Zhao et al., 2011).

Genes	Description
Oct4	Transcription factor expressed in undifferentiated pluripotent embryonic stem cells and germ cells during normal development. Together with Nanog and Sox 2, is required for the maintenance of pluripotent potential.
Sox2	Transcription factor expressed in undifferentiated pluripotent embryonic stem cells and germ cells during development. Together with Oct4 and Nanog, is necessary for the maintenance of pluripotent potential.
Myc family	Proto-oncogenes, including c-Myc, first used for generation of human and mouse iPSCs.
Klf family	Zinc-finger-containing transcription factor Kruppel-like factor 4 (KLF4) was first used for generation of human and mouse iPSCs
Nanog	Homeodomain-containing transcription factor essential for maintenance of pluripotency and self-renewal in embryonic stem cells. Expression is controlled by a network of factors including the key pluripotency regulator Oct4.
Lin 28	Conserved RNA binding protein and stem cell marker. Inhibitor of microRNA processing in embryonic stem (ES) and carcinoma (EC) cells.

Table 1. Combinations of the genes that have been used to obtain the induced pluripotent state in human somatic cells

2.1 Differentiation of iPSCs into cells of the heart

After the cells have been reprogrammed, it will be possible to differentiate them towards a wide range of specialized cells, using existing protocols for differentiation of hESCs. Differentiation of beating heart cells, the cardiomyocytes, from hESCs has now been achievable through various protocols for a decade (Kehat et al., 2001; Mummery et al., 2002). In 2007, human iPSCs were first reported to differentiate into cardiomyocytes (Takahashi et al., 2007), using a protocol including activin A and BMP4 which was described for differentiation of hESCs the same year (Laflamme et al., 2007). A comparison between the cardiac differentiation potential of hESCs and iPSCs concluded that the difference between the two cell sources were no greater than the known differences between different hESC lines and that iPSCs thus should be a viable alternative as an autologous cell source (Zhang et al., 2009). Furthermore, a recent study demonstrated that reprogramming excluding c-MYC yielded iPSCs which efficiently up-regulated a cardiac gene expression pattern and showed spontaneous beating in contrast to iPSCs reprogrammed with four factors including c-MYC (Martinez-Fernandez et al., 2010). On the transcriptional level, beating clusters from both iPSCs and hESCs were found to be similarly enriched for cardiac genes, although a small difference in their global gene expression profile was noted (Gupta et al., 2010). Taken together, these results indicate that cardiomyocytes differentiated from both hESCs and iPSCs are highly similar, although differences exist.

2.2 Additional methods to achieve reprogramming- 1.cloning = Somatic Cell Nuclear Transfer (SCNT) 2.cell fusion 3.egg extract

In addition to the iPSC procedure other ways exist to reprogram somatic cells including: 1) somatic cell nuclear transfer (SCNT), 2) cell fusion of somatic adult cells with pluripotent ESCs to generate hybrid cells and 3) cell extract from ESCs or embryo carcinoma cells (ECs). From the time when successful SCNT experiments, more commonly known as cloning, in the frog *Xenopus Laevis* (Gurdon et al., 1958) to the creation of the sheep Dolly (Wilmut et al., 1997), it has been proven that an adult cell nucleus transplanted into an unfertilized egg can support development of a new individual, and researchers have focused on identifying the molecular mechanisms that take place during this remarkable process. Even though SCNT has been around for 50 years, the molecular mechanisms that take place inside the egg remain largely unknown. The gigantic egg cell receiving a tiny nucleus is extremely difficult to study. Single cell analysis are required and gene knock-out of egg proteins is very challenging. In 2007 a report that the first primate ESCs were isolated from SCNT blastula embryos of the species Rhesus Monkey was published (Byrne et al., 2007). The reason why it took so long to perform successful SCNT in Rhesus Monkey was a technical issue; to enucleate the egg, modified polarized light was used instead of traditional methods using either mechanical removal of DNA or UV light mediated DNA destruction. The first reliable publication of successful human SCNT reported generation of a single cloned blastocyst (Stojkovic et al., 2005). Unfortunately, the dramatic advances in human SCNT reported by Hwang and colleagues in South Korea were largely a product of fraud (Cho et al., 2006). In human SCNT reports, left over eggs from IVF (*in vitro* fertilization) that failed to fertilize have been used, indicating poor egg quality. However, human SCNT using 29 donated eggs (oocytes) of good quality, and not leftovers from IVF, from three young women were reported to develop into cloned blastocysts, at a frequency as high as 23% (French et al., 2008). Theoretically, hESC lines can be derived *in vitro* from SCNT generated blastocysts. However, so far no established hESC line using the SCNT procedure has been reported. The shortage of donated high quality human eggs for research is a significant impediment for this field.

Other methods that have been used to elucidate the molecular mechanism of reprogramming are 2) fusion of somatic adult cells with pluripotent ESCs to generate hybrid cells or 3) cell extract from ESCs or ECs (Bhutani et al., 2010; Cowan et al., 2005; Freberg et al., 2007; Taranger et al., 2005; Yamanaka and Blau, 2010).

3. Molecular mechanisms of reprogramming

The mechanisms of nuclear reprogramming are not yet completely understood. The crucial event during reprogramming is the activation of ES- and the silencing of differentiation markers, while the genetic code remains intact. Major reprogramming of gene expression takes place inside the egg and genes that have been silenced during embryo development are awakened. In contrast, genes that are expressed in, and are specific for, the donated cell nucleus become inactivated most of the time, however some SCNT embryos remember their heritage and fail to inactivate somatic-specific genes (Ng and Gurdon, 2008). It has been reported that reprogramming involves changes in chromatin structure and chromatin components (Jullien et al., 2010; Kikyo et al., 2000). Importantly, initiation of Oct4 expression has been found to be crucial for successful nuclear transfers (Boiani et al., 2002; Byrne et al., 2003) and important for iPSC creation; all other reprogramming iPSC transcription factors have been replaced with other factors or chemical compounds, but only one report so far could exclude Oct4. In murine ES cells, Oct4 must hold a precise level to maintain them as just ES cells (Niwa et al., 2000) and therefore understanding the control of the Oct4 level will be key if one wants to understand pluripotency and reprogramming at the molecular level. A recent report demonstrated that Oct4 expression is regulated by scaffold attachment factor A (SAF-A). SAF-A was found on the Oct4 promoter only when the gene is actively transcribed in murine ESCs, depending on LIF, and gene silencing of SAF-A in ESCs resulted in down regulation of Oct4 (Vizlin-Hodzic et al., 2011). Other Oct4 modulators have been reported that in similarity with SAF-A are in complex with RNA polymerase II (Ding et al., 2009; Ponnusamy et al., 2009). Post-translational modifications have been shown to be able to modify the activity of Oct4, such as sumoylation (Wei et al., 2007) and ubiquitination (Xu et al., 2004). During the reprogramming process epigenetic marks are changed such as the removal of methyl groups on DNA (DNA demethylation) of the Oct4 promoter which has been shown during SCNT (Simonsson and Gurdon, 2004) and has also been observed in mouse (Yamazaki et al., 2006). The growth arrest and DNA damage inducible protein Gadd45a and deaminase Aid was shown to promote DNA demethylation of the Oct4 and Nanog promoters (Barreto et al., 2007; Bhutani et al., 2010). Consistent with those findings is that Aid together with Gadd45 and Mbd4 has been shown to promote DNA demethylation in zebrafish (Rai et al., 2008). Translational tumor protein (Tpt1) has been proposed to control Oct4 and shown to interact with nucleophosmin (Npm1) during mitosis of ESCs and such complexes are involved in cell proliferation (Johansson et al., 2010b; Koziol et al., 2007). Furthermore, phosphorylated nucleolin (Ncl-P) interacts with Oct4 during interphase in both murine and human ESCs (Johansson et al., 2010a). Core transcription factors, Oct4, Sox2 and Nanog, were shown to individually form complexes with nucleophosmin (Npm1) to control ESCs (Johansson and Simonsson, 2010). ESCs also display high levels of telomerase activity which maintain the length of the telomeres. The telomerase activity or Tert gene expression is rapidly down regulated during differentiation and are much lower or absent in somatic cells. Therefore, reestablishment of high telomerase activity (or reactivation of Tert gene) is important for reprogramming. In SCNT animals, telomere length in somatic cells has been reported to be comparable to that in normally fertilized animals (Betts et al., 2001; Lanza et al., 2000; Tian et al., 2000). A telomere length-resetting mechanism has been identified in the *Xenopus* egg (Vizlin-Hodzic et al., 2009).

When iPSCs first were introduced many thought that the molecular mechanism of reprogramming was solved once and for all. It was soon shown that to generate iPSC colonies one could use different combinations of transcription factors most efficiently together with retroviruses or more recently, exposure to chemical compounds together with the transcription factors, Oct4 and Klf4, and with retroviruses (Zhu et al., 2010) or retroviruses alone (Kane et al., 2010). What retroviruses do for the reprogramming process is unknown and the efficiency by which the egg reprograms the somatic cells is far more efficient than the iPSC procedure. Moreover, mutagenic effects have been documented in both laboratory and clinical gene therapy studies, principally as a result of a dysregulated host gene expression in the proximity of gene integration sites. So the first question to ask is whether all iPSC experiments so far forgot the obvious control of using only virus. The answer is probably no because the efficiency is very low with viruses alone as compared to using transcription factors combined with virus or identified reprogramming compounds. Reprogramming an adult somatic frog cell nucleus to generate a normal "clonal" new individual is far less efficient (0.1-3%) than reprogramming to create a blastocyst, from which ESCs are isolated (efficiency 20-40%) (Gurdon, 2008) and is comparable with blastula formation after human SCNT (23%). This number could be compared with iPSC procedure that has reported 0.5 % success rate at most with human cells (table 1). The low efficiency and slow kinetics of iPSC derivation suggest that there are other procedures that are more efficient, yet to decipher. There is a belief that there are different levels of pluripotency when it comes to ESC and also that reprogramming follows an organized sequence of events, beginning with downregulation of somatic markers and activation of pluripotency markers alkaline phosphatase, SSEA-4, and Fbxo15 before pluripotency endogenous genes such as Oct4, Nanog, Tra1-60 and Tra-1-80 become expressed and cells gain independence from exogenous transcription factor expression (Brambrink et al., 2008; Stadtfeld et al., 2008a). Only a small subset of somatic cells expressing the reprogramming factors down-regulates somatic markers and activates pluripotency genes (Wernig et al., 2008a).

3.1 History of reprogramming

SCNT has been around for more than fifty years although it was already proposed in 1938 by Hans Spemann (Spemann, 1938), an embryologist who received the Nobel Prize in Medicine for his development of new embryological micro surgery techniques. Spemann anticipated that "transplanting an older nucleus into an egg would be a fantastic experiment". Later on, Robert Briggs and Thomas King were the first to put the nuclear transfer technique into practice. However, they only managed to obtain viable offspring through nuclear transfer of undifferentiated cells in the frog species *Rana pipiens* (Briggs and King, 1952). During the 1950s to the 1970s a series of pioneering somatic nuclear transfer experiments performed by John Gurdon showed that nuclei from differentiated amphibian cells, for example tadpole intestinal or adult skin cells could generate cloned tadpoles (Gurdon, 1962; Gurdon et al., 1958; Gurdon et al., 1975). In 1997, the successful cloning of a mammal was first achieved. The sheep Dolly was produced by using the nuclei of cells cultured from an adult mammary gland (Wilmut et al., 1997). Following the cloning of Dolly, researchers have reported successful cloning of a number of species including cow, pig, mouse, rabbit, cat (named Copycat) and monkey. In 2006, reprogrammed murine iPSCs were reported by Takahashi and Yamanaka (Takahashi and Yamanaka, 2006) and in 2007 human iPSCs were reported (Takahashi et al., 2007; Yu et al., 2009).

4. Producing iPSCs from other cell types than fibroblasts

The most studied somatic cell type that has been reprogrammed into iPSCs is fibroblasts. The different human somatic cell types that have been transformed into iPSCs so far are summarized in table 2. The efficiency of fibroblast reprogramming does not exceed 1-5% but generally is extremely inefficient (0.001-0.1%) and occurs at a slow speed (> 2 weeks). In order to use iPSCs in clinical applications, improved efficiency, suitable factor delivery techniques and identification of true reprogrammed cells are crucial. In the fast growing field of regenerative medicine, patient-specific iPSCs offer a unique source of autologous cells for clinical applications. Although promising, using somatic cells of an adult individual as starting material for reprogramming in this context has also raised concern. Acquired somatic mutations that have been accumulated during an individual's life time will be transferred to the iPSCs, and there is a fear that these mutations may be associated with adverse events such as cancer development. As an alternative, iPSCs have been generated from human cord blood. These cells have been shown to differentiate into all three germ layers including spontaneous beating cardiomyocytes (Haase et al., 2009). Reprogrammed cells from cord blood have not only the advantage to come from a juvenescent cell source. In addition, cord blood is already routinely harvested for clinical use.

Another issue that has been raised in this field is a wish to harvest cells for reprogramming without surgical intervention. Therefore, reprogramming experiments have also been performed using plucked human hair follicle keratinocytes. These iPSCs were also able to differentiate into cells from all three germ layers including cardiomyocytes (Novak et al., 2010).

Human Origin Somatic Cell type	Efficiency	Reprogramming Factors	Reference
Fibroblasts	0.02%	OKSM	(Takahashi et al., 2007)
	0.02%	OSLN	(Yu et al., 2007)
	0.002%	OKS	(Nakagawa et al., 2008)
Hepatocytes	0.1%	OKSM	(Liu et al., 2010)
Keratinocytes	ND	OKSM	(Aasen et al., 2008)
	ND	OKS	(Aasen et al., 2008)
Neural stem cells	<0.004%	O	(Kim et al., 2008)
Amniotic cells	0.05-1.5%	OKSM	(Li et al., 2009)
	0.1%	OSN	(Zhao et al., 2010)
Adipose-derived stem cells	0.5%	OKSM	(Sugii et al., 2010)
	<0.1%	OKS	(Aoki et al., 2010)
Cord blood stem cells	ND	OKSM	(Eminli et al., 2009)
	<0.01%	OS	(Giorgetti et al., 2009)
Cord blood endothelial cells	<0.01%	OSLN	(Haase et al., 2009)
Mobilized peripheral blood	0.01%	OKSM	(Loh et al., 2009)

Table 2. Different somatic cell types that human iPSCs have been generated from

4.1 iPSC as a disease model

The introduction of iPSC technology holds a great promise for disease modelling. By differentiating iPSCs from patients into various cell lineages there is hope to be able to follow the disease progression and to identify new prognostic markers as well as to use the differentiated cells for drug screening in both toxicological testing and the development of new treatment. This approach has already been tested for monogenic diseases using genetically modified hESCs or hESCs from embryos carrying these diseases (reviewed in (Stephenson et al., 2009)). However, diseases with a more complex genetic background involving several or unknown genes have not been able to be studied in this way before iPSCs became available. An additional advantage with iPSCs is that since many diseases differ in both clinical symptoms and penetrance between patients, iPSCs derived from patients will offer the opportunity to reveal a clinical history as well. It could also provide a model for late-onset degenerative diseases such as Alzheimer's disease or osteoarthritis.

Recent work on cardiac arrhythmias has fully shown the potential of disease modelling using iPSCs. Long QT syndrome (LQTS) is characterized by rapid irregular heart beats due to abnormal ion channel function and the condition can lead to sudden death. So far, various mutations in at least 12 different genes have been associated with LQTS and the disease is subdivided into different types depending on which gene is affected (reviewed in (Bokil et al., 2010)). Fibroblasts from patients with LQTS1 (Moretti et al., 2010) and LQTS2 (Itzhaki et al., 2011; Matsa et al., 2011) were reprogrammed and differentiated into the cardiac lineage. These cells displayed the electrophysiological pattern characteristic to the disease. Moreover, the cells responded appropriately when treated with pharmacological compounds, which further extends the usability of these cells.

iPSCs have also been generated from fibroblasts from patients suffering from the LEOPARD syndrome, an autosomal-dominant developmental disorder where one of the major disease phenotypes includes hyperthropic cardiomyopathy. The authors showed that cardiomyocytes derived from those iPSCs were larger with another intracellular organization compared to cardiomyocytes derived from hESCs or iPSCs generated from a healthy sibling (Carvajal-Vergara et al., 2010). Today many laboratories and hospitals worldwide are producing iPSC lines from patients with various diseases. Patient-specific iPSC lines can be used as 1) a human modelling system for studying the molecular cause of, and in the long run for 2) the treatment of, degenerative diseases with autologous transplantation, which refers to the transplantation to a patient of his/her own cells. The therapeutic potential of iPSCs in combination with genetic repair has already been successfully shown in mouse models of sickle cell anemia (Hanna et al., 2007), Duchenne muscular dystrophy (DMD) (Kazuki et al., 2010), hemophilia A (Xu et al., 2009) and, in a rat model, Parkinson's disease (Wernig et al., 2008c). For diseases where animal and human physiology differ, disease-specific iPSC lines capable of differentiation into the tissue affected by the disease could recapitulate tissue formation and thereby enable determination of the cause of the disease and could provide cues to drug targets. Therefore iPSC lines from patients suffering from a variety of genetic diseases with either Mendelian or complex inheritance have been secured for future research, and include deaminase deficiency-related severe combined immunodeficiency (ADA-SCID), Shwachman-Bodian-Diamond syndrome (SBDS), Gaucher disease (GD) type III, Duchenne (DMD) and Becker muscular dystrophy (BMD), Parkinson disease (PD), Huntington disease (HD), juvenile-onset (type1) diabetes mellitus (JDM), Downs syndrome (DS)/trisomy21 and Lesch-Nyhan syndrome (Park et al., 2008a). Furthermore, iPSCs derived from amyotrophic lateral sclerosis (ALS) patients were terminally differentiated into motor neurons (Dimos et al., 2008).

4.2 Procedures to produce iPSCs

In the first iPSC reprogramming studies, retroviral or lentiviral vectors were used to introduce the transcription factors into somatic cells. By using these viral delivery systems,

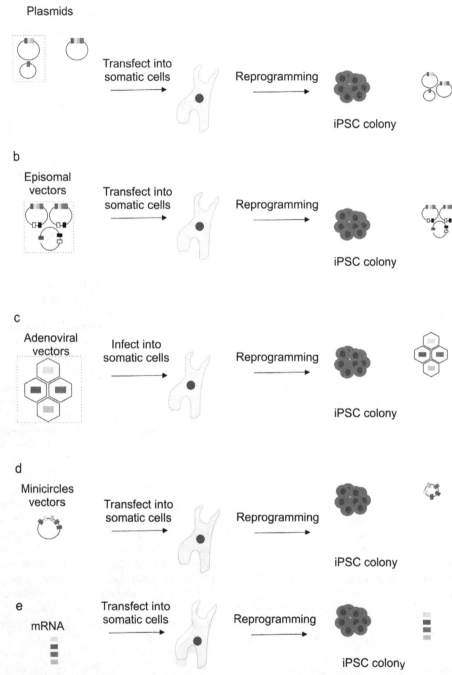

Fig. 2. Methods for producing induced pluripotent stem cells (iPSCs) by non-integrating vectors. Several different methods exist to generate iPSCs by non-integrating vectors: for

example by plasmid, episomal, adenoviral minicircle vectors and mRNA. a) A combination of expression plasmid vectors for defined reprogramming factors is transfected into somatic cells. Plasmid vectors are not integrated into the genome of transfected cells and are gradually lost during reprogramming. This method therefore requires multiple transfection steps. b) Somatic cells can be transfected by episomal vectors expressing defined reprogramming factors. These vectors can replicate themselves autonomously in cells during reprogramming under drug selection and are not integrated into the genome. Upon withdrawal of drug selection, the episomal vectors are lost. c) Adenovirus carrying defined reprogramming factors can be infected into somatic cells to transiently express these factors. This method requires multiple transductions since adenoviral vectors are lost upon celldivision. d) The minicircle vector method is based on PhiC31-vector intra molecular recombinant system that allows the bacterial elements of the vector to be degraded in bacteria. Minicircle vector containing only defined reprogramming factors is not degraded and is delivered into somatic cells by nucleofection. This strategy requires multiple transfection steps since minicircle vectors are lost upon cell division. e) Reprogramming using mRNA reprogramming factors have been achieved.

the transduced viral vectors and transgenes are randomly and permanently integrated into the genome of infected somatic cells and remains in the iPSCs. The vector integration into the host genome is a limitation of this technology if it is going to be used in human therapeutic applications due to increased risk of tumor formation (Okita et al., 2007). Approaches to derive transgene-free iPSCs are therefore critical. The first strategy was by using non-integrating (Figure 2) vectors. Efforts have been made to derive iPSCs by repeated plasmid transfections (Gonzalez et al., 2009; Okita et al., 2008) (Figure 2a), adenoviral (Stadtfeld et al., 2008b) (Figure 2b) and episomal vectors (Yu et al., 2009) (Figure 2c). Recently, minicircle vectors (Figure 2d) have been used to generate iPSCs (Jia et al., 2010). Unfortunately, reprogramming with these techniques has extremely low efficiency as compared to integrating viral vectors. Another promising alternative is the use of excisable integrating vectors, allowing for the generation of transgene-free iPSCs. A classical expression-excision system uses vectors with inserts flanked with recognition sites, loxP sites, for Cre-recombinase (Figure 3a). Consequently, DNA is excised upon Cre-recombinase expression in the cells. Cre-loxP-based approaches have been used to reprogram human somatic cells from individuals with Parkinson's disease by four different vectors (Soldner et al., 2009) or by a single, polycistronic lentiviral vector encoding reprogramming factors (Chang et al., 2009). Though, a potential limitation of Cre-loxP-based approaches is that a long terminal repeat (LTR) will remain after Cre-mediated excision which may interfere with the expression of endogenous genes. An alternative integration-free strategy is based on the piggy-Bac transposon (Figure 3b), a mobile genetic element from insects that integrates into the genome of mammalian cells and, most importantly, can be entirely removed by a transposase. Two research teams generated iPSCs using this system to deliver a single polycistron encoding four reprogramming factors into somatic cells (Woltjen et al., 2009; Yusa et al., 2009). Interestingly, the latest development indicates that gene transfection may not even be needed for the generation of iPSCs and that direct delivery of four recombinant reprogramming proteins that can penetrate the plasma membrane of somatic cells is sufficient (Zhou et al., 2009), or mRNA (Angel &Yanik, 2010; Plews et al., 2010; Warren et al. 2010; Yakoba et al., 2010; Zhou et al.,2009).

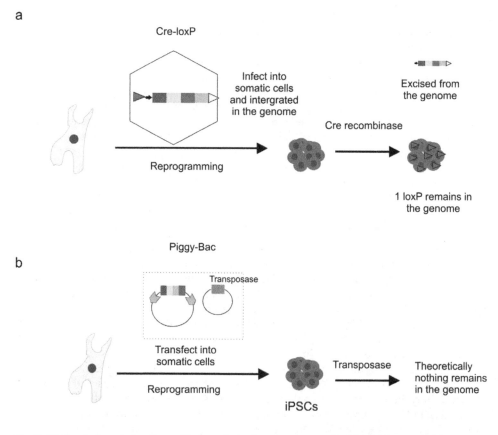

Fig. 3. Methods for production of induced pluripotent stem cells (iPSCs) by excisable integrating vectors. Two different methods exist today to generate iPSCs by excisable integrating vectors: by Cre-loxP and Piggy-Bac vectors. a) In the Cre-loxP viral delivery system, defined reprogramming factors are cloned into vectors flanked by recognition sites, loxP sites, for Cre-recombinase. Upon transduction into somatic cells, the loxP site is duplicated and reprogramming factos are stably integrated into the genome flanked by loxP sites. When Cre-recombinase is expressed, the integrated reprogramming factors are excised from the genome but one loxP site is left behind integrated into the genome of iPSCs. b) The Piggy-Bac transposon gene delivery system is based on a mobile genetic element that efficiently integrates into the genome of mammalian cells. When fusion gene encoding defined reprogramming factors in the transposon expression vector as well as transposase expression vector are transfected into somatic cells, the fusion gene is stably integrated into the genome. When transposase is expressed, the interated genetic material is excised from the genome resulting in transgene- and vector free iPSCs.

The therapeutic application of iPSCs is limited by another concern due to the use of potential oncogenes when iPSCs are produced. C-Myc is an oncogene and as such causes tumor formation, which has been observed in iPSC-derived chimeric mice (Okita et al., 2007). As a major step towards solving this issue, several studies have demonstrated that mouse and human iPSCs can be derived without C-Myc but the efficiency of reprogramming is reduced (Nakagawa et al., 2008; Wernig et al., 2008b; Yu et al., 2007). Although the oncogenic potential of C-Myc is mostly discussed, Oct4, Sox2 and Klf4 are also associated with multiple types of cancer (Bass et al., 2009; Gidekel et al., 2003; Wei et al., 2006). To circumvent this problem, a recent trend is to avoid the transduction of some of the oncogenes by 1) reprogramming somatic cells which already endogenously express sufficient levels of some of the reprogramming factors (Tsai et al., 2010), 2) replacing one or more reprogramming factors by small molecules like histone deacetylase inhibitor vaporic acid, the DNA methyltransferase inhibitor 5-aza-cytidine, the Wnt signaling component WNT3a, the L-channel calcium channel agonist Bayk8644 (Huangfu et al., 2008a; Huangfu et al., 2008b), or 3) dual inhibition of mitogen activated protein kinase signaling and glycogen synthase kinase-3 (Silva et al., 2008). It has been reported that Sox2 can be replaced by Sox1, Klf4 by Klf2 and c-Myc by N-myc or L-myc indicating that they are not fundamentally required for generation of iPSCs (Yamanaka, 2009). Tet-on™ technology has been used to express exogenously reprogramming factors in presence of Doxycycline. Removal of Doxycycline results in that iPSC colonies that endogenously express pluripotent genes and colonies that are truly reprogrammed remains.

5. Transplanting cells

In order to make cell therapy (route 1 in Figure 1) using iPSCs a reality in medicine many obstacles need to be overcome. Organ transplantation between individuals is complicated due to the limited availability of matched tissues and consequently the requirement for life-long treatment with immunosuppressive drugs that can cause serious side effects. The hope is that iPSCs that are already genetically matched with the patient would circumvent these issues. Another advantage of iPSCs over current transplantation approaches is the opportunity of repairing mutations that cause the disease by homologous recombination, which has not been very successful in adult stem cells due to difficulties in propagating those cells *in vitro*. In mouse, iPSC technology combined with correction of a known disease-causing mutation has been proven successful. In human autologous cell therapy has been used since the mid 90´s for the treatment of focal cartilage lesions, using the patient's chondrocytes transplanted into the injured knee (Brittberg et al., 1994), thereby alleviated osteoarthritic symptoms and induction of tissue repair. The cell therapy gives stable long-term results up to 20 years after surgery in some patients but is less successful in others (Lindahl et al., 2003; Peterson et al., 2010). One drawback with this technique is the supply of cells. Large injuries require large amounts of cells, and there is a limit of the size of the biopsies that can be taken out from the patient. Introducing the iPSC technique in such system might improve the process. Since the iPSCs have theoretically an unlimited proliferation capacity, these cells can be used to reach larger quantities of cells. When sufficient numbers have been produced, the iPSCs are differentiated into chondrocytes and transplanted to the lesion. In this case, no biopsy would need to be harvested, since iPSCs can be made from a regular skin fibroblast. Before this somewhat futuristic scenario can come true, rigorous characterization of the iPSC is needed, since these cells, as all stem cells, can form teratoma *in vivo* (Fairchild, 2010). The iPSCs have however, been shown to retain their epigenic memory from the tissue from which they originate. It would therefore be easier to differentiate an iPSC to a chondrocyte if the donor cell was a chondrocyte (Kim et al., 2010), and maybe terminally so, thus avoiding risk for terratoma formation. A biopsy would thus be needed, but a relatively small cell harvest could with the iPSC technique result in the treatment of larger injuries. The iPSC procedure could also lead to a therapy-outcome that is more predicted and constant due to that chondrogenic differentiation of iPSC probably result in a more homogeneous cell-population. Since cartilage lacks vascularisation and thus is immunoprivileged the derivation of a universal donor chondrocytes cell line based on the iPSC technology could be an interesting option. If such cells are combined with a suitable matrix scaffold a cartilage regeneration therapy could potentially have a much wider application and be more cost effective than current autologous procedures.

5.1 Directprogramming of somatic cells into another cell type
Switching from one somatic cell type into another cell type, not necessarily via a pluripotent cell state was first demonstrated when fibroblasts formed myofibers after transduction with retroviral vectors expressing the skeletal muscle factor MyoD (Davis et al., 1987). Further, it has been reported that pancreatic acinar cells could be transformed into insulin-producing β cells by overexpression of the pancreatic factors Pdx1, MafA and Ngn3 *in vivo* (Zhou et al., 2008) as well as that ESCs could be directly differentiated into specific dopamine neurons by overexpression of only one factor, Lmx1 (Friling et al., 2009). These experiments proved that transdifferentiation do not require reprogramming into a pluripotent state, although all such experiments have used some kind of retroviruses and if only virus in itself can contribute to pluripotency as has recently been shown one cannot completely rule out that the switch hasn't passed via a pluripotent state.

6. Final remarks

To date, clinically valid iPSCs do not yet exist, but are under development worldwide. Some will argue that the complexity of reprogramming is solved by the iPSC technology, however apart from the defined reprogramming factors, retroviruses help in the reprogramming process in an unknown way, and is still inefficient compared to SCNT which argues for that more can be learnt about reprogramming. Also the fact that different combinations of reprogramming factors, or replacement with chemicals, have been used successfully indicates that there exist reprogramming molecules yet to be discovered. Therefore, further investigations are needed to learn more about the molecular mechanisms of iPSCs and how to prevent tumor formation following *in vivo* transplantation. Awaiting *in vivo* safety, these techniques offer exciting possibilities for mapping mechanisms of different diseases and screening for patient-specific therapies and drugs. To derive iPSCs from the patient's own cells following differentiation into the disease-causing cells means recapitulating the disease in a test tube for genomic, proteomic and epigenomic analysis. The iPSC as a human *in vitro* disease modeling system is a new promising and fast expanding research area.

7. References

Aasen, T., Raya, A., Barrero, M.J., Garreta, E., Consiglio, A., Gonzalez, F., Vassena, R., Bilic, J., Pekarik, V., Tiscornia, G., *et al.* (2008). Efficient and rapid generation of induced pluripotent stem cells from human keratinocytes. Nat Biotechnol 26, 1276-1284.

Angel, M. & Yanik, M. F. (2010). Innate immune suppression enables frequent transfection with RNA encoding reprogramming proteins. *PLoS One* 5, e11756.

Aoki, T., Ohnishi, H., Oda, Y., Tadokoro, M., Sasao, M., Kato, H., Hattori, K., and Ohgushi, H. (2010). Generation of induced pluripotent stem cells from human adipose-derived stem cells without c-MYC. Tissue Eng Part A 16, 2197-2206.

Barreto, G., Schafer, A., Marhold, J., Stach, D., Swaminathan, S.K., Handa, V., Doderlein, G., Maltry, N., Wu, W., Lyko, F., *et al.* (2007). Gadd45a promotes epigenetic gene activation by repair-mediated DNA demethylation. Nature 445, 671-675.

Bass, A.J., Watanabe, H., Mermel, C.H., Yu, S., Perner, S., Verhaak, R.G., Kim, S.Y., Wardwell, L., Tamayo, P., Gat-Viks, I., *et al.* (2009). SOX2 is an amplified lineage-survival oncogene in lung and esophageal squamous cell carcinomas. Nat Genet 41, 1238-1242.

Betts, D., Bordignon, V., Hill, J., Winger, Q., Westhusin, M., Smith, L., and King, W. (2001). Reprogramming of telomerase activity and rebuilding of telomere length in cloned cattle. Proc Natl Acad Sci U S A 98, 1077-1082.

Bhutani, N., Brady, J.J., Damian, M., Sacco, A., Corbel, S.Y., and Blau, H.M. (2010). Reprogramming towards pluripotency requires AID-dependent DNA demethylation. Nature 463, 1042-1047.

Boiani, M., Eckardt, S., Scholer, H.R., and McLaughlin, K.J. (2002). Oct4 distribution and level in mouse clones: consequences for pluripotency. Genes Dev 16, 1209-1219.

Bokil, N.J., Baisden, J.M., Radford, D.J., and Summers, K.M. (2010). Molecular genetics of long QT syndrome. Mol Genet Metab 101, 1-8.

Brambrink, T., Foreman, R., Welstead, G.G., Lengner, C.J., Wernig, M., Suh, H., and Jaenisch, R. (2008). Sequential expression of pluripotency markers during direct reprogramming of mouse somatic cells. Cell Stem Cell 2, 151-159.

Briggs, R., and King, T.J. (1952). Transplantation of Living Nuclei From Blastula Cells into Enucleated Frogs' Eggs. Proc Natl Acad Sci U S A 38, 455-463.

Brittberg, M., Lindahl, A., Nilsson, A., Ohlsson, C., Isaksson, O., and Peterson, L. (1994). Treatment of deep cartilage defects in the knee with autologous chondrocyte transplantation. N Engl J Med 331, 889-895.

Byrne, J.A., Pedersen, D.A., Clepper, L.L., Nelson, M., Sanger, W.G., Gokhale, S., Wolf, D.P., and Mitalipov, S.M. (2007). Producing primate embryonic stem cells by somatic cell nuclear transfer. Nature 450, 497-502.

Byrne, J.A., Simonsson, S., Western, P.S., and Gurdon, J.B. (2003). Nuclei of adult mammalian somatic cells are directly reprogrammed to oct-4 stem cell gene expression by amphibian oocytes. Curr Biol 13, 1206-1213.

Carvajal-Vergara, X., Sevilla, A., D'Souza, S.L., Ang, Y.S., Schaniel, C., Lee, D.F., Yang, L., Kaplan, A.D., Adler, E.D., Rozov, R., *et al.* (2010). Patient-specific induced pluripotent stem-cell-derived models of LEOPARD syndrome. Nature 465, 808-812.

Chang, C.W., Lai, Y.S., Pawlik, K.M., Liu, K., Sun, C.W., Li, C., Schoeb, T.R., and Townes, T.M. (2009). Polycistronic lentiviral vector for "hit and run" reprogramming of adult skin fibroblasts to induced pluripotent stem cells. Stem Cells 27, 1042-1049.

Cho, M.K., McGee, G., and Magnus, D. (2006). Research conduct. Lessons of the stem cell scandal. Science 311, 614-615.

Cowan, C.A., Atienza, J., Melton, D.A., and Eggan, K. (2005). Nuclear reprogramming of somatic cells after fusion with human embryonic stem cells. Science 309, 1369-1373.

Davis, R.L., Weintraub, H., and Lassar, A.B. (1987). Expression of a single transfected cDNA converts fibroblasts to myoblasts. Cell 51, 987-1000.

Dimos, J.T., Rodolfa, K.T., Niakan, K.K., Weisenthal, L.M., Mitsumoto, H., Chung, W., Croft, G.F., Saphier, G., Leibel, R., Goland, R., et al. (2008). Induced pluripotent stem cells generated from patients with ALS can be differentiated into motor neurons. Science 321, 1218-1221.

Ding, L., Paszkowski-Rogacz, M., Nitzsche, A., Slabicki, M.M., Heninger, A.K., de Vries, I., Kittler, R., Junqueira, M., Shevchenko, A., Schulz, H., et al. (2009). A genome-scale RNAi screen for Oct4 modulators defines a role of the Paf1 complex for embryonic stem cell identity. Cell Stem Cell 4, 403-415.

Eminli, S., Foudi, A., Stadtfeld, M., Maherali, N., Ahfeldt, T., Mostoslavsky, G., Hock, H., and Hochedlinger, K. (2009). Differentiation stage determines potential of hematopoietic cells for reprogramming into induced pluripotent stem cells. Nat Genet 41, 968-976.

Fairchild, P.J. (2010). The challenge of immunogenicity in the quest for induced pluripotency. Nat Rev Immunol 10, 868-875.

Freberg, C.T., Dahl, J.A., Timoskainen, S., and Collas, P. (2007). Epigenetic reprogramming of OCT4 and NANOG regulatory regions by embryonal carcinoma cell extract. Mol Biol Cell 18, 1543-1553.

French, A.J., Adams, C.A., Anderson, L.S., Kitchen, J.R., Hughes, M.R., and Wood, S.H. (2008). Development of human cloned blastocysts following somatic cell nuclear transfer with adult fibroblasts. Stem Cells 26, 485-493.

Friling, S., Andersson, E., Thompson, L.H., Jonsson, M.E., Hebsgaard, J.B., Nanou, E., Alekseenko, Z., Marklund, U., Kjellander, S., Volakakis, N., et al. (2009). Efficient production of mesencephalic dopamine neurons by Lmx1a expression in embryonic stem cells. Proc Natl Acad Sci U S A 106, 7613-7618.

Gidekel, S., Pizov, G., Bergman, Y., and Pikarsky, E. (2003). Oct-3/4 is a dose-dependent oncogenic fate determinant. Cancer Cell 4, 361-370.

Giorgetti, A., Montserrat, N., Aasen, T., Gonzalez, F., Rodriguez-Piza, I., Vassena, R., Raya, A., Boue, S., Barrero, M.J., Corbella, B.A., et al. (2009). Generation of induced pluripotent stem cells from human cord blood using OCT4 and SOX2. Cell Stem Cell 5, 353-357.

Gonzalez, F., Barragan Monasterio, M., Tiscornia, G., Montserrat Pulido, N., Vassena, R., Batlle Morera, L., Rodriguez Piza, I., and Izpisua Belmonte, J.C. (2009). Generation of mouse-induced pluripotent stem cells by transient expression of a single nonviral polycistronic vector. Proc Natl Acad Sci U S A 106, 8918-8922.

Gupta, M.K., Illich, D.J., Gaarz, A., Matzkies, M., Nguemo, F., Pfannkuche, K., Liang, H., Classen, S., Reppel, M., Schultze, J.L., et al. (2010). Global transcriptional profiles of beating clusters derived from human induced pluripotent stem cells and embryonic stem cells are highly similar. BMC Dev Biol 10, 98.

Gurdon, J. (2008). Primate therapeutic cloning in practice. Nat Biotechnol 26, 64-65.

Gurdon, J.B. (1962). The developmental capacity of nuclei taken from intestinal epithelium cells of feeding tadpoles. J Embryol Exp Morphol 10, 622-640.

Gurdon, J.B., Elsdale, T.R., and Fischberg, M. (1958). Sexually mature individuals of Xenopus laevis from the transplantation of single somatic nuclei. Nature 182, 64-65.

Gurdon, J.B., Laskey, R.A., and Reeves, O.R. (1975). The developmental capacity of nuclei transplanted from keratinized skin cells of adult frogs. J Embryol Exp Morphol 34, 93-112.

Haase, A., Olmer, R., Schwanke, K., Wunderlich, S., Merkert, S., Hess, C., Zweigerdt, R., Gruh, I., Meyer, J., Wagner, S., et al. (2009). Generation of induced pluripotent stem cells from human cord blood. Cell Stem Cell 5, 434-441.

Hanna, J., Wernig, M., Markoulaki, S., Sun, C.W., Meissner, A., Cassady, J.P., Beard, C., Brambrink, T., Wu, L.C., Townes, T.M., et al. (2007). Treatment of sickle cell anemia mouse model with iPS cells generated from autologous skin. Science 318, 1920-1923.

Heng, J.C., Feng, B., Han, J., Jiang, J., Kraus, P., Ng, J.H., Orlov, Y.L., Huss, M., Yang, L., Lufkin, T., et al. (2010). The nuclear receptor Nr5a2 can replace Oct4 in the reprogramming of murine somatic cells to pluripotent cells. Cell Stem Cell 6, 167-174.

Huangfu, D., Maehr, R., Guo, W., Eijkelenboom, A., Snitow, M., Chen, A.E., and Melton, D.A. (2008a). Induction of pluripotent stem cells by defined factors is greatly improved by small-molecule compounds. Nat Biotechnol 26, 795-797.

Huangfu, D., Osafune, K., Maehr, R., Guo, W., Eijkelenboom, A., Chen, S., Muhlestein, W., and Melton, D.A. (2008b). Induction of pluripotent stem cells from primary human fibroblasts with only Oct4 and Sox2. Nat Biotechnol 26, 1269-1275.

Itzhaki, I., Maizels, L., Huber, I., Zwi-Dantsis, L., Caspi, O., Winterstern, A., Feldman, O., Gepstein, A., Arbel, G., Hammerman, H., et al. (2011). Modelling the long QT syndrome with induced pluripotent stem cells. Nature 471, 225-229.

Jia, F., Wilson, K.D., Sun, N., Gupta, D.M., Huang, M., Li, Z., Panetta, N.J., Chen, Z.Y., Robbins, R.C., Kay, M.A., et al. (2010). A nonviral minicircle vector for deriving human iPS cells. Nat Methods 7, 197-199.

Johansson, H., and Simonsson, S. (2010). Core transcription factors, Oct4, Sox2 and Nanog, individually form complexes with nucleophosmin (Npm1) to control embryonic stem (ES) cell fate determination. Aging (Albany NY) 2, 815-822.

Johansson, H., Svensson, F., Runnberg, R., Simonsson, T., and Simonsson, S. (2010a). Phosphorylated nucleolin interacts with translationally controlled tumor protein during mitosis and with Oct4 during interphase in ES cells. PLoS One 5, e13678.

Johansson, H., Vizlin-Hodzic, D., Simonsson, T., and Simonsson, S. (2010b). Translationally controlled tumor protein interacts with nucleophosmin during mitosis in ES cells. Cell Cycle 9.

Jullien, J., Astrand, C., Halley-Stott, R.P., Garrett, N., and Gurdon, J.B. (2010). Characterization of somatic cell nuclear reprogramming by oocytes in which a linker histone is required for pluripotency gene reactivation. Proc Natl Acad Sci U S A 107, 5483-5488.

Kane, N.M., Nowrouzi, A., Mukherjee, S., Blundell, M.P., Greig, J.A., Lee, W.K., Houslay, M.D., Milligan, G., Mountford, J.C., von Kalle, C., et al. (2010). Lentivirus-mediated reprogramming of somatic cells in the absence of transgenic transcription factors. Mol Ther *18*, 2139-2145.

Kazuki, Y., Hiratsuka, M., Takiguchi, M., Osaki, M., Kajitani, N., Hoshiya, H., Hiramatsu, K., Yoshino, T., Kazuki, K., Ishihara, C., *et al.* (2010). Complete genetic correction of ips cells from Duchenne muscular dystrophy. Mol Ther *18*, 386-393.

Kehat, I., Kenyagin-Karsenti, D., Snir, M., Segev, H., Amit, M., Gepstein, A., Livne, E., Binah, O., Itskovitz-Eldor, J., and Gepstein, L. (2001). Human embryonic stem cells can differentiate into myocytes with structural and functional properties of cardiomyocytes. J Clin Invest *108*, 407-414.

Kikyo, N., Wade, P.A., Guschin, D., Ge, H., and Wolffe, A.P. (2000). Active remodeling of somatic nuclei in egg cytoplasm by the nucleosomal ATPase ISWI. Science *289*, 2360-2362.

Kim, J.B., Zaehres, H., Wu, G., Gentile, L., Ko, K., Sebastiano, V., Arauzo-Bravo, M.J., Ruau, D., Han, D.W., Zenke, M., *et al.* (2008). Pluripotent stem cells induced from adult neural stem cells by reprogramming with two factors. Nature *454*, 646-650.

Kim, K., Doi, A., Wen, B., Ng, K., Zhao, R., Cahan, P., Kim, J., Aryee, M.J., Ji, H., Ehrlich, L.I., *et al.* (2010). Epigenetic memory in induced pluripotent stem cells. Nature *467*, 285-290.

Koziol, M.J., Garrett, N., and Gurdon, J.B. (2007). Tpt1 activates transcription of oct4 and nanog in transplanted somatic nuclei. Curr Biol *17*, 801-807.

Laflamme, M.A., Chen, K.Y., Naumova, A.V., Muskheli, V., Fugate, J.A., Dupras, S.K., Reinecke, H., Xu, C., Hassanipour, M., Police, S., *et al.* (2007). Cardiomyocytes derived from human embryonic stem cells in pro-survival factors enhance function of infarcted rat hearts. Nat Biotechnol *25*, 1015-1024.

Lanza, R.P., Cibelli, J.B., Blackwell, C., Cristofalo, V.J., Francis, M.K., Baerlocher, G.M., Mak, J., Schertzer, M., Chavez, E.A., Sawyer, N., *et al.* (2000). Extension of cell life-span and telomere length in animals cloned from senescent somatic cells. Science *288*, 665-669.

Li, C., Zhou, J., Shi, G., Ma, Y., Yang, Y., Gu, J., Yu, H., Jin, S., Wei, Z., Chen, F., *et al.* (2009). Pluripotency can be rapidly and efficiently induced in human amniotic fluid-derived cells. Hum Mol Genet *18*, 4340-4349.

Lindahl, A., Brittberg, M., and Peterson, L. (2003). Cartilage repair with chondrocytes: clinical and cellular aspects. Novartis Found Symp *249*, 175-186; discussion 186-179, 234-178, 239-141.

Liu, H., Ye, Z., Kim, Y., Sharkis, S., and Jang, Y.Y. (2010). Generation of endoderm-derived human induced pluripotent stem cells from primary hepatocytes. Hepatology *51*, 1810-1819.

Loh, Y.H., Agarwal, S., Park, I.H., Urbach, A., Huo, H., Heffner, G.C., Kim, K., Miller, J.D., Ng, K., and Daley, G.Q. (2009). Generation of induced pluripotent stem cells from human blood. Blood *113*, 5476-5479.

Lowry, W.E., Richter, L., Yachechko, R., Pyle, A.D., Tchieu, J., Sridharan, R., Clark, A.T., and Plath, K. (2008). Generation of human induced pluripotent stem cells from dermal fibroblasts. Proc Natl Acad Sci U S A *105*, 2883-2888.

Martinez-Fernandez, A., Nelson, T.J., Ikeda, Y., and Terzic, A. (2010). c-MYC independent nuclear reprogramming favors cardiogenic potential of induced pluripotent stem cells. J Cardiovasc Transl Res *3*, 13-23.

Matsa, E., Rajamohan, D., Dick, E., Young, L., Mellor, I., Staniforth, A., and Denning, C. (2011). Drug evaluation in cardiomyocytes derived from human induced pluripotent stem cells carrying a long QT syndrome type 2 mutation. Eur Heart J *32*, 952-962.

Meissner, A., Wernig, M., and Jaenisch, R. (2007). Direct reprogramming of genetically unmodified fibroblasts into pluripotent stem cells. Nat Biotechnol *25*, 1177-1181.

Moretti, A., Bellin, M., Welling, A., Jung, C.B., Lam, J.T., Bott-Flugel, L., Dorn, T., Goedel, A., Hohnke, C., Hofmann, F., *et al.* (2010). Patient-specific induced pluripotent stem-cell models for long-QT syndrome. N Engl J Med *363*, 1397-1409.

Mummery, C., Ward, D., van den Brink, C.E., Bird, S.D., Doevendans, P.A., Opthof, T., Brutel de la Riviere, A., Tertoolen, L., van der Heyden, M., and Pera, M. (2002). Cardiomyocyte differentiation of mouse and human embryonic stem cells. J Anat *200*, 233-242.

Nakagawa, M., Koyanagi, M., Tanabe, K., Takahashi, K., Ichisaka, T., Aoi, T., Okita, K., Mochiduki, Y., Takizawa, N., and Yamanaka, S. (2008). Generation of induced pluripotent stem cells without Myc from mouse and human fibroblasts. Nat Biotechnol *26*, 101-106.

Ng, R.K., and Gurdon, J.B. (2008). Epigenetic memory of an active gene state depends on histone H3.3 incorporation into chromatin in the absence of transcription. Nat Cell Biol *10*, 102-109.

Niwa, H., Miyazaki, J., and Smith, A.G. (2000). Quantitative expression of Oct-3/4 defines differentiation, dedifferentiation or self-renewal of ES cells. Nat Genet *24*, 372-376.

Novak, A., Shtrichman, R., Germanguz, I., Segev, H., Zeevi-Levin, N., Fishman, B., Mandel, Y.E., Barad, L., Domev, H., Kotton, D., *et al.* (2010). Enhanced reprogramming and cardiac differentiation of human keratinocytes derived from plucked hair follicles, using a single excisable lentivirus. Cell Reprogram *12*, 665-678.

Okita, K., Ichisaka, T., and Yamanaka, S. (2007). Generation of germline-competent induced pluripotent stem cells. Nature *448*, 313-317.

Okita, K., Nakagawa, M., Hyenjong, H., Ichisaka, T., and Yamanaka, S. (2008). Generation of mouse induced pluripotent stem cells without viral vectors. Science *322*, 949-953.

Park, I.H., Arora, N., Huo, H., Maherali, N., Ahfeldt, T., Shimamura, A., Lensch, M.W., Cowan, C., Hochedlinger, K., and Daley, G.Q. (2008a). Disease-specific induced pluripotent stem cells. Cell *134*, 877-886.

Park, I.H., Zhao, R., West, J.A., Yabuuchi, A., Huo, H., Ince, T.A., Lerou, P.H., Lensch, M.W., and Daley, G.Q. (2008b). Reprogramming of human somatic cells to pluripotency with defined factors. Nature *451*, 141-146.

Peterson, L., Vasiliadis, H.S., Brittberg, M., and Lindahl, A. (2010). Autologous chondrocyte implantation: a long-term follow-up. Am J Sports Med *38*, 1117-1124.

Plews, J. R., Li, J., Jones, M., Moore, H. D., Mason, C., Andrews, P. W. & Na, J. (2010). Activation of pluripotency genes in human fibroblast cells by a novel mRNA based approach. *PLoS One* 5, e14397.

Ponnusamy, M.P., Deb, S., Dey, P., Chakraborty, S., Rachagani, S., Senapati, S., and Batra, S.K. (2009). RNA polymerase II associated factor 1/PD2 maintains self-renewal by its interaction with Oct3/4 in mouse embryonic stem cells. Stem Cells *27*, 3001-3011.

Rai, K., Huggins, I.J., James, S.R., Karpf, A.R., Jones, D.A., and Cairns, B.R. (2008). DNA demethylation in zebrafish involves the coupling of a deaminase, a glycosylase, and gadd45. Cell 135, 1201-1212.

Redmer, T., Diecke, S., Grigoryan, T., Quiroga-Negreira, A., Birchmeier, W., and Besser, D. (2011). E-cadherin is crucial for embryonic stem cell pluripotency and can replace OCT4 during somatic cell reprogramming. EMBO Rep 12, 720-726.

Shi, Y., Do, J.T., Desponts, C., Hahm, H.S., Scholer, H.R., and Ding, S. (2008). A combined chemical and genetic approach for the generation of induced pluripotent stem cells. Cell Stem Cell 2, 525-528.

Silva, J., Barrandon, O., Nichols, J., Kawaguchi, J., Theunissen, T.W., and Smith, A. (2008). Promotion of reprogramming to ground state pluripotency by signal inhibition. PLoS Biol 6, e253.

Simonsson, S., and Gurdon, J. (2004). DNA demethylation is necessary for the epigenetic reprogramming of somatic cell nuclei. Nat Cell Biol 6, 984-990.

Soldner, F., Hockemeyer, D., Beard, C., Gao, Q., Bell, G.W., Cook, E.G., Hargus, G., Blak, A., Cooper, O., Mitalipova, M., et al. (2009). Parkinson's disease patient-derived induced pluripotent stem cells free of viral reprogramming factors. Cell 136, 964-977.

Spemann, H. (1938). Embryonic Development and Induction. New Haven: Yale University Press.

Stadtfeld, M., Maherali, N., Breault, D.T., and Hochedlinger, K. (2008a). Defining molecular cornerstones during fibroblast to iPS cell reprogramming in mouse. Cell Stem Cell 2, 230-240.

Stadtfeld, M., Nagaya, M., Utikal, J., Weir, G., and Hochedlinger, K. (2008b). Induced pluripotent stem cells generated without viral integration. Science 322, 945-949.

Stephenson, E.L., Mason, C., and Braude, P.R. (2009). Preimplantation genetic diagnosis as a source of human embryonic stem cells for disease research and drug discovery. BJOG 116, 158-165.

Stojkovic, M., Stojkovic, P., Leary, C., Hall, V.J., Armstrong, L., Herbert, M., Nesbitt, M., Lako, M., and Murdoch, A. (2005). Derivation of a human blastocyst after heterologous nuclear transfer to donated oocytes. Reprod Biomed Online 11, 226-231.

Sugii, S., Kida, Y., Kawamura, T., Suzuki, J., Vassena, R., Yin, Y.Q., Lutz, M.K., Berggren, W.T., Izpisua Belmonte, J.C., and Evans, R.M. (2010). Human and mouse adipose-derived cells support feeder-independent induction of pluripotent stem cells. Proc Natl Acad Sci U S A 107, 3558-3563.

Takahashi, K., Tanabe, K., Ohnuki, M., Narita, M., Ichisaka, T., Tomoda, K., and Yamanaka, S. (2007). Induction of pluripotent stem cells from adult human fibroblasts by defined factors. Cell 131, 861-872.

Takahashi, K., and Yamanaka, S. (2006). Induction of pluripotent stem cells from mouse embryonic and adult fibroblast cultures by defined factors. Cell 126, 663-676.

Taranger, C.K., Noer, A., Sorensen, A.L., Hakelien, A.M., Boquest, A.C., and Collas, P. (2005). Induction of dedifferentiation, genomewide transcriptional programming, and epigenetic reprogramming by extracts of carcinoma and embryonic stem cells. Mol Biol Cell 16, 5719-5735.

Tian, X.C., Xu, J., and Yang, X. (2000). Normal telomere lengths found in cloned cattle. Nat Genet 26, 272-273.

Tsai, S.Y., Clavel, C., Kim, S., Ang, Y.S., Grisanti, L., Lee, D.F., Kelley, K., and Rendl, M. (2010). Oct4 and klf4 reprogram dermal papilla cells into induced pluripotent stem cells. Stem Cells 28, 221-228.

Vizlin-Hodzic, D., Johansson, H., Ryme, J., Simonsson, T., and Simonsson, S. (2011). SAF-A Has a Role in Transcriptional Regulation of Oct4 in ES Cells Through Promoter Binding. Cell Reprogram.

Vizlin-Hodzic, D., Ryme, J., Simonsson, S., and Simonsson, T. (2009). Developmental studies of Xenopus shelterin complexes: the message to reset telomere length is already present in the egg. FASEB J 23, 2587-2594.

Warren, L., Manos, P. D., Ahfeldt, T., Loh, Y. H., Li, H., Lau, F., Ebina, W., Mandal, P. K., Smith, Z. D. & other authors (2010). Highly efficient reprogramming to pluripotency and directed differentiation of human cells with synthetic modified mRNA. Cell Stem Cell 7, 618-630.

Wei, D., Kanai, M., Huang, S., and Xie, K. (2006). Emerging role of KLF4 in human gastrointestinal cancer. Carcinogenesis 27, 23-31.

Wei, F., Scholer, H.R., and Atchison, M.L. (2007). Sumoylation of Oct4 enhances its stability, DNA binding, and transactivation. J Biol Chem 282, 21551-21560.

Wernig, M., Lengner, C.J., Hanna, J., Lodato, M.A., Steine, E., Foreman, R., Staerk, J., Markoulaki, S., and Jaenisch, R. (2008a). A drug-inducible transgenic system for direct reprogramming of multiple somatic cell types. Nat Biotechnol 26, 916-924.

Wernig, M., Meissner, A., Cassady, J.P., and Jaenisch, R. (2008b). c-Myc is dispensable for direct reprogramming of mouse fibroblasts. Cell Stem Cell 2, 10-12.

Wernig, M., Meissner, A., Foreman, R., Brambrink, T., Ku, M., Hochedlinger, K., Bernstein, B.E., and Jaenisch, R. (2007). In vitro reprogramming of fibroblasts into a pluripotent ES-cell-like state. Nature 448, 318-324.

Wernig, M., Zhao, J.P., Pruszak, J., Hedlund, E., Fu, D., Soldner, F., Broccoli, V., Constantine-Paton, M., Isacson, O., and Jaenisch, R. (2008c). Neurons derived from reprogrammed fibroblasts functionally integrate into the fetal brain and improve symptoms of rats with Parkinson's disease. Proc Natl Acad Sci U S A 105, 5856-5861.

Wilmut, I., Schnieke, A.E., McWhir, J., Kind, A.J., and Campbell, K.H. (1997). Viable offspring derived from fetal and adult mammalian cells. Nature 385, 810-813.

Woltjen, K., Michael, I.P., Mohseni, P., Desai, R., Mileikovsky, M., Hamalainen, R., Cowling, R., Wang, W., Liu, P., Gertsenstein, M., et al. (2009). piggyBac transposition reprograms fibroblasts to induced pluripotent stem cells. Nature 458, 766-770.

Xu, D., Alipio, Z., Fink, L.M., Adcock, D.M., Yang, J., Ward, D.C., and Ma, Y. (2009). Phenotypic correction of murine hemophilia A using an iPS cell-based therapy. Proc Natl Acad Sci U S A 106, 808-813.

Xu, H.M., Liao, B., Zhang, Q.J., Wang, B.B., Li, H., Zhong, X.M., Sheng, H.Z., Zhao, Y.X., Zhao, Y.M., and Jin, Y. (2004). Wwp2, an E3 ubiquitin ligase that targets transcription factor Oct-4 for ubiquitination. J Biol Chem 279, 23495-23503.

Yakubov, E., Rechavi, G., Rozenblatt, S. & Givol, D. (2010). Reprogramming of human fibroblasts to pluripotent stem cells using mRNA of four transcription factors. Biochem Biophys Res Commun 394, 189-193.

Yamanaka, S. (2009). A fresh look at iPS cells. Cell *137*, 13-17.

Yamanaka, S., and Blau, H.M. (2010). Nuclear reprogramming to a pluripotent state by three approaches. Nature *465*, 704-712.

Yamazaki, Y., Fujita, T.C., Low, E.W., Alarcon, V.B., Yanagimachi, R., and Marikawa, Y. (2006). Gradual DNA demethylation of the Oct4 promoter in cloned mouse embryos. Mol Reprod Dev *73*, 180-188.

Yu, J., Hu, K., Smuga-Otto, K., Tian, S., Stewart, R., Slukvin, II, and Thomson, J.A. (2009). Human induced pluripotent stem cells free of vector and transgene sequences. Science *324*, 797-801.

Yu, J., Vodyanik, M.A., Smuga-Otto, K., Antosiewicz-Bourget, J., Frane, J.L., Tian, S., Nie, J., Jonsdottir, G.A., Ruotti, V., Stewart, R., *et al.* (2007). Induced pluripotent stem cell lines derived from human somatic cells. Science *318*, 1917-1920.

Yusa, K., Rad, R., Takeda, J., and Bradley, A. (2009). Generation of transgene-free induced pluripotent mouse stem cells by the piggyBac transposon. Nat Methods *6*, 363-369.

Zhang, J., Wilson, G.F., Soerens, A.G., Koonce, C.H., Yu, J., Palecek, S.P., Thomson, J.A., and Kamp, T.J. (2009). Functional cardiomyocytes derived from human induced pluripotent stem cells. Circ Res *104*, e30-41.

Zhao, H.X., Li, Y., Jin, H.F., Xie, L., Liu, C., Jiang, F., Luo, Y.N., Yin, G.W., Wang, J., Li, L.S., *et al.* (2010). Rapid and efficient reprogramming of human amnion-derived cells into pluripotency by three factors OCT4/SOX2/NANOG. Differentiation *80*, 123-129.

Zhao, T., Zhang, Z.N., Rong, Z., and Xu, Y. (2011). Immunogenicity of induced pluripotent stem cells. Nature *474*, 212-215.

Zhao, X.Y., Li, W., Lv, Z., Liu, L., Tong, M., Hai, T., Hao, J., Guo, C.L., Ma, Q.W., Wang, L., *et al.* (2009). iPS cells produce viable mice through tetraploid complementation. Nature *461*, 86-90.

Zhou, H., Wu, S., Joo, J.Y., Zhu, S., Han, D.W., Lin, T., Trauger, S., Bien, G., Yao, S., Zhu, Y., *et al.* (2009). Generation of induced pluripotent stem cells using recombinant proteins. Cell Stem Cell *4*, 381-384.

Zhou, Q., Brown, J., Kanarek, A., Rajagopal, J., and Melton, D.A. (2008). In vivo reprogramming of adult pancreatic exocrine cells to beta-cells. Nature *455*, 627-632.

Zhu, S., Li, W., Zhou, H., Wei, W., Ambasudhan, R., Lin, T., Kim, J., Zhang, K., and Ding, S. (2010). Reprogramming of human primary somatic cells by OCT4 and chemical compounds. Cell Stem Cell *7*, 651-655.

2

Relevance of HLA Expression Variants in Stem Cell Transplantation

Britta Eiz-Vesper and Rainer Blasczyk
Institute for Transfusion Medicine, Hannover Medical School, Hannover
Germany

1. Introduction

Matching the donor and recipient for class I and II human leukocyte antigens (HLA) is pivotal to the success of allogeneic hematopoietic stem cell transplantation (HSCT). Transplantation across HLA barriers will lead to the development of T-cell responses to the mismatched HLA molecules, resulting in T-cell–mediated graft-versus-host disease (GvHD) or graft rejection in patients with insufficient immune suppression. The accuracy of testing and matching criteria has an important impact on the transplant outcome, but exact matching across multiple HLA loci (e.g., HLA-A, HLA-B, HLA-C, and HLA-DRB1) is a challenging task. Today, serological HLA diagnostic tests are being replaced by DNA-based typing methods considering only selected regions of the genes. Therefore, HLA null alleles or expression variants bearing their variation outside of these regions may be misdiagnosed as normally expressed variants, resulting in HLA mismatches that are highly likely to stimulate allogeneic T cells and trigger GvHD. This chapter will address the relevance, genetics, prevalence and diagnosis of HLA expression, variants of HLA class I loci and will discuss their clinical implications for transplantation.

2. The human major histocompatibility complex

The human major histocompatibility complex (MHC), also referred to as the human leukocyte antigen (HLA) complex, is encoded on the short arm of chromosome 6 (6p21) and is extremely polymorphic (Parham et al. 1988). HLA class I molecules are expressed on most nucleated cells. The HLA class I region comprises the gene loci for the heavy chains of the three classical human leukocyte antigens, HLA-A, -B, and -C. They consist of a heavy chain (44 kDa) and a non-covalently bound $\beta2$ microglobulin ($\beta2$m) light chain (12 kDa) encoded by chromosome 15. The heavy chain is made up of three extracellular domains: $\alpha1$, $\alpha2$, and $\alpha3$. The highly polymorphic region of HLA class I molecules is located in the DNA and amino acid sequences of the $\alpha1$ and $\alpha 2$ domains, which form the peptide-binding groove. Endogenous 8 to 12 amino acid peptides are presented to CD8+ cytotoxic T lymphocytes (CTLs) (Natarajan et al. 1999). The $\alpha3$ domain is mainly invariant and contains the binding site for the co-receptor CD8. Because of the MHC's role in recognizing pathogenic and cancerous peptides, these genes are under high environmental pressure to be very polymorphic. A total of 4,946 HLA class I alleles have been identified to date (http://www.ebi.ac uk/imgt/hla; released April 2011).

HLA class I molecules are stabilized by disulfide bonds located in the α2 and α3 domains between cysteine (C) residues at amino acid positions 101/164 and 203/259. These bonds are essential for the correct processing and function of the molecules (Solheim 1999). Amino acid substitutions in these crucial C residues are likely to cause aberrant expression of the respective HLA class I molecules and may also change the affinity of the peptide-binding groove towards endogenous peptides (Warburton et al. 1994; Hirv et al. 2006; Hinrichs et al. 2009; Hinrichs et al. 2010).

HLA class II molecules (DR, DQ, DP) are mainly expressed on hematopoietic cells (macrophages, dendritic cells, T cells and B cells). The heterodimers are formed by two membrane-bound chains (α and β), each consisting of two domains (α1/α2 or β1/β2, respectively) encoded by two genes co-located in the centromeric part of the MHC. The antigenic peptide (up to 30 amino acids) is presented to CD4+ T helper cells (T_h cells) in a cleft formed by the outermost α1 and β1 domains. Nearly all of the polymorphisms occur at exon 2 of the respective A or B genes. Peptides presented by HLA class II molecules are derived from exogenous proteins as well as from epitopes of plasma membranes or endosomes (Rudensky et al. 1991; Chicz et al. 1993; Sant 1994). The nonpolymorphic β2 domain contains the binding site for the T cell co-receptor CD4. More than 1,457 HLA class II alleles have been identified to date (http://www.ebi.ac uk/imgt/hla; released April 2011).

2.1 Peptide presentation by HLA

The ability to recognize and distinguish between self and non-self is primarily mediated by T lymphocytes, which survey the protein environment of cell surfaces for binding partners, i.e. for signs of foreign invasion. T cells do not recognize proteins directly; instead, they recognize imprints of ongoing protein metabolism in the form of peptides presented by HLA molecules. This phenomenon is called MHC restriction. The biological function of HLA molecules is to present antigenic peptides to T cells. Therefore, HLA molecules play a central role in T cell-mediated adoptive immunity. MHC class I molecules present peptides from endogenously synthezised proteins, whereas MHC class II molecules present peptides from incorporated exogenous proteins. All of these peptides originate from foreign or host cell proteins and are generated by proteasomal cleavage (class I pathway) or lysosomal processing (class II pathway). It has been estimated that about 0.5% of presented peptides are bound to MHC molecules, whereas more than 99% are ignored. Consequently, peptide binding to HLA is the single most selective event involved in antigen processing and presentation (Yewdell, Norbury, and Bennink 1999; Yewdell and Bennink 2001). A T cell-mediated immune response occurs when the T-cell receptor recognizes a specific peptide-MHC complex and thus identifies cells that have been infected by intracellular parasites or viruses or cells containing abnormal proteins (e.g., tumor cells). The peptides beeing part of a certain peptide-MHC complex triggering T-cell recognition are important tools for diagnosis and treatment of infectious, autoimmune, allergic and neoplastic diseases (Ferrari et al. 2000; Haselden, Kay, and Larche 2000; Singh 2000; Wang, Phan, and Marincola 2001).

Different polymorphic HLA molecules have different peptide binding specificities (Falk et al. 1991; Sette et al. 1994; Bade-Doeding et al. 2007; Bade-Doeding et al. 2011). Peptides presented by MHC class I molecules are derived from cytoplasmic proteins by proteolytic degradation in the proteasome. Therefore, the MHC class I presentation pathway is often called the cytosolic or endogenous pathway. The MHC class I crystal structure features a unique peptide-binding groove at the outer polymorphic α2 and α3 domains (Bjorkman et al. 1987, Madden et al. 1991). This groove can be subdivided into six pockets (A-F) of different size, shape, and function (Garrett et al. 1989; Matsumura et al. 1992). A pocket is defined as a unit having an affinity for a certain peptide side chain (e.g., affinity of pocket A for peptide position P1 and pocket B for P2). Some pockets have a well-shaped structure with an affinity for only one side chain, whereas others have an affinity for a group of side chains. In some cases, the boundaries between pockets are unclear. The most important residues and positions of a peptide are known as anchor residues and anchor positions. The identity and spacing of these primary anchors constitutes the peptide motif of an HLA specificity (Sette et al. 1987; Sette et al. 1989; Jardetzky et al. 1991; Ruppert et al. 1994; Rammensee, Friede, and Stevanoviic 1995). A typical peptide is 8 to 12 amino acids in length and binds in the peptide-binding groove, exhibiting an extended conformation with its terminal amino group bound to a pocket at one end of the groove and its terminal carboxyl group bound to a pocket at the other end of the groove.

Peptide binding motifs generally contain two to three anchor positions (Rammensee, Friede, and Stevanoviic 1995). Other features such as secondary anchors and disfavored residues have also been described as playing an important role in defining the peptide-MHC interaction (Ruppert et al. 1993). The peptide-binding cleft of HLA class II molecules is formed by the outer α1 and β1 domains. Since it does not narrow at the ends, it can accommodate longer peptides containing up to 30 but usually 13 to 17 amino acids. The peptides presented by class II molecules are derived from extracellular proteins internalized by endophagocytosis and degraded in an endocytic compartment. Hence, the MHC class II-dependent pathway of antigen presentation is called the endocytic or exogenous pathway.

2.2 HLA nomenclature and typing methods

According to the World Health Organization (WHO) Committee on Nomenclature for Factors of the HLA System (Holdsworth et al. 2009), each HLA allele name has a unique number corresponding to up to four sets of digits separated by colons. The 2-digits before the first colon describe the type, which often corresponds to the serological antigen carried by an allotype. The next set of digits are used to list the subtypes, numbers being assigned in the order in which DNA sequences have been determined. Broad families of alleles are clustered into serotypes (e.g., HLA-A1).

There are two levels of typing: low-resolution (2-digits) and high-resolution (at least 4-digits). Low-resolution typing delivers results equivalent to serological typing and can be achieved by serological (microlymphocytotoxicity test) or molecular techniques. Due to its simplicity and low cost, serologic typing is still used in some laboratories. High-resolution typing can only be achieved by DNA-based techniques allowing classification of the individual alleles within each serotype (e.g., HLA-A*01:01). A number of HLA typing methods based on PCR technology have been developed. PCR with sequence-specific primers (PCR-SSP), PCR followed by sequence-specific oligonucleotide probing (PCR-SSO) and PCR followed by sequencing-based typing (PCR-SBT) are currently the most commonly used molecular methods for low- and high-resolution HLA typing. These methods have displaced serology in most laboratories because of a much greater accuracy.

2.2.1 Types and nomenclature of HLA expression variants

To label HLA alleles with an alternative expression pattern the WHO Nomenclature Committee for Factors of the HLA System defined suffixes ('N', 'L', 'S', 'C', 'A', 'Q'), that are added to an allele name to indicate its expression status (Holdsworth et al. 2009). Alleles shown to be not expressed ('Null' alleles) are given the suffix 'N'. The alteration does not necessarily imply the lack of production of an internal partial product which might be a T-cell target (Elsner and Blasczyk 2004). HLA alleles with 'Low' cell surface expression of an intact antigen compared to normal levels are indicated using the suffix 'L'. The suffix 'S' is used to denote an allele specifying a protein which is exclusively expressed as a 'Secreted' molecule but not as a cell surface protein. A 'Q' suffix is used when the expression of an allele is 'Questionable' given that the mutation seen in the allele has previously been shown to affect normal expression levels. The suffix 'C' is used to denote an allele product found in the 'Cytoplasm' but not on the cell surface, and the suffix 'A' indicates 'Aberrant' expression.

Currently, 197 HLA class I alleles (168 N, 5 L, 24 Q and 1 S allele) and 21 HLA class II alleles (all null alleles) with variant expression are listed in the IMGT/HLA database on the HLA nomenclature website (www.ebi.ac.uk/imgt/hla; released April 2011). As of April 2011, no alleles have been named with a 'C' or 'A' suffix. Most of these alleles carry mutations causing stop codons, leaving no doubt about their non-expression. Examples include HLA-A*02:82N, HLA-A*23:08N, HLA-A*24:132N, HLA-B*14:07N, HLA-B*39:40N, HLA-B*46:07N, HLA-B*56:190N, or HLA-C*06:49N. In the case of HLA-A*03:03N, a frame deletion is responsible for non-expression (Lienert et al. 1996).

Only four HLA-A alleles (HLA-A*01:01:38L, HLA-A*02:01:01:02L, HLA-A*24:02:01:02L, HLA-A*30:14L) and one HLA-B allele (HLA-B*39:01:01:02L) with low-expression patterns have been identified up to now (Balas et al. 1994; Magor et al. 1997; Laforet et al. 1997; Dunn et al. 2004; Hirv et al. 2006; Perrier et al. 2006). Low expression of these alleles is usually associated with a low expression of the corresponding mRNA. However, the alteration causing the low expression of HLA*A-30:14L is not associated with a reduced mRNA level, but rather seems to result from the loss of the disulfide bond between the cysteine residues at positions 101 and 164 in the α2 domain (Hirv et al. 2006; Hinrichs et al. 2009).

The only soluble secreted allele (S) known so far is HLA-B*44:02:01:02S (Dubois et al. 2004). This HLA-B44 variant was typed as a null allele by microlymphocytotoxicity, whereas the B*44:02:01:01 allele was identified by PCR-SSP. DNA sequencing revealed a single nucleotide difference at the end of intron 4 in the acceptor splicing site, leading to a splicing error characterized by the deletion of exon 5 (transmembrane domain of the HLA antigen).

All known HLA class I Q alleles (7 HLA-A, 9 HLA-B and 8 HLA-C) and the HLA-A*30:14L allele have cysteine residue mutations at amino acid position 101 or 164 affecting the 101/164 disulfide bridge in the α2 domain. Point mutations altering codon 101 have been described for HLA-C*02:25Q and HLA-C*03:22Q (Middleton et al. 2006). In the case of HLA-A*02:293Q, HLA-A*11:50Q, HLA-A*30:14L (Hirv et al. 2006), HLA-A*32:11Q (Tang et al. 2006), HLA-B*15:218Q, HLA-B*35:65Q (Elsner et al. 2006), HLA-B*37:16Q, HLA-B*39:38Q (Tang et al. 2006), HLA-B*40:133Q, HLA-C*04:59Q, HLA-C*07:121Q, HLA-C*12:42Q, HLA-C*15:32Q and HLA-C*16:16Q, point mutations in codon 164 result in a replacement of the Cys residue, causing disruption of the disulfide bond in the α2 domain. HLA-A*30:14L is the only one of these alleles described as having a low expression pattern not affecting the corresponding mRNA levels (Hirv et al. 2006; Hinrichs et al. 2009). There are no known alleles with an amino acid mutation at positions 203 or 259 affecting the bridge in the α3 domain.

2.3 HLA in transplantation

The best donor is an HLA genotypically matched sibling identified by family typing. When no identical sibling donor is available, transplantation of stem cells from an HLA-matched unrelated donor can result in comparable disease–free survival, particularly for good-risk patients (Petersdorf et al. 2004; Petersdorf 2007; 2008). Nevertheless, unrelated transplantation is associated with a higher frequency of post-transplant complications than in genotypically matched sibling HSCT, mainly because of undefined HLA incompatibilities. The negative impact of HLA mismatches on the outcome of hematopoietic stem cell transplantation has been demonstrated in a variety of studies (Mickelson et al. 2000; Ottinger et al. 2003; Schaffer et al. 2003). Most allele mismatches affect differences in the T-cell receptor contact area of the heavy chain or the peptide-binding site causing a change in the peptide binding repertoire both leading to a T cell-mediated allorecognition.

HistoCheck (www.histocheck.org) is an online tool which helps clinicians and researchers visualize the amino acid substitutions of HLA alleles so that they can make informed judgments about their functional similarity (Elsner et al. 2004). Because exact HLA matching is often not possible, it is important to understand which alleles are the most similar. *HistoCheck* provides crystallography-based 3-dimensional (3D) visualizations of the allelic mismatches by highlighting amino acid mismatches, positions, and functions. The user is provided with dissimilarity scores (DSSs) for the amino acids involved as well as an over-all DSS for the two alleles. However, scoring HLA mismatches by HistoCheck has not been shown to predict clinical outcome in unrelated hematopoietic stem cell transplantation.

Several large-scale studies have shown that high-resolution matching of patients and unrelated donors significantly improves post-transplant survival (Bray et al. 2008), the incidence and severity of acute and chronic GVHD (Morishima et al. 2002; Morishima et al. 2007), and engraftment (Petersdorf et al. 2001; Flomenberg et al. 2004; Lee et al. 2007; Petersdorf 2008). Regarding cord blood transplantation, several studies have shown that the degree of HLA match is important as well, but a large cell dose may be at least equally important (Laughlin et al. 2004; Rocha, Sanz, and Gluckman 2004; Arcese et al. 2006; Eapen et al. 2007).

The National Marrow Donor Program (NMDP, www.marrow.org) proposed minimum HLA matching requirements for adult donors for HLA-A, -B, -C and -DRB1 (8/8) typed, at high resolution by DNA-based methods and cord blood units (CBU) for HLA-A, -B, (low resolution) and -DRB1 (high resolution) (Table 1) (Bray et al. 2008; Kamani et al. 2008).

Considering HLA allele and haplotype frequencies can be very useful when interpreting typing results and finding appropriate donors. Simply knowing that a patient's haplotype is extremely rare can prevent futile registry searches. Considering allele frequency alone is insufficient, because a rare allele can be acceptable when it is found in its most common haplotype. Being aware of rare alleles and haplotypes is also an important factor in quality control. Furthermore, typing results in registries are often incomplete. In the case where there are two matching donors, but each donor typing is incomplete with respect to different alleles, then haplotype frequencies can help choose the donor who is most likely to be an exact match. To overcome these limitations the new matching algorithm *HapLogic* (www.marrow.org) and *Haplocheck* (www.haplocheck.org) were developed. *HapLogic* a new enhanced matching algorithm that automatically identifies the donors or CBUs with the highest potential to match the patient, was established by the NMDP to accelerate and improve the efficiency of searches. The new matching algorithm analyzes the haplotypes of millions of donors on NMDP's *Be The Match Registry*. HapLogic uses advanced logic to predict a donor's or CBU's high-resolution match and builds upon mathematical formulas that predict DR match in AB donors (Hurley et al. 2006).

HLA locus	Tissue type patient?	Match donor and patient?
A	Yes, allele level	Yes
B	Yes, allele level	Yes
C	Yes, allele level	Yes
DRA	No	No
DRB1	Yes, allele level	Yes
DRB3, 4, and 5	Yes (DRB1 association)	Unknown
DQA1	No	No
DQB1	Yes (DRB1 association)	Uncertain
DPA1	No	No
DPB1	No	Uncertain

Table 1. HLA tissue typing recommended by the NMDP (from www.marrow.org) (Bray et al. 2008; Kamani et al. 2008)

The web tool *HaploCheck* is addressing this chance by ranking typing results based upon haplotype frequencies. The user enters the typing results for a patient, for which the cis/trans phase is unknown. The result is a list of separated haplotypes, ordered by frequency. Very rare alleles and associations are highlighted to inform the user of potential problems when searching registries, or to identify potential typing errors. For the case that a single mismatch is unavoidable, the user is presented with a list of mismatch-containing haplotypes and their frequencies. This can not only prevent futile registry searches, but also enable the clinician to make decisions about accepted mismatches before initiating a registry search.

3. Prevalence and allogenicity of HLA class I expression variants

Few investigators have systematically addressed the prevalence of HLA null and alternatively expressed alleles, which has been shown to be about 0.003% and 0.3%, respectively (Noreen et al. 2001; Elsner and Blasczyk 2004; Smith et al. 2005). Considering that most studies indicate that the prevalence of these alleles is around 1 per 1000 individuals, these alleles are not particularly rare. Consequently, it was recommended that laboratories typing unrelated bone marrow patients and donors should have a strategy to identify these expression variants (Elsner and Blasczyk 2004).

HLA null and expression variants are typically identified by the discrepancy between serological and molecular typing results. As molecular typing techniques have nearly displaced serological methods and are focusing on selected regions of the HLA genes many expression variants are likely to be overlooked. In solid organ transplantation, HLA expression variants are not considered in the matching procedure. In allogeneic HSCT, expression variants make an essential difference and can strongly affect transplant-related mortality since HLA mismatches are the major cause of severe GvHD or graft rejection. Thus, in contrast to solid organ transplantation, excluding HLA expression variants is required in the matching process for HSCT (Elsner and Blasczyk 2004; Hirv et al. 2006; Hinrichs et al. 2009).

Overlooking an HLA null allele in the donor would result in a T cell-mediated allorecognition of the recipient's HLA and may lead to the development of acute severe GvHD (Elsner and Blasczyk 2004). In the reverse setting (recipient null allele, donor expressed allele), allogeneic recognition of the recipient's stem cells may lead to their destruction and subsequent graft failure. Accordingly, mismatches between expressed and non-expressed HLA variants should be avoided in HSCT. In case of a recipient with an HLA null allele having no HLA-identical donor with the same null variant, matching must be performed as if the patient would be homozygous for the expressed allele of the respective HLA locus (Figure 1).

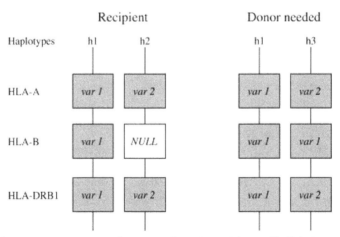

Fig. 1. Haplotypes in a recipient-donor combination with a null allele in one of the recipient's haplotypes. Shadowed boxes indicate normally expressed variants. The recipient carries an HLA-B null allele (white box). In the donor search the recipient's haplotype h2 has to be 'replaced' by haplotype (h3) containing the expressed HLA-B allele (var1). However, such a haplotype may be rare and a matching donor hard to find (Elsner and Blasczyk 2004).

On the other hand, an incomplete HLA molecule may be generated, as has been shown for HLA-B*44:02:01:02S, which might be presented via the indirect allogeneic recognition pathway (Magor et al. 1997; Dubois et al. 2004). Provided that the HLA-derived peptides fit into the peptide-binding groove and are capable of triggering a strong T-cell response, they may act as minor histocompatibility antigens (mHags). This could also apply to those HLA expression variants where the transcription of a truncated mRNA is known and/or translation is probable. It also shows that premature stop codons do not automatically lead to the interruption of transcription (Balas et al. 1994; Laforet et al. 1997; Magor et al. 1997; Dunn et al. 2004; Hirv et al. 2006; Perrier et al. 2006; Eiz-Vesper, Blasczyk, and Horn 2007). In the light of countless non-HLA mHags this is probably of inferior importance.

4. Characterization of HLA expression variants by cytokine-induced HLA secretion

Because of the clinical importance of expresion variants an HLA secretion assay was designed capable of discriminating between low-expression (L) and non-expressed (N) HLA variant alleles and assigning questionably expressed (Q) alleles to either group (Hinrichs et al. 2009).

All of the aforementioned HLA class I alleles with an unknown expression profile (Q alleles; 7 HLA-A, 9 HLA-B and 8 HLA-C) and HLA-A*30:14L, have a mutation of cysteine residue 101 or 164 affecting disulfide bridge 101/164 in the α2 domain. Because HLA-A*30:14L is the only one of these alleles described to have a low expression pattern with no effect on mRNA levels (Hirv et al. 2006; Hinrichs et al. 2009), A*30:14L was used as an expression model. HLA-A*30:14L was reported to be non-expressed under normal conditions and to show weak aberrant expression after cultivation of the corresponding B-lymphoblastoid cell line at 30°C (Hirv et al. 2006).

HLA-A*30:14L was originally identified in a patient suffering from chronic myeloid leukemia (Hirv et al. 2006). The sequence of this allele is identical to that of HLA-A*30:01 except for a transversion at nucleotide position 563 in exon 3 (guanine to cytosine substitution), resulting in a replacement of cysteine by serine at position 164, impairing disulfide bridge formation in the α2 domain of the mature polypeptide. This alteration of the secondary structure presumably decreases expression, rendering HLA-A*30:14L basically undetectable by serology.

Human cell lines (HEK293, C1R and K562) expressing recombinant soluble HLA (sHLA) molecules (Table 2) were incubated with interferon (IFN)-γ and/or tumor necrosis factor (TNF)-α (Hinrichs et al. 2009). These pro-inflammatory cytokines are known to enhance the expression of HLA molecules by affecting the interaction of DNA-binding proteins with the HLA-A promoter regions, resulting in the increased transcription of heavy and light chain genes (Girdlestone 1996; Gobin et al. 1997; Gobin et al. 1998; Gobin et al. 1999; Johnson 2003). In addition, these cytokines induce the transcription of proteasome subunits, peptide transporters and chaperones that promote the expresson of HLA class I molecules by providing peptides for presentation (Ma et al. 1997; Lankat-Buttgereit and Tampe 2002).

Expression of soluble HLA-A*30:14L and HLA-A*30:01 was measured in the supernatants of transfected and untransfected cells incubated with or without IFN-γ and/or TNF-α using a W6/32 and anti-β2-microglobulin-based sandwich ELISA (Figure 1) (Bade-Doeding et al. 2007). HLA-A*30:14L was not detected in the supernatant of unstimulated transfectants. Stimulation with IFN-γ and/or TNF-α increased HLA-A*30:14L secretion to detectable levels and increased HLA-A*30:01 expression up to 8-fold, but did not result in any difference between mRNA levels of HLA-A*30:14L and A*30:01 (Figure 2).

Day		Expression level (ng/ml)		
		HEK293	C1R	K562
1	HLA-A*30:01	31.3 ± 10.3	98.0 ± 14.7	155.8 ± 73.9
	HLA-A*30:14L	0	3.2 ± 1.7	0
3	HLA-A*30:01	383.2 ± 56.5	225.8 ± 177.5	143.5 ± 40.8
	HLA-A*30:14L	1.8 ± 1.4	0	0
7	HLA-A*30:01	160.4 ± 3.2	253.6 ± 16.1	175.9 ± 74.7
	HLA-A*30:14L	0	9.7 ± 4.9	0

Table 2. Soluble HLA-A*30:01 and HLA-A*30:14L expression levels (ng/ml) in the supernatant of three transfected cell lines (HEK293, C1R and K562) after 1, 3 and 7 days of incubation.

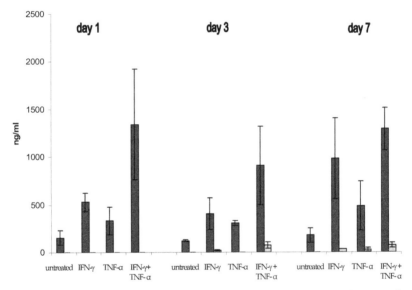

Fig. 2. Secretion of soluble HLA-A*30:01 and HLA-A*30:14L by transfected K562 cells

Expression of mRNA transcripts of both alleles was determined by real-time PCR. For control, Epstein-Barr virus (EBV)-transformed B-lymphoblastoid cell line (B-LCL) expressing HLA-A*30:14L was established from cells of the patient's mother (genotype HLA-A*30:14L,*02:01) (Hirv et al. 2006). The positive control was a B-LCL expressing HLA-A*30:01 (genotype HLA-A*30:01,*02:01). In both B-LCLs and HEK293 cells, the mRNA level of HLA-A*30:14L was nearly identical to that of HLA-A*30:01 (Figure 3). This finding suggests that the mRNA transcription rate of sHLA-A*30:14L is not affected by the mutation at nucleotide position 563 (G->C). The mRNA levels of both alleles clearly increased in response to combined stimulation with IFN-γ and TNF-α. In view of this lack of any difference in mRNA transcription, the protein expression defect is most likely caused by the missing disulfide bond in the α2 domain.

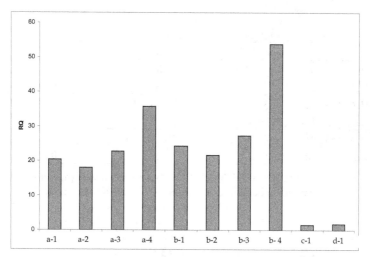

Fig. 3. Detection of mRNA levels of HLA-A*30 alleles in B-LCLs and HEK293 cells

mRNA expression of the HLA-A*30 alleles in transfected cell lines and B-LCLs was determined by real-time PCR. Shown are representative results for HEK293 cells measured after 3 days of culture in the presence ("treated") or absence ("untreated") of the cytokines IFN-γ and/or TNF-α. Data were acquired using a probe specific for the HLA-A30 sequence. Similar results were achieved for all transfected cell lines. Lanes: a) sHLA-A*30:01-transfected HEK293, b) sHLA-A*30:14L-transfected HEK293, c) EBRCC-256 (HLA-A*30:01), d) EBRCC-1818 (HLA-A*30:14L), 1 untreated, 2 IFN-γ-treated, 3 TNF-α-treated, 4 IFN-γ plus TNF-α-treated

The observation that HLA-A*30:14L protein accumulates inside the cells indicates that HLA-A*30:14L translation is not affected. Consequently, the lack of protein secretion in the supernatant is best explained by post-translational instability of the HLA-A*30:14L molecules because of the missing disulfide bridge (Hinrichs et al. 2009). Based on these findings, it is likely that the intracellular enriched HLA-A*30:14L protein is a major substrate for proteasomal cleavage and that it provides a flood of peptide fragments presented to cytotoxic T lymphocytes. As a result of this indirect surface expression by the presentation of peptide fragments, it is possible that GvHD or graft rejection might be promoted in the event of mismatching (Benichou 1999). Consequently, considering HLA-A*30:14L as null allele is, in case of a mismatch with any other HLA-A allele, potentially more dangerous in terms of GvHD and graft rejection than a mismatch with its most related allele HLA-A*30:01. Indeed, mistyping HLA-A*30:14L as an N allele has led to a severe GvHD in a patient transplanted with hematopoietic stem cells from an HLA-A*02:01 homozygous donor (Hirv et al. 2006).

In recent studies, the cytokine-based HLA secretion assay was used to classify the expression patterns of HLA-A*32:11Q (Tang et al. 2006) and HLA-B*35:65Q (Elsner et al. 2006). Both alleles undergo cysteine substitution at amino acid position 164 and thus lack the disulfide bond between the cysteine residues at amino acid positions 101 and 164 in the α2 domain of the mature protein. This interferes with HLA maturation inside the ER and therefore impairs cell surface expression. In concordance with the results of Hinrichs et al. (Hinrichs et al. 2009), IFN-γ and TNF-α increased the expression of the HLA expression variants, making HLA-A*32:11Q and HLA-B*35:65Q distinctly detectable. Compared to HLA-A*32:01 and HLA-B*35:01, the variants have very weak protein levels, indicating a low expression status. Consequently, they should be handled as low expression variants (L alleles).

5. The nature of peptides presented by HLA class I expression variants

The functional integrity of HLA low-expression variants is a prerequisite for considering them as essential in hematopoietic stem cell donor and recipient matching to diminish the risk of serious complications such as GvHD or graft rejection. HLA class I molecules present endogenous peptides 8-12 amino acids in length to CD8+ cytotoxic T lymphocytes (Natarajan et al. 1999). Most amino acid polymorphisms of different HLA class I molecules are located in the peptide-binding region shaped by parts of the α1 and α2 domains; these polymorphisms determine the characteristics of presented peptides. Peptide motifs have been reported for the most common HLA-A and B alleles and for some rare variants. Importantly, differences in peptide binding among the alleles of a serological group have also been described (Prilliman et al. 1999; Bade-Doeding et al. 2011,). Identification and comparison of allele-specific peptide-binding motifs provide important information for donor-recipient matching and prediction of HLA subtype allogenicity in allogeneic HSCT.

In order to determine the functionality of HLA low-expression alleles, peptides from recombinant truncated HLA-A*30:14L molecules secreted in the supernatant of a human cell line were eluted and sequenced (Hinrichs et al 2010). The suitability of the monoclonal anti-HLA class I antibody W6/32 for purifying recombinant HLA-A*30:14L molecules suggested its proper folding and assembly. Presumably, more soluble HLA-A*30:14L is produced and secreted into the supernatant that might not be correctly folded because of the lack of a disulfide bridge in the α2 domain.

Edman pool sequencing of eluted peptides corroborated the hypothesis that peptides are presented by HLA low expression variants and showed idential peptide motifs in HLA-A*30:01 and HLA-A*30:14L confirming the previously described peptide motif of A*30:01 (Lamberth et al. 2008; Sidney et al. 2008). The C-terminal position (PΩ) was identified as a primary anchor position. The preferred residues of the HLA-A*30 peptide epitopes at this position are lysine (K), valine (V) or arginine (R). The preference for lysine as the top amino acid at the PΩ position of the bound peptides, like described by positional scanning combinatorial peptide libraries (PSCPL) analysis, could be consolidated by the obtained peptide sequence data (Lamberth et al. 2008; Sidney et al. 2008). Position P3 of the peptides was identified as a primary-secondary anchor showing a high preference for the basic amino acids K and R. Six amino acids are reportedly favored at position P2: phenylalanine (F), serine (S), threonine (T), valine (V), isoleucine (I) or leucine (L).

The size of the obtained peptides ranged from 8 to 14 amino acids, but most had a length of 9 to 10 aa. The sequences of 200 HLA-A*30:01 ligands and of 100 HLA-A*30:14L ligands were identified. The following three peptide epitopes (3%) were presented by both HLA-A*30:01 and HLA-A*30:14L: 1) VLDTPGPPV, a nonameric peptide derived from titin (isoform N2-A, aa position 19783-19791), a protein of human muscle ultrastructure and elasticity; 2) EITALAPSTMK, an 11-mer peptide derived from human muscle protein ACTA1 (actin, alpha 1, skeletal muscle; aa position 301-311); and 3) DNIQGITKPAIR, a 12-mer peptide derived from a histone protein (HIST2H4A; aa position 25-36) (Table 3).

Peptide position	1	2	3	4	5	6	7	8	9	10	11	12	Source
Ligand	V	L	D	T	P	G	P	P	V				Titin (TTN titin isoform N2-A)
	E	I	T	A	L	A	P	S	T	M	K		Actin (ACTA1)
	D	N	I	Q	G	I	T	K	P	A	I	R	Histone (HIST2H4A)

Table 3. Shared peptide epitopes of HLA-A*30:14L and HLA-A*30:01

To verify the presentation of naturally presented peptides from recombinant HLA-A*30:01/30:14L molecules, peptide binding was analyzed by flow cytometry (Storkus et al. 1993; Zeh et al. 1994; Maeurer et al. 1996) in three EBV-transformed B-LCLs expressing either HLA-A*30:14L,*02:01 (Ulm-241539), HLA-A*30:01,*02:01 (EBRCC-256) or HLA-A*02:01 (EBRCC-2296) (Warburton et al. 1994; Hirv et al. 2006; Hinrichs et al. 2009; 2010). Acid treatment of the cell lines resulted in the dissociation of the naturally bound peptides and the release of β2 microglobulin from the HLA class I heavy chain. The HLA class I molecules were then reconstituted by adding fluorescein isothiocyanate (FITC)-labeled HLA peptide ligands and recombinant β2 microglobulin. The synthetic FITC-labeled peptide EITALAK(FITC)PSTMK (HLA-A*30:01/30:14L) and the immunodominant HLA-A*02:01-restricted CMVpp65$_{495-503}$ peptide (NLVPMK(FITC)VATV) were used. Reconstitution of HLA with the HLA-A*30 ligand mounted up to 51% (Ulm-241539) and 74% (EBRCC-256), respectively, compared to 25% for the HLA-A*02:01 homozygous cell line (EBRCC-2296). Binding on cells expressing the normal HLA-A*30:01 allele was higher than on those expressing HLA-A*30:14L, the low expression variant (Figure 4). The results confirm that the A*30 peptide previously isolated binds to HLA-A*30 on the cell surface. Peptide binding was found for the A*30:01 specific peptide on the HLA-A*30:14L-expressing cell line (Ulm-241539), indicating the stability of HLA-A*30:14L cell surface expression.

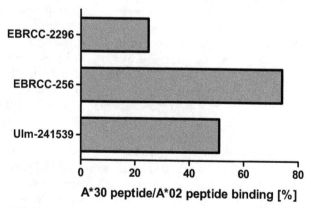

Fig. 4. Relative A*30/A*02:01 peptide-binding intensities for different HLA-expressing B-LCLs

Homology-based modeling for each HLA-A*30 alleles with the shared 9, 11 and 12-mer peptide epitopes revealed only marginal differences between the two HLA-A*30 alleles. The HLA-A*30:01 and HLA-A*30:14L models were essentially identical with the Cys164 Ser substitution, but simply adopted an alternate rotamer conformation upon breakage of the disulfide bond. Therefore, only the HLA-A*30:14L model is illustrated (Figure 5).

Although the models look identical and the alleles appear to bind identical peptides, the Cys164Ser variation could potentially generate additional flexibility within the peptide-binding groove, thereby influencing binding kinetics, particularly in peptides of lower affinity. Such an effect could stimulate a T-cell immune response and have serious implications in allogeneic HSCT.

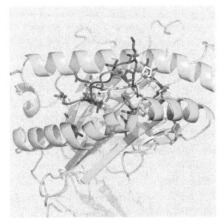

Fig. 5. Homology-based model of HLA-A*30:14L with the three shared peptide ligands

Modeling of the HLA-A*30:01 and HLA-A*30:14L structures was carried out using the SCWRL homology-based modeling server (Wang, Canutescu, and Dunbrack 2008) while employing the crystal structure of the closely related HLA-A*11:01 (1Q94) as a template. Peptide templates for 9-mer (1Q94), 11-mer (2BVO) and 12-mer (3BW9) were superimposed and merged with the HLA-A*30:14L model. Peptide mutagenesis was then performed using DeepView (Guex and Peitsch 1997) and the rotamer library to find the best side chain orientations with minimum steric clashes. Each model was then subjected to energy minimization using DeepView software. The graphics program PyMOL (http://www.pymol.org) was used to generate the structural models.

6. Conclusions

Since HLA mismatches are the main cause of severe GvHD and graft rejection, misinterpretation of HLA null alleles and expression variants as irrelevant could strongly affect transplant-related mortality.

The cytokine-based HLA secretion assay can be used to distinguish between low-expressed and non-expressed HLA alleles in order to classify alleles with a currently undefined expression status (questionable alleles, Q) as well as to re-classify certain alleles which have been assigned as null variants (N). Additionally, discrimination between cytokine inducible and non-inducible defect alleles may be important in allotransplant settings in which a cytokine storm usually occurs following pre-transplant myeloablative conditioning or post-transplant immunosuppressive therapy.

The fact that the monoclonal anti-HLA class I antibody W6/32 is a conformational antibody implies that only correctly folded, β2 microglobulin-assembled and peptide-loaded MHC complexes can be detected. This suggests that parts of soluble HLA-A*30:14L molecules are assembled correctly and secreted by transfectants. Presumably, more soluble HLA-A*30:14L is produced and secreted into the supernatant, but it might not be correctly folded because of the lack of the disulfide bridge in the α2 domain. Therefore, these molecules are not detected by the conformational anti-HLA-ABC mAb. This assumption arose after comparing mRNA and associated protein levels of HLA-A*30:14L and HLA-A*30:01 alleles (Hinrichs et al. 2009). Additionally, it was found that HLA-A*30:14L accumulates inside the cells; therefore, it might be a major substrate for proteasomal cleavage and could provide a flood of peptide fragments presented to cytotoxic T lymphocytes. As a result of this indirect allorecognition pathway, GvHD or graft rejection might be promoted in the event of a severe mismatch.

It was shown for the first time that an HLA low expression allele (HLA-A*30:14L) presents peptides with identical features to those of its most closely related relative, HLA-A*30:01 (Hinrichs et al. 2010). The results indicate that a mismatch at amino acid position 164 might be permissive. Therefore, mismatching of these alleles will presumably be of low allogenicity in allogeneic HSCT. The fact that a low expression variant is not only functional and able to present peptides, but also shares epitopes with its related variant leads to the conclusion that low expression variants need to be considered in donor selection as permissive or non-permissive mismatches, respectively. Increasing knowledge of the expression behavior of HLA expression variants, such as L and Q alleles, will help to improve HLA allogenicity prediction algorithms by delivering proof that these variants are fully functional. Taking all relevant factors into account, the results shown allow to predict the immunogenicity of aberrantly expressed alleles in a transplant setting.

In the case of HLA-A*30:14L misinterpreting it as a null allele is, in case of a mismatch with any other HLA-A allele, potentially more dangerous in terms of GvHD and graft rejection according to the direct and indirect allo-recognition pathway than a mismatch with its most related allele HLA-A*30:01. Indeed, mistyping HLA-A*30:14L as an N allele has led to a severe GvHD in a patient transplanted with hematopoietic stem cells from an HLA-A*02:01 homozygous donor (Hirv et al. 2006).

In order to predict the relevance of similar alleles with disulfide bridge rearrangements (e.g., HLA-A*32:11Q and B*35:65Q) in allogeneic HSCT, it is important to know their surface expression as well as their peptide binding of HLA variants. From a clinical perspective, HLA variants with similar disulfide bridge variations need to be considered as functionally active in an allogeneic HSCT setting as long as the opposite has not been shown.

7. Acknowledgments

The authors would like to thank Jan Hinrichs and Daniel Föll for performing the experiments and contributing helpful discussions. The authors are grateful to Christina Bade-Döding, Nektarios Ladas and Trevor Huyton for help in peptide data analysis and homology–based modeling. This work is supported in part by funding from the Deutsche Forschungsgemeinschaft (DFG, German Research Foundation) for the Cluster of Excellence

REBIRTH (From Regenerative Biology to Reconstructive Therapy) and by the German Federal Ministry of Education and Research (reference number: 01EO0802).

8. References

Arcese, W., V. Rocha, M. Labopin, G. Sanz, A. P. Iori, M. de Lima, A. Sirvent, A. Busca, S. Asano, I. Ionescu, P. Wernet, and E. Gluckman. 2006. Unrelated cord blood transplants in adults with hematologic malignancies. *Haematologica* 91 (2):223-30.

Bade-Doeding, C., A. Theodossis, S. Gras, L. Kjer-Nielsen, B. Eiz-Vesper, A. Seltsam, T. Huyton, J. Rossjohn, J. McCluskey, and R. Blasczyk. 2011. The impact of human leukocyte antigen (HLA) micropolymorphism on ligand specificity within the HLA-B*41 allotypic family. *Haematologica* 96 (1):110-8.

Bade-Doeding, C., D. S. DeLuca, A. Seltsam, R. Blasczyk, and B. Eiz-Vesper. 2007. Amino acid 95 causes strong alteration of peptide position Pomega in HLA-B*41 variants. *Immunogenetics* 59 (4):253-9.

Balas, A., F. Garcia-Sanchez, F. Gomez-Reino, and J. L. Vicario. 1994. HLA class I allele (HLA-A2) expression defect associated with a mutation in its enhancer B inverted CAT box in two families. *Hum Immunol* 41 (1):69-73.

Benichou, G. 1999. Direct and indirect antigen recognition: the pathways to allograft immune rejection. *Front Biosci* 4:D476-80.

Bjorkman, P. J., M. A. Saper, B. Samraoui, W. S. Bennett, J. L. Strominger, and D. C. Wiley. 1987. The foreign antigen binding site and T cell recognition regions of class I histocompatibility antigens. *Nature* 329 (6139):512-8.

Bjorkman P.J., M. A. Saper , B. Samraoui , W. S. Bennett, J. L.Strominger, and D. C. Wiley. 1987. Structure of the human class I histocompatibility antigen, HLA-A2. *Nature* 329 (6139):506-12.

Bray, R. A., C. K. Hurley, N. R. Kamani, A. Woolfrey, C. Muller, S. Spellman, M. Setterholm, and D. L. Confer. 2008. National marrow donor program HLA matching guidelines for unrelated adult donor hematopoietic cell transplants. *Biol Blood Marrow Transplant* 14 (9 Suppl):45-53.

Chicz, R. M., R. G. Urban, J. C. Gorga, D. A. Vignali, W. S. Lane, and J. L. Strominger. 1993. Specificity and promiscuity among naturally processed peptides bound to HLA-DR alleles. *J Exp Med* 178 (1):27-47.

Dubois, V., J. M. Tiercy, M. P. Labonne, A. Dormoy, and L. Gebuhrer. 2004. A new HLA-B44 allele (B*440201025) with a splicing mutation leading to a complete deletion of exon 5. *Tissue Antigens* 63 (2):173-80.

Dunn, P. P., J. R. Turton, J. Downing, S. Williams, C. V. Navarrete, and C. Darke. 2004. HLA-A*24020102L in the UK blood donor population. *Tissue Antigens* 63 (6):589-91.

Eapen, M., P. Rubinstein, M. J. Zhang, C. Stevens, J. Kurtzberg, A. Scaradavou, F. R. Loberiza, R. E. Champlin, J. P. Klein, M. M. Horowitz, and J. E. Wagner. 2007. Outcomes of transplantation of unrelated donor umbilical cord blood and bone marrow in children with acute leukaemia: a comparison study. *Lancet* 369 (9577):1947-54.

Eiz-Vesper, B., R. Blasczyk, and P. A. Horn. 2007. Description of the first HLA-DRB1 null allele. *Immunogenetics* 59 (6):507-10.

Elsner, H. A., and R. Blasczyk. 2004. Immunogenetics of HLA null alleles: implications for blood stem cell transplantation. *Tissue Antigens* 64 (6):687-95.

Elsner, H. A., D. DeLuca, J. Strub, and R. Blasczyk. 2004. HistoCheck: rating of HLA class I and II mismatches by an internet-based software tool. *Bone Marrow Transplant* 33 (2):165-9.

Elsner, H. A., P. A. Horn, C. Schoenemann, W. W. Altermann, and R. Blasczyk. 2006. Aberrant expression of HLA-B*3565Q is associated with a disrupted disulfide bond. *Immunogenetics* 58 (11):929-31.

Falk, K., O. Rotzschke, S. Stevanovic, G. Jung, and H. G. Rammensee. 1991. Allele-specific motifs revealed by sequencing of self-peptides eluted from MHC molecules. *Nature* 351 (6324):290-6.

Ferrari, G., D. D. Kostyu, J. Cox, D. V. Dawson, J. Flores, K. J. Weinhold, and S. Osmanov. 2000. Identification of highly conserved and broadly cross-reactive HIV type 1 cytotoxic T lymphocyte epitopes as candidate immunogens for inclusion in Mycobacterium bovis BCG-vectored HIV vaccines. *AIDS Res Hum Retroviruses* 16 (14):1433-43.

Flomenberg, N., L. A. Baxter-Lowe, D. Confer, M. Fernandez-Vina, A. Filipovich, M. Horowitz, C. Hurley, C. Kollman, C. Anasetti, H. Noreen, A. Begovich, W. Hildebrand, E. Petersdorf, B. Schmeckpeper, M. Setterholm, E. Trachtenberg, T. Williams, E. Yunis, and D. Weisdorf. 2004. Impact of HLA class I and class II high-resolution matching on outcomes of unrelated donor bone marrow transplantation: HLA-C mismatching is associated with a strong adverse effect on transplantation outcome. *Blood* 104 (7):1923-30.

Garrett, T. P., M. A. Saper, P. J. Bjorkman, J. L. Strominger, and D. C. Wiley. 1989. Specificity pockets for the side chains of peptide antigens in HLA-Aw68. *Nature* 342 (6250):692-6.

Girdlestone, J. 1996. Transcriptional regulation of MHC class I genes. *Eur J Immunogenet* 23 (5):395-413.

Gobin, S. J., V. Keijsers, M. van Zutphen, and P. J. van den Elsen. 1998. The role of enhancer A in the locus-specific transactivation of classical and nonclassical HLA class I genes by nuclear factor kappa B. *J Immunol* 161 (5):2276-83.

Gobin, S. J., A. Peijnenburg, V. Keijsers, and P. J. van den Elsen. 1997. Site alpha is crucial for two routes of IFN gamma-induced MHC class I transactivation: the ISRE-mediated route and a novel pathway involving CIITA. *Immunity* 6 (5):601-11.

Gobin, S. J., M. van Zutphen, A. M. Woltman, and P. J. van den Elsen. 1999. Transactivation of classical and nonclassical HLA class I genes through the IFN-stimulated response element. *J Immunol* 163 (3):1428-34.

Guex, N., and M. C. Peitsch. 1997. SWISS-MODEL and the Swiss-PdbViewer: an environment for comparative protein modeling. *Electrophoresis* 18 (15):2714-23.

Haselden, B. M., A. B. Kay, and M. Larche. 2000. Peptide-mediated immune responses in specific immunotherapy. *Int Arch Allergy Immunol* 122 (4):229-37.

Hinrichs, J., C. Figueiredo, K. Hirv, J. Mytilineos, R. Blasczyk, P. A. Horn, and B. Eiz-Vesper. 2009. Discrimination of HLA null and low expression alleles by cytokine-induced secretion of recombinant soluble HLA. *Mol Immunol* 46 (7):1451-7.

Hinrichs, J., D. Foll, C. Bade-Doeding, T. Huyton, R. Blasczyk, and B. Eiz-Vesper. 2010. The nature of peptides presented by an HLA class I low expression allele. *Haematologica* 95 (8):1373-80.

Hirv, K., U. Pannicke, J. Mytilineos, and K. Schwarz. 2006. Disulfide bridge disruption in the alpha2 domain of the HLA class I molecule leads to low expression of the corresponding antigen. *Hum Immunol* 67 (8):589-96.

Holdsworth, R., C. K. Hurley, S. G. Marsh, M. Lau, H. J. Noreen, J. H. Kempenich, M. Setterholm, and M. Maiers. 2009. The HLA dictionary 2008: a summary of HLA-A, -B, -C, -DRB1/3/4/5, and -DQB1 alleles and their association with serologically defined HLA-A, -B, -C, -DR, and -DQ antigens. *Tissue Antigens* 73 (2):95-170.

Hurley, C. K., J. E. Wagner, M. I. Setterholm, and D. L. Confer. 2006. Advances in HLA: practical implications for selecting adult donors and cord blood units. *Biol Blood Marrow Transplant* 12 (1 Suppl 1):28-33.

Jardetzky, T. S., W. S. Lane, R. A. Robinson, D. R. Madden, and D. C. Wiley. 1991. Identification of self peptides bound to purified HLA-B27. *Nature* 353 (6342):326-9.

Johnson, D. R. 2003. Locus-specific constitutive and cytokine-induced HLA class I gene expression. *J Immunol* 170 (4):1894-902.

Kamani, N., S. Spellman, C. K. Hurley, J. N. Barker, F. O. Smith, M. Oudshoorn, R. Bray, A. Smith, T. M. Williams, B. Logan, M. Eapen, C. Anasetti, M. Setterholm, and D. L. Confer. 2008. State of the art review: HLA matching and outcome of unrelated donor umbilical cord blood transplants. *Biol Blood Marrow Transplant* 14 (1):1-6.

Laforet, M., N. Froelich, A. Parissiadis, H. Bausinger, B. Pfeiffer, and M. M. Tongio. 1997. An intronic mutation responsible for a low level of expression of an HLA-A*24 allele. *Tissue Antigens* 50 (4):340-6.

Lamberth, K., G. Roder, M. Harndahl, M. Nielsen, C. Lundegaard, C. Schafer-Nielsen, O. Lund, and S. Buus. 2008. The peptide-binding specificity of HLA-A*3001 demonstrates membership of the HLA-A3 supertype. *Immunogenetics* 60 (11):633-43.

Lankat-Buttgereit, B., and R. Tampe. 2002. The transporter associated with antigen processing: function and implications in human diseases. *Physiol Rev* 82 (1):187-204.

Laughlin, M. J., M. Eapen, P. Rubinstein, J. E. Wagner, M. J. Zhang, R. E. Champlin, C. Stevens, J. N. Barker, R. P. Gale, H. M. Lazarus, D. I. Marks, J. J. van Rood, A. Scaradavou, and M. M. Horowitz. 2004. Outcomes after transplantation of cord blood or bone marrow from unrelated donors in adults with leukemia. *N Engl J Med* 351 (22):2265-75.

Lee, S. J., J. Klein, M. Haagenson, L. A. Baxter-Lowe, D. L. Confer, M. Eapen, M. Fernandez-Vina, N. Flomenberg, M. Horowitz, C. K. Hurley, H. Noreen, M. Oudshoorn, E. Petersdorf, M. Setterholm, S. Spellman, D. Weisdorf, T. M. Williams, and C. Anasetti. 2007. High-resolution donor-recipient HLA matching contributes to the success of unrelated donor marrow transplantation. *Blood* 110 (13):4576-83.

Lienert, K., G. Russ, S. Lester, G. Bennett, X. Gao, and J. McCluskey. 1996. Stable inheritance of an HLA-"blank" phenotype associated with a structural mutation in the HLA-A*0301 gene. *Tissue Antigens* 48 (3):187-91.

Ma, W., P. J. Lehner, P. Cresswell, J. S. Pober, and D. R. Johnson. 1997. Interferon-gamma rapidly increases peptide transporter (TAP) subunit expression and peptide transport capacity in endothelial cells. *J Biol Chem* 272 (26):16585-90.

Madden, D. R., J. C. Gorga, J. L. Strominger, and D. C. Wiley. 1991. The structure of HLA-B27 reveals nonamer self-peptides bound in an extended conformation. *Nature* 353 (6342):321-5.

Maeurer, M. J., D. Martin, E. Elder, W. J. Storkus, and M. T. Lotze. 1996. Detection of naturally processed and HLA-A1-presented melanoma T-cell epitopes defined by CD8(+) T-cells' release of granulocyte-macrophage colony-stimulating factor but not by cytolysis. *Clin Cancer Res* 2 (1):87-95.

Magor, K. E., E. J. Taylor, S. Y. Shen, E. Martinez-Naves, N. M. Valiante, R. S. Wells, J. E. Gumperz, E. J. Adams, A. M. Little, F. Williams, D. Middleton, X. Gao, J. McCluskey, P. Parham, and K. Lienert-Weidenbach. 1997. Natural inactivation of a common HLA allele (A*2402) has occurred on at least three separate occasions. *J Immunol* 158 (11):5242-50.

Matsumura, M., D. H. Fremont, P. A. Peterson, and I. A. Wilson. 1992. Emerging principles for the recognition of peptide antigens by MHC class I molecules. *Science* 257 (5072):927-34.

Mickelson, E. M., E. Petersdorf, C. Anasetti, P. Martin, A. Woolfrey, and J. A. Hansen. 2000. HLA matching in hematopoietic cell transplantation. *Hum Immunol* 61 (2):92-100.

Middleton, D., A. Meenagh, S. G. Marsh, and J. Martin. 2006. A HLA-Cw*03 allele, Cw*0322Q with limited or no expression. *Tissue Antigens* 67 (4):343-5.

Morishima, Y., T. Kawase, M. Malkki, and E. W. Petersdorf. 2007. Effect of HLA-A2 allele disparity on clinical outcome in hematopoietic cell transplantation from unrelated donors. *Tissue Antigens* 69 Suppl 1:31-5.

Morishima, Y., T. Sasazuki, H. Inoko, T. Juji, T. Akaza, K. Yamamoto, Y. Ishikawa, S. Kato, H. Sao, H. Sakamaki, K. Kawa, N. Hamajima, S. Asano, and Y. Kodera. 2002. The clinical significance of human leukocyte antigen (HLA) allele compatibility in patients receiving a marrow transplant from serologically HLA-A, HLA-B, and HLA-DR matched unrelated donors. *Blood* 99 (11):4200-6.

Natarajan, K., H. Li, R. A. Mariuzza, and D. H. Margulies. 1999. MHC class I molecules, structure and function. *Rev Immunogenet* 1 (1):32-46.

Noreen, H. J., N. Yu, M. Setterholm, M. Ohashi, J. Baisch, R. Endres, M. Fernandez-Vina, U. Heine, S. Hsu, M. Kamoun, Y. Mitsuishi, D. Monos, L. Perlee, S. Rodriguez-Marino, A. Smith, S. Y. Yang, K. Shipp, J. Hegland, and C. K. Hurley. 2001. Validation of DNA-based HLA-A and HLA-B testing of volunteers for a bone marrow registry through parallel testing with serology. *Tissue Antigens* 57 (3):221-9.

Ottinger, H. D., S. Ferencik, D. W. Beelen, M. Lindemann, R. Peceny, A. H. Elmaagacli, J. Husing, and H. Grosse-Wilde. 2003. Hematopoietic stem cell transplantation: contrasting the outcome of transplantations from HLA-identical siblings, partially HLA-mismatched related donors, and HLA-matched unrelated donors. *Blood* 102 (3):1131-7.

Parham, P., C. E. Lomen, D. A. Lawlor, J. P. Ways, N. Holmes, H. L. Coppin, R. D. Salter, A. M. Wan, and P. D. Ennis. 1988. Nature of polymorphism in HLA-A, -B, and -C molecules. *Proc Natl Acad Sci U S A* 85 (11):4005-9.

Perrier, P., A. Dormoy, C. Andre-Botte, and N. Froelich. 2006. HLA-A*02010102L: a laborious assignment. *Tissue Antigens* 68 (5):442-5.

Petersdorf, E. W. 2007. Risk assessment in haematopoietic stem cell transplantation: histocompatibility. *Best Pract Res Clin Haematol* 20 (2):155-70.

Petersdorf, E. W. 2008. Optimal HLA matching in hematopoietic cell transplantation. *Curr Opin Immunol* 20 (5):588-93.

Petersdorf, E. W., C. Anasetti, P. J. Martin, T. Gooley, J. Radich, M. Malkki, A. Woolfrey, A. Smith, E. Mickelson, and J. A. Hansen. 2004. Limits of HLA mismatching in unrelated hematopoietic cell transplantation. *Blood* 104 (9):2976-80.

Petersdorf, E. W., J. A. Hansen, P. J. Martin, A. Woolfrey, M. Malkki, T. Gooley, B. Storer, E. Mickelson, A. Smith, and C. Anasetti. 2001. Major-histocompatibility-complex class I alleles and antigens in hematopoietic-cell transplantation. *N Engl J Med* 345 (25):1794-800.

Prilliman, K. R., K. W. Jackson, M. Lindsey, J. Wang, D. Crawford, and W. H. Hildebrand. 1999. HLA-B15 peptide ligands are preferentially anchored at their C termini. *J Immunol* 162 (12):7277-84.

Rammensee, H. G., T. Friede, and S. Stevanoviic. 1995. MHC ligands and peptide motifs: first listing. *Immunogenetics* 41 (4):178-228.

Rocha, V., G. Sanz, and E. Gluckman. 2004. Umbilical cord blood transplantation. *Curr Opin Hematol* 11 (6):375-85.

Rudensky, AYu, P. Preston-Hurlburt, S. C. Hong, A. Barlow, and C. A. Janeway, Jr. 1991. Sequence analysis of peptides bound to MHC class II molecules. *Nature* 353 (6345):622-7.

Ruppert, J., R. T. Kubo, J. Sidney, H. M. Grey, and A. Sette. 1994. Class I MHC-peptide interaction: structural and functional aspects. *Behring Inst Mitt* (94):48-60.

Ruppert, J., J. Sidney, E. Celis, R. T. Kubo, H. M. Grey, and A. Sette. 1993. Prominent role of secondary anchor residues in peptide binding to HLA-A2.1 molecules. *Cell* 74 (5):929-37.

Sant, A. J. 1994. Endogenous antigen presentation by MHC class II molecules. *Immunol Res* 13 (4):253-67.

Schaffer, M., A. Aldener-Cannava, M. Remberger, O. Ringden, and O. Olerup. 2003. Roles of HLA-B, HLA-C and HLA-DPA1 incompatibilities in the outcome of unrelated stem-cell transplantation. *Tissue Antigens* 62 (3):243-50.

Sette, A., S. Buus, E. Appella, J. A. Smith, R. Chesnut, C. Miles, S. M. Colon, and H. M. Grey. 1989. Prediction of major histocompatibility complex binding regions of protein antigens by sequence pattern analysis. *Proc Natl Acad Sci U S A* 86 (9):3296-300.

Sette, A., S. Buus, S. Colon, J. A. Smith, C. Miles, and H. M. Grey. 1987. Structural characteristics of an antigen required for its interaction with Ia and recognition by T cells. *Nature* 328 (6129):395-9.

Sette, A., J. Sidney, M. F. del Guercio, S. Southwood, J. Ruppert, C. Dahlberg, H. M. Grey, and R. T. Kubo. 1994. Peptide binding to the most frequent HLA-A class I alleles measured by quantitative molecular binding assays. *Mol Immunol* 31 (11):813-22.

Sidney, J., E. Assarsson, C. Moore, S. Ngo, C. Pinilla, A. Sette, and B. Peters. 2008. Quantitative peptide binding motifs for 19 human and mouse MHC class I molecules derived using positional scanning combinatorial peptide libraries. *Immunome Res* 4:2.

Singh, R. R. 2000. The potential use of peptides and vaccination to treat systemic lupus erythematosus. *Curr Opin Rheumatol* 12 (5):399-406.

Smith, D. M., J. E. Baker, W. B. Gardner, G. W. Martens, and E. D. Agura. 2005. HLA class I null alleles and new alleles affect unrelated bone marrow donor searches. *Tissue Antigens* 66 (2):93-8.

Solheim, J. C. 1999. Class I MHC molecules: assembly and antigen presentation. *Immunol Rev* 172:11-9.

Storkus, W. J., H. J. Zeh, 3rd, R. D. Salter, and M. T. Lotze. 1993. Identification of T-cell epitopes: rapid isolation of class I-presented peptides from viable cells by mild acid elution. *J Immunother Emphasis Tumor Immunol* 14 (2):94-103.

Tang, T. F., L. Hou, B. Tu, W. Y. Hwang, A. E. Yeoh, J. Ng, and C. K. Hurley. 2006. Identification of nine new HLA class I alleles in volunteers from the Singapore stem cell donor registries. *Tissue Antigens* 68 (6):518-20.

Wang, E., G. Q. Phan, and F. M. Marincola. 2001. T-cell-directed cancer vaccines: the melanoma model. *Expert Opin Biol Ther* 1 (2):277-90.

Wang, Q., A. A. Canutescu, and R. L. Dunbrack, Jr. 2008. SCWRL and MolIDE: computer programs for side-chain conformation prediction and homology modeling. *Nat Protoc* 3 (12):1832-47.

Warburton, R. J., M. Matsui, S. L. Rowland-Jones, M. C. Gammon, G. E. Katzenstein, T. Wei, M. Edidin, H. J. Zweerink, A. J. McMichael, and J. A. Frelinger. 1994. Mutation of the alpha 2 domain disulfide bridge of the class I molecule HLA-A*0201. Effect on maturation and peptide presentation. *Hum Immunol* 39 (4):261-71.

Yewdell, J. W., and J. R. Bennink. 2001. Cut and trim: generating MHC class I peptide ligands. *Curr Opin Immunol* 13 (1):13-8.

Yewdell, J. W., C. C. Norbury, and J. R. Bennink. 1999. Mechanisms of exogenous antigen presentation by MHC class I molecules in vitro and in vivo: implications for generating CD8+ T cell responses to infectious agents, tumors, transplants, and vaccines. *Adv Immunol* 73:1-77.

Zeh, H. J., 3rd, G. H. Leder, M. T. Lotze, R. D. Salter, M. Tector, G. Stuber, S. Modrow, and W. J. Storkus. 1994. Flow-cytometric determination of peptide-class I complex formation. Identification of p53 peptides that bind to HLA-A2. *Hum Immunol* 39 (2):79-86.

3

Importance of Non-HLA Gene Polymorphisms in Hematopoietic Stem Cell Transplantation

Jeane Visentainer and Ana Sell
Maringa State University
Brazil

1. Introduction

In the last 10 years, non-HLA genotypes have been investigated for their potential roles in the occurrence and severity of graft-versus-host disease (GvHD) as well as for their contribution to overall transplant-related mortality, infectious episodes, and overall survival.

These non-HLA-encoded genes include polymorphisms within the regulatory sequences of the cytokine genes, or genes associating with innate immunity: *KIR* (killer immunoglobulin-like receptor) genes, *MIC* (MHC class I chain-related) genes, and others.

The first studied non-HLA genes were polymorphisms in regulatory cytokine genes because of cytokine role in GvHD immunopathogenesis. Single nucleotide polymorphisms in several regions of cytokine genes were correlated with the transplant overcome in several studies (Kim et al., 2005; Laguila Visentainer et al., 2005; Lin et al., 2003; Mlynarczewska et al., 2004; Viel et al., 2007; reviewed in Dickinson, 2008).

2. Role of cytokines in graft-versus-host disease after allogeneic stem cell transplantation

The pathophysiology of acute GvHD can be considered a cytokine storm (Ferrara, 2000), initializing with the transplant conditioning regimen that damages and activates host tissues. Activated host cells secrete inflammatory cytokines, such as tumor necrosis factor (TNF)-α and interleukin (IL)-1. This initial cytokine release is further amplified in the second phase by presentation of host antigens to donor T cells and the subsequent proliferation and differentiation of these activated T cells. These cells secrete a variety of cytokines, such as IL-2, TNF-α, interferon (IFN)-γ, IL-4, IL-6, IL-10, and transforming growth factor-beta (TGF)-β1. Several reports have demonstrated the increase of these cytokines in the serum from patients with acute GvHD (Kayaba et al., 2000; Liem et al., 1998; Sakata et al., 2001; Visentainer et al., 2003).

Although chronic GvHD remains a frequent complication of hematopoietic stem cell transplantation (HSCT), the pathogenesis is still unclear. However, it is known that cytokines also play an important role in its development (Iwasaki, 2004; Letterio & Roberts, 1998; Liem et al., 1999; Margolis & Vogelsang, 2000; Zhang et al., 2006). Chronic GvHD is a multisystem alloimmune and autoimmune disorder characterized by immune dysregulation, immunodeficiency, impaired organ function and decreased survival (Baird & Pavletic, 2006). It starts with the expansion of donor T cells in response to allo or auto-antigens that escape assessment thymus and the mechanisms of deletion. T cells induce damage in target organs by attacking cytolytic, inflammatory cytokines and fibrosis by activating B cells, with production of autoantibodies (Pérez-Simón et al., 2006).

Thus multiple cytokines are important in GvHD pathogenesis and regulation (Ferrara & Krenger, 1998; Jung et al., 2006; Kappel et al., 2009; Reddy et al., 2003; Tawara et al., 2008; Visentainer et al., 2005; Yi et al., 2008). Furthermore, the timing and duration of cytokine expression may be a critical factor determining the induction of the graft-versus-host (GvH) reaction, and cytokine dysregulation could potentially contribute to the severity of GvHD.

Recently, Choi et al. (2010) and Paczesny et al. (2010) reviewed the biology of acute GvHD, and concluded that the underlying mechanisms of GvHD have emerged as a complex network of immune interactions where the key players are the naive T cells, the host and donor APCs, CTLs and regulatory T cells, along with new players such as Plasmacytoid DCs (pDCs), B cells and Th17 cells.

2.1 Cytokine gene polymorphisms

The production of some cytokines is under genetic control. Polymorphisms in the regulatory regions of several cytokine genes may cause inter-individual differences in cytokine production (Wilson et al., 1997; Turner et al., 1997; Awad et al., 1998; Fishman et al., 1998; Pravica et al., 1999). As these polymorphisms segregate independently, each person is a mosaic of high-, intermediate-, and low-producing phenotypes. These cytokine polymorphisms are known to have functional relevance in post-transplant outcome, rejection and GvHD, following solid organ (Benza et al., 2009; Fernandes et al., 2002; Hahn et al., 2001; Karimi et al., 2011; Reviron et al., 2001) and hematopoietic stem cell transplantation (Ambruzova et al., 2009; Karimi et al., 2010; Laguila Visentainer et al., 2005; Leffell et al., 2001; Takahashi et al., 2000; Tambur et al., 2001), respectively.

2.2 Impact of cytokine gene polymorphisms on graft-vs-host disease

Many studies in recent years have focused on correlating donor and/or recipient genotype with GvHD risk. Table 1 summarizes the various polymorphisms in genes encoding both pro- and anti-inflammatory factors and their receptors that have been studied in GvHD.

3. Killer immunoglobulin-like receptors and hematopoietic stem cell transplantation

Natural killer (NK) cell effector function is regulated by a balance between activating receptors and inhibitory receptors for major histocompatibility complex (MHC) class I molecules (Joyce & Sun, 2011; Parham et al., 2006; Yokoyama et al., 2006). In the setting of allogeneic HSCT, donor NK cells may attack recipient cells that lack the appropriate HLA class I ligands for the donor KIR. Several studies have shown that certain combinations of killer immunoglobulin-like receptors and human leukocyte antigens (in both donors and recipients) can affect the chances of survival of transplant patients, particularly in relation to the graft-versus-leukemia effect, which may be associated to decreased relapse rates in certain groups (reviewed in Franceschi et al., 2011).

GvHD		References
Acute	**Chronic**	
SNP/Genotype		**References**
	IL1A-889*2	Cullup et al. (2003)
IL6-174 G/C	IL6-174 GG	Lin et al. (2003)
	IL6-174 CC	Laguila Visentainer et al. (2005)
TNF-308 GG/GA		Takahashi et al. (2000)
	TNF-238 GA	Viel et al. (2007)
IL2-330 GT		Macmillan et al. (2003)
	IL10-1082,-819,-592 ATA/ATA	Kim et al. (2005)
IL10-592 A/A		Lin et al. (2003)
IL-10RB A/A	IL-10RB A/A	Sivula et al. (2009)
TGFB1+869,+915 TG/GG		Leffell et al. (2001)
TGFB1+869 T		Hattori et al. (2002)
TGF- beta1 codon 25 GG		Rashidi-Nezhad et al. (2010)
IFN-γ T+874A		Karimi et al. (2010)
IL-7RA		Shamim et al. (2011)

Table 1. Polymorphisms in genes encoding both pro- and anti-inflammatory factors and their receptors in GvHD

3.1 Killer immunoglobulin-like receptors

The group of *KIR* genes comprises a region of approximately 150 Kb in the leukocyte receptor complex (LRC) on chromosome 19q13.4 (Uhrberg et al., 1997). KIRs are members of a group of regulatory molecules on the surface of NK cells, in subgroups of Tγδ+ lymphocytes, effector Tαβ+ lymphocytes and memory lymphocytes (Rajagopalan & Long, 2005). The KIR family includes activating and inhibitory molecules. Inhibitory KIRs (2DL and 3DL) have a long cytoplasmic tail containing tyrosine-based inhibitory motifs (ITIMs) that trigger inhibitory events of cytotoxicity. In contrast, activating KIRs (2DS and 3DS) interact with the DAP12 molecule, which has tyrosine-based activation motifs (ITAMs) that cause a cascade that results in an increase in cytoplasmic granulation and the production of cytokines and chemokines, thereby initiating immune response (McVicar et al., 2001).

The balance between activation and inhibition of NK cells occurs through the binding of KIRs with HLA class I molecules present in all nucleated cells of an individual. Most KIRs bind to HLA-C molecules. It is worth remembering the importance of the dimorphism of amino acids, such as residue 80 of α-helix-1, in the definition of this HLA receptor. On this basis, HLA-C alleles may be defined as "Group 1" or "Group 2": C1 – HLA-Cw*01, *03, *07, *08, *12, *13, *14, and *16 and C2 – HLA-Cw*02, *04, *05, *06, *07, *15, *17, and *18, which are specific for KIR2DL2/2DL3/2DS2 and KIR2DL1/2DS1, respectively (Boyton & Altmann, 2007). Evidence suggests that HLA-Cw4 is a receptor for KIR2DS4 (Katz et al., 2001). The KIR2DL4, for example, specificity binds to the HLA-G molecule (Rajagopalan & Long, 1999), while the KIR3DL1 receptor binds to a subset of HLA molecules with the Bw4 epitope, present in approximately one third of all HLA-B molecules. The KIR3DS1 is highly homologous with 3DL1 and seems to share the Bw4 epitope as ligand, although this needs to be experimentally verified. The KIR3DL2 receptor is still being discussed, but studies suggest that HLA-A3 and HLA-A11 perform this role (O'Connor et al., 2006).

Based on the genetic content and pattern of segregation at the population level, *KIR* haplotypes are divided into two groups, A and B, varying in the type and number of genes present. The *KIR* group A haplotype is uniform in terms of gene content (*3DL3, 2DL3, 2DL1, 2DP1, 3DP1, 2DL4, 3DL1, 2DS4,* and *3DL2*), of which all but 1 encode inhibitory receptors. In contrast, the *KIR* group B haplotype is more diverse in the *KIR* genes it contains, has more activating receptors, and is characterized by the *2DL2, 2DS1, 2DS2, 2DS3,* and *2DS5* genes (Uhrberg et al., 1997).

3.2 Impact of killer immunoglobulin-like receptors and hematopoietic stem cell transplantation

Previous studies have examined the effect of donor and recipient *KIR* genotypes on the outcome of allogeneic HSCT (Bishara et al., 2004; Gagne et al., 2002; Sun et al., 2005). One study found a 100% risk of GvHD after unrelated donor BMT, when the donor contained *KIR* genes absent in the recipient, compared to a 60% risk of GvHD with other combinations (Gagne et al., 2002).

In 2004, one study carried out *KIR-HLA* genotyping of 220 related HLA identical donor-recipient pairs (112 for myeloid diseases and 108 lymphoid diseases) (Cook et al., 2004). For patients with myeloid diseases, survival was lower in those homozygous for Group 2 (C2) HLA-C compared to patients with Group 1 (C1). This effect was observed only when the donor had the *KIR2DS2* gene. As *KIR2DS2* is in strong linkage disequilibrium with *KIR2DL2* (receptor inhibited by C1), this would indirectly indicate lower survival in patients who do not have the receptor for *KIR2DL2*, an opposite result to the model in which this lack of inhibition could result in NK cell alloreactivity with a consequent elimination of residual leukemic cells (Witt et al., 2006). In 178 patients with AML, CML, ALL and primary myelodysplastic syndrome (MDS) who received HSCT with T cell depletion from HLA-identical related donors, some authors observed that the disease-free survival was significantly higher in patients with AML and MDS that did not have the HLA ligand for the inhibitory KIR of the donor (Hsu et al., 2005). Moreover, the relapse rate was lower in these individuals, which may be related to higher survival rates. The results differ from a study in which T cell depletion was not performed (Cook et al., 2004). In another study (Schellekens et al., 2008) involving 83 patients with different types of hematologic malignancies who received HSCT from related HLA-identical donors without T cell depletion, a high relapse rate was found when high numbers of activating KIRs were present in both the patient and donor. According to the authors, a consequence of this finding may be an increased alloreactivity of the host against graft, impairing the response of donor cells resulting in an insufficient graft-versus-leukemia effect and increased risk of leukemic relapse.

Nowadays, there is no unequivocal evidence that polymorphic genes for KIR involved in innate immunity sufficiently influence GvHD and transplant outcome to change clinical practice (Davies et al., 2002; Cooley et al., 2009; Giebel et al., 2003; Hsu et al., 2005; Ludajic et al., 2009; Miller et al., 2007; Moretta et al., 2009; Schellekens et al., 2008; Symons et al., 2010; Witt et al., 2006).

Using a large cohort of patients, Venstrom et al. (2010) demonstrated that individual donor activating KIR, recipient HLA class I ligands, and donor *KIR* gene copy number all impact KIR-driven NK effects. They also showed that not all *KIR* B haplotypes have equivalent clinical impact, and they proposed that future studies consider specific B haplotype subsets or individual *KIR* genes in their analyses.

However, there are conflicting results in many studies, which may be due to the heterogeneity in HSCT protocols employed, differences in inclusion criteria, the HSCT preparative regimen and graft content, the degree of donor HLA-incompatibility, and posttransplant immunosuppression. Beside of this, according to early studies, Symons et al. (2010) have described 4 models of NK cell alloreactivity to predict HSCT outcomes: 1) KIR ligand incompatibility; 2) receptor-ligand model; 3) missing ligand model; and 4) *KIR* gene-gene model. And, contradictory results obtained from these models have made it difficult to conclude which model is most predictive of transplant outcome.

4. *MICA* and *MICB* matching in bone marrow transplantation

Retrospective and prospective studies have shown that matching donors and recipients for non-HLA DNA sequences in the MHC (beta and delta block matching) can result in improved patient survival and less severe GvHD (Tay et al., 1995; Witt et al., 2000). One of these blocks, the beta block, spans about 300 kb and contains the immunologically relevant *HLA-B, HLA-C, MICA,* and *MICB* genes (Kitcharoen et al., 2006). The polymorphic MICA molecule likely may be a target for specific antibodies and T cells in solid organ grafts or in GvHD (Zhang & Stastny, 2006).

4.1 *MICA* and *MICB* genes
In 1994, two new polymorphic families of MHC class I related genes, termed MHC class I-related chain A (*MICA*) and B (*MICB*) were described (Bahram et al., 1994). These genes are highly polymorphic with at least 76 alleles for *MICA* and 31 alleles for *MICB* (IMGT/HLA database; http://www.ebi.ac.uk/imgt/hla/stats.html), and are located in the MHC classical class I region (Horton et al., 2004), 46.4 and 141.2 kb centromeric to *HLA-B*, respectively (Bahram et al., 1994; Bahram et al., 2000; Leelayuwat et al., 1994). They encode cell surface glycoproteins that do not associate with β_2-microglobulin. These molecules function as restriction elements for intestinal $\gamma\delta$ T cells and they behave as cell stress molecules. MICA is expressed in endothelial cells, keratinocytes and monocytes, but not in CD4+, CD8+ or CD19+ lymphocytes (Zwirner et al., 1999).

The MICA gene products have been shown to play a role in some aspects of antigen presentation and T-cell recognition, and appear to be important in innate immunity as ligands to NKG2D receptor expressed on most $\gamma\delta$ T cells, CD8 $\alpha\beta$ T cells, and NK cells (Tieng et al., 2002).

4.2 *MICA* and *MICB* and relevance to stem cell transplantation outcome
Several studies have shown that the highly polymorphic MIC antigens are expressed in transplanted organs and may cause early graft rejection (Hankey et al., 2002; Mizutani et al., 2006; Narayan et al., 2011; Panigrahi et al., 2007; Sumitran-Holgersson, 2008; Terasaki et al., 2007). The polymorphisms of MICA and MICB may be involved in allogeneic BMT and GvHD (Gannage et al., 2008; Murai et al., 2003; Parmar et al. 2009; Przepiorka et al., 1995) because they are augmented by stress in epithelia (Groh et al., 1996) and are recognized by a subpopulation of intestinal $\gamma\delta$ T cells (Zou et al. 2007). In addition to classical HLA class I and II matching, matches at *MICA* and *MICB* loci have been shown to increase patient survival (Kitcharoen et al., 2006).

Recent review has discussed the genetics and biology of the *MICA* gene and its products, and their importance in disease related to NK activity and allograft rejection or GvHD

(Choy & Phipps, 2010). According to Parmar et al. (2009), some HSCT cases with matched *HLA* but mismatched *MICA* showed an increased incidence of GvHD, and according to Boukouaci et al. (2009), MICA-129 valine and soluble MICA are risk factors for chronic GvHD, whereas the presence of anti-MICA antibodies that can neutralize soluble MICA confers protection.

A methionine to valine change at position 129 of the α2-heavy chain domain categorized the *MICA* alleles into strong (MICA-129 met) and weak (MICA-129 val) binders of NKG2D receptor (Steinle et al., 2001). Varying affinities of *MICA* alleles for NKG2D may affect thresholds of NK-cell triggering and T-cell modulation. According to Boukouaci et al. (2009), in the context of cGVHD, the weak engagement of NKG2D receptors by the weak binder MICA-129 val allele may impair NK/cytotoxic T lymphocyte cell activation/costimulation, possibly skewing the TH1 pathway toward TH2 with consequent B-cell activation and Ab production.

5. Conclusion

Analysis of non-HLA genetics may permit more accurate assessment of transplant-related complications, improve donor selection and individualized prophylaxis, and aid in the development of a prognostic risk index. Overall, this type of analysis could potentially define high- and low-risk patient groups, and to result in effective therapeutic strategies for GvHD.

6. References

Ambruzova, Z.; Mrazek, F.; Raida, L.; Jindra, P.; Vidan-Jeras, B.; Faber, E.; Pretnar, J.; Indrak, K. & Petrek, M. (2009). Association of IL6 and CCL2 gene polymorphisms with the outcome of allogeneic haematopoietic stem cell transplantation. *Bone Marrow Transplantation*, Vol.44, No.4, (August 2009), pp.227-235, ISSN 0268-3369

Awad, M.R.; El-Gamel, A.; Hasleton, P.; Turner, D.M.; Sinnott, P.J. & Hutchinson, I.V. (1998). Genotypic variation in the transforming growth factorb1 gene. *Transplantation*, Vol.66, No.8, (October 1998), pp.1014-1020, ISSN 0041-1337

Bahram, S. (2000). MIC genes: from genetics to biology. *Advances in Immunology*, Vol.76, (2000), pp.1-60, ISSN 0065-2776

Bahram, S.; Bresnahan, M.; Geraghty, D.E. & Spies, T. (1994). A second lineage of mammalian major histocompatibility complex class I genes. *Proceedings of the National Academy of Sciences of the United States of America*, Vol.91, No.14, (Jul 1994), pp. 6259-6263, ISSN 0027-8424

Baird, K. & Pavletic, S.Z. Chronic graft versus host disease. (2006). *Current Opinion in Hematology*, Vol.13, No.6, (November 2006), pp. 426-435, ISSN 1065-6251

Benza, R.L.; Coffey, C.S.; Pekarek, D.M.; Barchue J.P.; Tallaj, J.A.; Passineau, M.J. & Grenett, H.E. (2009). Transforming growth factor-beta polymorphisms and cardiac allograft rejection. *The Journal of Heart and Lung Transplantation*, Vol.28, No.10, (October 2009), pp.1057-1062, ISSN 1053-2498

Bishara, A; De Santis, D.; Witt C.C.; Brautbar, C.; Christiansen, F.T.; Or, R.& Nagler, A.; Slavin, S. (2004). The beneficial role of inhibitory KIR genes of HLA class I NK epitopes in haploidentically mismatched stem cell allografts may be masked by residual donor-alloreactive T cells causing GVHD. *Tissue Antigens*, Vol.63, (March 2004), pp.204-211, ISSN 0001-2815

Boukouaci, W.; Busson, M.; Peffault de Latour, R.; Rocha, V.; Suberbielle, C.; Bengoufa, D.; Dulphy, N.; Haas, P.; Scieux, C.; Amroun, H.; Gluckman, E.; Krishnamoorthy, R.; Toubert, A.; Charron, D.; Socié, G. & Tamouza, R. (2009). MICA-129 genotype, soluble MICA, and anti-MICA antibodies as biomarkers of chronic graft-versus-host disease. *Blood*, Vol.114, No.25, (December 2009), pp.5216–5224, ISSN 0006-4971

Boyton, R.J. & Altmann, D.M. (2007). Natural killer cells, killer immunoglobulin like receptors and human leukocyte antigen class I in disease. *Clinical of Experimental Immunology*, Vol.149, No.1, (January 2007), pp.1-8, ISSN 0009-9104

Choi, S.W.; Levine, J.E. & Ferrara, J.L. (2010). Pathogenesis and Management of Graft-versus-Host Disease. *Immunology and Allergy Clinics of North America*, Vol.30, No.1, (February 2010), pp.75–101, ISSN 0889-8561

Choy, M.K. & Phipps, M.E. (2010). MICA polymorphism: biology and importance in immunity and disease. *Trends in Molecular Medicine*, Vol.16, No.3, (March 2010), pp.97-106, ISSN 1471-4914

Cook, M.A.; Milligan, D.W.; Fegan, C.D.; Darbyshire, P.J.; Mahendra, P.; Craddock, C.F.; Moss, P.A. & Briggs, D.C. (2004). The impact of donor KIR and patient HLA-C genotypes on outcome following HLA-identical sibling hematopoietic stem cell transplantation for myeloid leukemia. *Blood*, Vol.103, No.4, (February 2004), pp.1521-1526, ISSN 0006-4971

Cullup, H.; Dickinson, A.M.; Cavet, J.; Jackson, G.H. & Middleton, P.G. (2003). Polymorphisms of interleukin-1alpha constitute independent risk factors for chronic graft-versus-host disease after allogeneic bone marrow transplantation. *British Journal of Haematology*, Vol.122, No.5, (September 2003), pp.778-787, ISSN 0007-1048

Davies, S.M.; Ruggieri, L.; DeFor, T.; Wagner, J.E.; Weisdorf, D.J.; Miller, J.S.; Velardi, A. & Blazar, B.R. (2002). Evaluation of KIR ligand incompatibility in mismatched unrelated donor hematopoietic transplants. *Blood*, Vol.100, No.10, (November 2002), pp.3825-3827, ISSN 0006-4971

Fernandes, H.; Koneru, B.; Fernandes, N.; Hameed, M.; Cohen, MC.; Raveche, E. & Cohen, S. (2002). Investigation of promoter polymorphisms in the tumor necrosis factor-a and interleukin-10 genes in liver transplant patients. *Transplantation*, Vol.73, No.12, (June 2002), pp.1886-1891, ISSN 0041-1337

Ferrara, J.L. & Krenger, W. (1998). Graft-versus-host disease: the influence of type 1 and type 2 T cell cytokines. *Transfusion Medicine Reviews*, Vol.12, No.1, (January 1998), pp.1–17, ISSN 0887-7963

Ferrara, J.L. (2000). Pathogenesis of acute graft-versus-host disease: cytokines and cellular effectors. *Journal of Hematotherapy & Stem Cell Research*, Vol.9, No.3, (June 2000), pp. 299-306, ISSN 1061-6128

Fishman, D.; Faulds, G.; Jeffery, R.; Mohamedali, V.; Yudkin, J.S.; Humphries, S. & Woo, P. (1998). The effect of novel polymorphisms in the interleukin-6 (IL-6) gene on IL-6 transcription and plasma IL-6 levels, and an association with systemic-onset juvenile chronic arthritis. *The Journal of Clinical Investigation*, Vol.102, No.7, (October 1998), pp.1369-1376, ISSN 0021-9738

Franceschi, D.S.;de Souza, C.A.; Aranha, F.J.; Cardozo, D.M.; Sell, A.M. & Visentainer, J.E. (2011). Importance of killer immunoglobulin-like receptors in allogeneic hematopoietic stem cell transplantation. *Revista Brasileira de Hematologia e Hemoterapia*, Vol.33, No.2, (April 2011), ISSN 1516-8484

Gagne, K.; Brizard, G.; Gueglio. B.; Milpied, N. ; Herry, P.; Bonneville, F.; Chéneau, M.L.; Schleinitz, N.; Cesbron, A.; Folléa, G.; Harrousseau, J.L & Bignon, J.D. (2002). Relevance of KIR gene polymorphisms in bone marrow transplantation outcome. *Human Immunology*, Vol.63, (April 2002), pp.271-280, ISSN 0198-8859

Gannage, M.; Buzyn, A. ; Bogiatzi, S.I.; Lambert, M.; Soumelis, V; Dal Cortivo, L.; Cavazzana-Calvo, M.; Brousse, N. & Caillat-Zucman, S. (2008). Induction of NKG2D ligands by gamma radiation and tumor necrosis factor-alpha may participate in the tissue damage during acute graft-versus-host disease. *Transplantation*, Vol.85, No.6, (March 2008), pp.911-915, ISSN 0041-1337

Gasser, S. & Raulet, D.H. (2006). Activation and self-tolerance of natural killer cells. *Immunological Reviews*, Vol.214, No.1, (December 2006), pp.130-142, ISSN: 0105-2896

Giebel, S.; Locatelli, F.; Lamparelli, T.; Velardi, A.; Davies, S.; Frumento, G.; Maccario, R.; Bonetti, F.; Wojnar, J.; Martinetti, M.; Frassoni, F.; Giorgiani, G.; Bacigalupo, A. & Holowiecki, J. (2003). Survival advantage with KIR ligand incompatibility in hematopoietic stem cell transplantation from unrelated donors. *Blood*, Vol.102, No.3, (August 2003), pp.814-819, ISSN 0006-4971

Groh, V.; Bahram, S; Bauer, S.; Herman, A.; Beauchamp, M. & Spies T. (1996). Cell stress-regulated human major histocompatibility complex class I gene expressed in gastrointestinal epithelium. *Proceedings of the National Academy of Sciences of the United States of America*, Vol.93, No.22 (October 1996), pp. 12445-12450, ISSN 0027-8424

Hahn, A.B.; Kasten-Jolly, J.C.; Constantino, D.M.; Graffunder, E. & Conti, D.J. (2001). TNF-alpha, IL-6, IFN-gamma, and IL-10 gene expression polymorphisms and the IL-4 receptor a-chain variant Q576R: effects on renal allograft outcome. *Transplantation*, Vol.72, No.4, (August 2001), pp.660-665, ISSN 0041-1337

Hankey, K.G.; Drachenberg, C.B.; Papadimitriou, J.C.; Klassen, D.K.; Philosophe, B.; Bartlett, S.T.; Groh, V.; Spies, T. & Mann, D.L. (2002). MIC expression in renal and pancreatic allografts. *Transplantation* Vol.73, No.2, (January 2002), pp. 304-306, ISSN 0041-1337

Hattori, H.; Matsuzaki, A.; Suminoe, A.; Ihara, K.; Nagatoshi, Y.; Sakata, N.; Kawa, K.; Okamura, J. & Hara, T. (2002). Polymorphisms of transforming growth factor-beta1 and transforming growth factor-beta1 type II receptor genes are associated with acute graft-versus-host disease in children with HLA matched sibling bone marrow transplantation. *Bone Marrow Transplanation*, Vol.30, No.10, (November 2002), pp.665-671, ISSN 0268-3369

Horton, R.; Wilming, L.; Rand, V.; Lovering R.C.; Bruford, E.A.; Khodiyar, V.K.; Lush, M.; Povey, S.; Talbot, C.C. Jr.; Wright, M.W.; Wain, H.M.; Trowsdale, J.; Ziegler, A. & Beck, S. (2004). Gene map of the extended human MHC. *Nature Reviews Genetics*, Vol.5, No.12, (December 2004), pp.889-899, ISSN 1471-0056

Hsu, K.C.; Keever-Taylor, C.A.; Wilton, A.; Pinto, C.; Heller, G.; Arkun, K.; O'Reilly, R.J.; Horowitz, M.M. & Dupont, B. (2005). Improved outcome in HLA-identical sibling hematopoietic stem-cell transplantation for acute myelogenous leukemia predicted by KIR and HLA genotypes. *Blood*, Vol.105, No.12, (June 2005), pp.4878-4884, ISSN 0006-4971

Iwasaki, T. (2004). Recent advances in the treatment of graft-versus-host disease. *Clinical Medicine & Research*, Vol.2, No.4, (November 2004), pp.243-252, ISSN 1539-4182

Joyce, M.G. & Sun, P.D. (2011). The structural basis of ligand recognition by natural killer cell receptors. *Journal of Biomedicine and Biotechnology*, Vol.2011, (May 2011), pp.1-15, ISSN 1110-7243

Jung, U.; Foley, J.E.; Erdmann, A.A.; Toda, Y.; Borenstein, T.; Mariotti, J. & Fowler, D.H. (2006). Ex vivo rapamycin generates Th1/Tc1 or Th2/Tc2 effector T cells with enhanced in vivo function and differential sensitivity to post-transplant rapamycin therapy. *Biology of Blood and Marrow Transplantation*, Vol.12, No.9, (September 2006), pp.905–918, ISSN 1083-8791

Kappel, L.W.; Goldberg, G.L.; King, C.G.; Suh, D.Y.; Smith, O.M.; Ligh, C.; Holland, A.M.; Grubin, J.; Mark, N.M.; Liu, C.; Iwakura, Y.; Heller, G. & van den Brink, M.R. (2009). IL-17 contributes to CD4-mediated graft-versushost disease. *Blood*, Vol.113, No.4, (January 2009), pp.945–952, ISSN 0006-4971

Karimi, M.H.; Daneshmandi, S.; Pourfathollah, A.A.; Geramizadeh, B.; Ramzi, M.; Yaghobi, R. & Ebadi, P. (2010). The IFN-γ Allele Correlated to Moderate-to-Severe Acute Graft-Versus-Host Disease After Allogeneic Stem Cell Transplant. *Experimental and Clinical Transplantation*, Vol.8, No.2, (June 2010), pp.125-129, ISSN 1304-0855

Karimi, M.H.; Daneshmandi, S.; Pourfathollah, A.A.; Geramizadeh, B.; Yaghobi, R.; Rais-Jalali, G.A.; Roozbeh, J. & Bolandparvaz, S. (2011). A study of the impact of cytokine gene polymorphism in acute rejection of renal transplant recipients. *Molecular Biology Reports*, [Epub ahead of print], (May 2011), ISSN 0301-4851

Katz, G.; Markel, G.; Mizrahi, S.; Arnon, T.I. & Mandelboim, O. (2001). Recognition of HLA-Cw4 but not HLA-Cw6 by the NK cell receptor killer cell Ig-like receptor two-domain short tail number 4. *Journal of Immunology*, Vol.166, No.12, (June 2001), pp.7260-7267, ISSN 0022-1767

Kayaba, H.; Hirokawa, M.; Watanabe, A.; Saitoh, N.; Changhao, C.; Yamada, Y.; Honda, K.; Kobayashi, Y.; Urayama, O. & Chihara, J. (2000). Serum markers of graft-versus-host disease after bone marrow transplantation. *The Journal of Allergy and Clinical Immunology*, Vol.106, No.2, (July 2000), pp. S40-S44, ISSN 00917-6749

Kim, D.H.; Lee, N.Y.; Sohn, S.K.; Baek, J.H.; Kim, J.G.; Suh, J.S.; Lee, K.B. & Shin, I.H. (2005). IL-10 promoter gene polymorphism associated with the occurrence of chronic GVHD and its clinical course during systemic immunosuppressive treatment for chronic GVHD after allogeneic peripheral blood stem cell transplantation. *Transplantation*, Vol.79, No.11, (June 2005), pp.1615-1622, ISSN 0041-1337

Kitcharoen, K.; Witt, C.S.; Romphruk, A.V.; Christiansen, F.T. & Leelayuwat, C. (2006). MICA, MICB, and MHC beta block matching in bone marrow transplantation: relevance to transplantation outcome. *Human Immunology*, Vol.67, No.3, (March 2006), pp.238–246, ISSN 0198-8859

Laguila Visentainer, J.E.; Lieber, S.R.; Lopes Persoli, L.B.; Dutra Marques, S.B.; Vigorito, A.C.; Penteado Aranha, F.J.; de Brito Eid, K.A.; Oliveira, G.B.; Martins Miranda, E.C.; Bragotto, L. & de Souza, C.A. (2005). Relationship between cytokine gene polymorphisms and graft-versus-host disease after allogeneic stem cell transplantation in a Brazilian population. *Cytokine*, Vol.32, No.3-4, (November 2005), pp.171-177, ISSN: 1043-4666

Lanier, L.L. (2008). Up on the tightrope: natural killer cell activation and inhibition. *Nature Immunology*, Vol.9, No.5, (May 2008), pp.495-502, ISSN 1529-2908

Leelayuwat, C.; Townend, D.C.; Degli-Esposti, M.A.; Abraham, L.J. & Dawkins, R.L. (1994). A new polymorphic and multicopy RL: A new polymorphic and multicopy MHC gene family related to non mammalian class I. *Immunogenetics*, Vol.40, No.51, (1994), pp. 339-351, ISSN 0093-7711

Leffell, M.S.; Vogelsang, G.B.; Lucas, D.P.; Delaney, N.L. & Zachary, A.A. (2001). Association between TGF-beta expression and severe GVHD in allogeneic bone marrow transplantation. *Transplantation Proceedings*, Vol.33, No.1-2, (February-March 2001), pp.485-486, ISSN 0041-1345

Letterio, J.J. & Roberts, A.B. (1998). Regulation of immune responses by TGFbeta. *Annual Review of Immunology*, Vol.16, (April 1998), pp.137-161, ISSN 15453278

Liem, L.M.; Fibbe, W.E.; van Houwelingen, H.C. & Golmy, E. (1999). Serum transforming growth factor-b1 levels in bone marrow transplant recipients correlate with blood cell counts and chronic graft-versus-host disease. *Transplantation*, Vol.67, No.1, (January 1999), pp. 59-65, ISSN 0041-1337

Liem, L.M.; van Houwelingen, H.C. & Goulmy, E. (1998). Serum cytokine levels after HLA-identical bone marrow transplantation. *Transplantation*, Vol.66, No.7, (October 1998), pp.863-871, ISSN 0041-1337

Lin, M.T., Storer, B., Martin, P.J., Tseng, L.H., Gooley, T., Chen, P.J. & Hansen, J.A. (2003). Relation of an interleukin-10 promoter polymorphism to graft-versus-host disease and survival after hematopoietic-cell transplantation. *The New England Journal of Medicine*, Vol.349, No.23, (December 2003), pp.2201-2210, ISSN 0028-4793

Ludajic, K.; Balavarca, Y.; Bickeböller, H.; Rosenmayr, A.; Fae, I.; Fischer, G.F.; Kouba, M.; Pohlreich, D.; Kalhs, P. & Greinix, H.T. (2009). KIR genes and KIR ligands affect occurrence of acute GVHD after unrelated, 12/12 HLA matched, hematopoietic stem cell transplantation. *Bone Marrow Transplantation*, Vol.44, No.2, (July 2009), pp.97–103, ISSN 0268-3369

Macmillan, M.L.; Radloff, G.A.; Kiffmeyer, W.R.; Defor, T.E.; Weisdorf, D.J. & Davies, S.M. (2003). High-producer interleukin-2 genotype increases risk for acute graft-versus-host disease after unrelated donor bone marrow transplantation. *Transplantation*, Vol.76, No.12, (December 2003), pp.1758-1762, ISSN 0041-1337

Margolis, J. & Vogelsang, G. (2000). Chronic graft-versus-host disease. *Journal of Hematotherapy & Stem Cell Research*, Vol.9, No.3, (June 2000), pp.339-346, ISSN 1061-6128

McVicar, D.W. & Burshtyn, D.N. (2001). Intracellular signaling the killer immunoglobulin-like receptors and Ly49. *Sciences´s STKE: signal transduction knowledge environment*, Vol.2001, No.75, (March 2001), pp. re1, ISSN 1945-0877

Mlynarczewska, A.; Wysoczanska, B.; Karabon, L.; Bogunia-Kubik, K. & Lange, A. (2004) Lack of IFN-gamma 2/2 homozygous genotype independently of recipient age and intensity of conditioning regimen influences the risk of aGVHD manifestation after HLA-matched sibling haematopoietic stem cell transplantation. *Bone Marrow Transplantation*, Vol.34, No.4, (August 2004), pp.339-344, ISSN 0268-3369

Miller, J.S.; Cooley, S.; Parham, P.; Farag, S.S.; Verneris, M.R.; McQueen, K.L.; Guethlein, L.A.; Trachtenberg, E.A.; Haagenson, M.; Horowitz, M.M.; Klein, J.P. & Weisdorf, D.J. (2007). Missing KIR-ligands are associated with less relapse and increased graft versus host disease (GVHD) following unrelated donor allogeneic HCT. *Blood*, Vol.109, No.11, (June 2007), pp.5058–5061, ISSN 0006-4971

Mizutani, K.; Terasaki, P.I.; Shih, R.N.; Pei, R. Ozawa, M. & Lee, J. (2006). Frequency of MIC Antibody in Rejected Renal Transplant Patients without HLA Antibody. *Human Immunology*, Vol.67, No.3, (March 2006) pp. 223–229, ISSN 0198-8859

Moretta, A.; Pende, D.; Locatelli, F. & Moretta, L. (2009). Activating and inhibitory killer immunoglobulin-like receptors (KIR) in haploidentical haemopoietic stem cell transplantation to cure high-risk leukaemias. *Clinical Experimental of Immunology*, Vol.157, No.3, (September 2009), pp.325–331, ISSN 0093-9104

Murai, M.; Yoneyama, H.; Ezaki, T.; Suematsu, M.; Terashima, Y.; Harada, A.; Hamada, H.; Asakura, H.; Ishikawa, H & Matsushima, K. (2003). Peyer's patch is the essential site in initiating murine acute and lethal graft-versus-host reaction. *Nature Immunology*, Vol.4, No.2, (February 2003), pp. 3154-3160, ISSN 1529-2908

Narayan, S.; Tsai, E.W.; Zhang, Q.; Wallace, W.D.; Reed, E.F. & Ettenger, R.B. (2011). Acute rejection associated with donor specific anti-MICA antibody in a highly sensitized pediatric renal transplant recipient. *Pediatric Transplantation*, Vol.15, No.1, (February 2011), pp.E1-7, ISSN 1397-3142

O'Connor, G.M.; Hart, O.M. & Gardiner, C.M. (2006). Putting the natural killer cell in its place. *Immunology*, Vol.117, No.1, (January 2006), pp.1-10, ISSN 0019-2805

Paczesny, S.; Hanauer, D.; Sun, Y. & Reddy, P. (2010). New perspectives on the biology of acute GVHD. *Bone Marrow Transplantation*, Vol.45, No.1, (January 2010), pp.1–11, ISSN 0268-3369

Panigrahi, A.; Gupta, N.; Siddiqui, J.A.; Margoob, A.; Bhowmik, D.; Guleria, S. & Mehra, N.K. (2007). Post Transplant Development of MICA and Anti-HLA Antibodies is Associated with Acute Rejection Episodes and Renal Allograft Loss. *Human Immunology*, Vol.68, No.5, (May 2007), pp.362–367, ISSN 0198-8859

Parham, P. (2006). Taking license with natural killer cell maturation and repertoire development. *Immunological Reviews*, Vol.214, No.1, (December 2006), pp.155-160, ISSN 1529-2908

Parmar, S.; Del Lima, M.; Zou, Y.; Patah, P.A.; Liu, P.; Cano, P.; Rondon, G.; Pesoa, S.; de Padua Silva, L.; Qazilbash, M.H.; Hosing, C.; Popat, U.; Kebriaei, P.; Shpall, E.J.; Giralt, S.; Champlin, R.E.; Stastny, P. & Fernandez-Vina, M. (2009). Donor-recipient mismatches in MHC class I chain-related gene A in unrelated donor transplantation lead to increased incidence of acute graft-versus-host disease. *Blood*, (October 2009), Vol.114, No.14, pp.2884–2887, ISSN 0006-4971

Pérez-Simón, J.A.; Sánchez-Abarca, I.; Díezcampelo, M.; Caballero, D. & San Miguel, J. (2006). Chronic Graft-Versus-Host Disease Pathogenesis and Clinical Management. *Drugs*, Vol.66, No.8, (2006), pp. 1041-1057, ISSN 0012-6667

Pravica, V.; Asderakis, A.; Perrey, C.; Hajeer, A.; Sinnott, P.J. & Hutchinson, I.V. (1999). In vitro production of IFN-gamma correlates with CA repeat polymorphism in the human IFN-gamma gene. *European Journal of Immunogenetics*, Vol.26, No.1, (February 1999), pp.1-3, ISSN 0960-7420

Przepiorka, D.; Weisdorf, D.; Martin, P.; Klingemann, H.G.; Beatty, P.; Hows, J & Thomas, E.D. (1995). 1994 Consensus Conference on Acute GVHD Grading. Bone Marrow Transplantation, Vol.15, No.6, (June 1995), pp. 825-828, ISSN 0268-3369

Rajagopalan, S. & Long, E.O. (1999). A human histocompatibility leukocyte antigen (HLA)-G-specific receptor expressed on all natural killer cells. Journal of Experimental Medicine, Vol.189, No.7, (1999), pp.1093-1100. ISSN 0022-1007

Rajagopalan, S. & Long, E.O. (2005). Understanding how combinations of HLA and KIR genes influence disease. The Journal of Experimental Medicine, Vol.201, No.7, (April 2005), pp.1025-1029, ISSN 0022-1007

Rashidi-Nezhad, A.; Azimi, C.; Alimoghaddam, K.; Ghavamzadeh, A.; Hossein-Nezhad, A.; Izadi, P.; Sobhani, M.; Noori-Daloii, A.R. & Noori-Daloii, M.R. (2010). TGF-Beta codon 25 polymorphism and the risk of graft-versus-host disease after allogenic hematopoietic stem cell transplantation. Iranian Journal of Allergy, Asthma and Immunology, Vol.9, No.1, (March 2010), pp.1-6, ISSN 1735-1502

Reddy, P. & Ferrara, J.L. (2003). Immunobiology of acute graft-versus-host disease. Blood Reviews, (December 2003), Vol.17, No.4, pp.187–194, ISSN 0268-960X

Reviron, D.; Dussol, B.; Andre, M.; Brunet, P.; Mercier, P. & Berland, Y. (2001). TNF-alpha and IL-6 gene polymorphism and rejection in kidney transplantation recipients. Transplantation Proceedings, Vol.33, No.1-2, (February-March 2001), pp.350-351, ISSN 0041-1345

Sakata, N; Yasui, M.; Okamura, T.; Inoue, M.; Yumura-Yagi, K. & Kawa, K. (2001). Kinetics of plasma cytokines after hematopoietic stem cell transplantation from unrelated donors: the ratio of plasma IL-10/sTNFR level as a potential prognostic marker in severe acute graft-versus-host disease. Bone Marrow Transplantation, Vol.27, No.11, (June 2001), pp. 1153-1161, ISSN 0268-3369

Schellekens, J.; Rozemuller, E.H.; Petersen, E.J.; van den Tweel, J.G.; Verdonck, L.F. & Tilanus, M.G. (2008). Activating KIRs exert a crucial role on relapse and overall survival after HLA-identical sibling transplantation. Molecular Immunology, Vol.45, No.8, (April 2008), pp.2255-2261, ISSN 0161-5890

Shamim, Z.; Ryder, L.P.; Christensen, I.J.; Toubert, A.; Norden, J.; Collin, M.; Jackson, G.; Dickinson, A.M. & Müller, K. (2011). Prognostic Significance of Interleukin-7 Receptor-α Gene Polymorphisms in Allogeneic Stem-Cell Transplantation: A Confirmatory Study. Transplantation, (April 2011), Vol.91, No.7, pp.731–736, ISSN 0041-1337

Sivula, J.; Turpeinen, H.; Volin, L. & Partanen, J. (2009). Association of IL-10 and IL-10Rβ gene polymorphisms with graft-versus-host disease after haematopoietic stem cell transplantation from an HLA-identical sibling donor. BMC Immunology, Vol.10, (May 2009), pp.24-30, ISSN 1471-2172

Steinle, A.; Li, P.; Morris, D.L.; Groh, V.; Lanier, L.L.; Strong, R.K. & Spies, T. (2001). Interactions of human NKG2D with its ligands MICA, MICB, and homologs of the mouse RAE-1 protein family. Immunogenetics, Vol.53, No.4, (May-June 2001), pp.279-287, ISSN: 0093-7711

Sumitran-Holgersson, S. (2008). Relevance of MICA and other non- HLA antibodies in clinical transplantation. Current Opinion of Immunology, Vol.20, No.5 (October 2008), pp.607–613, ISSN 0952-7915

Sun, J.Y.; Gaidulis, L.; Dagis, A.; Palmer, J.; Rodriguez, R.; Miller, M.M.; Forman, S.J. & Senitzer, D. (2005). Killer Ig-like receptor (KIR) compatibility plays a role in the prevalence of acute GVHD in unrelated hematopoietic cell transplants for AML. Bone Marrow Transplantation, Vol.36, No.6, (September 2005), pp.525-530, ISSN 0268-3369

Symons, H.J.; Leffell, M.S.; Rossiter, N.D.; Zahurak, M.; Jones, R.J. & Fuchs, E.J. (2010). Improved Survival with Inhibitory Killer Immunoglobulin Receptor (KIR) Gene Mismatches and KIR Haplotype B Donors after Nonmyeloablative, HLA-Haploidentical Bone Marrow Transplantation. Biology of Blood and Marrow Transplantation, Vol.16, No.4, (April 2010), pp.533-542, ISSN 1083-8791

Takahashi, H.; Furukawa, T.; Hashimoto, S.; Susuki, N.; Yamazaki, F.; Inano, K.; Takahashi, M.; Aizawa, Y. & Koike, T. (2000). Contribution of TNF-alpha and IL-10 gene polymorphisms to graftversus-host disease following allo-hematopoietic stem cell transplantation. Bone Marrow Transplantation, Vol.26, No.12, (December 2000), pp.1317-1323, ISSN 0268-3369

Tambur, A.R.; Yaniv, I.; Stein, J.; Lapidot, M.; Shabtai, E.; Kfir, B. & Klein, T. (2001). Cytokine gene polymorphism in patients with graft-versus-host disease. Transplantation Proceedings, Vol.33, No.1-2, (February-March 2001), pp.502-503, ISSN 0041-1345

Tawara, I.; Maeda, Y.; Sun, Y.; Lowler, K.P.; Liu, C.; Toubai, T.; McKenzie, A.N & Reddy, P. (2008). Combined Th2 cytokine deficiency in donor T cells aggravates experimental acute graft-vs-host disease. Experimental Hematology, Vol.36, No.8, (August 2008), pp.988–996, ISSN 0301-472X

Tay, G.K.; Witt, C.S.; Christiansen, F.T.; Charron, D.; Baker, D.; Herrmann, R.; Smith, L.K.; Diepeveen, D.; Mallal, S. & McCluskey, J. (1995). Matching for MHC haplotypes results in improved survival following unrelated bone marrow transplantation. Bone Marrow Transplantation, Vol.15, No.3, (March 1995), pp.381–385, ISSN 0268-3369

Terasaki, P.I.; Ozawa, M. & Castro R. (2007). Four-year follow-up of a prospective trial of HLA an MICA antibodies on kidney graft survival. American Journal of Transplantation, Vol.7, No.2, (February 2007), pp. 408–415, ISSN 1600-6135

Tieng, V.; Le Bouguenec, C. ; du Merle, L.; Bertheau, P.; Desreumaux, P.; Janin, A.; Charron, D. & Toubert, A. (2002). Binding of Escherichia coli adhesin AfaE to CD55 triggers cell-surface expression of the MHC class I-related molecule MICA. Proceedings of the National Academy of Sciences of the United States of America, Vol.99, No.5, (March 2002), pp.2977-2982, ISSN 0027-8424

Turner, D.M.; Williams, D.M.; Sankaran, D.; Lazarus, M.; Sinnott, P.J. & Hutchinson, I.V. (1997). An investigation of polymorphism in the interleukin-10 gene promoter. European Journal of Immunogenetics, Vol.24, No.1, (February 1997), pp.1-8, ISSN 0960-7420

Uhrberg, M.; Valiante, N.M.; Shum, B.P.; Shilling, H.G.; Lienert-Weidenbach, K.; Corliss, B.; Tyan, D.; Lanier, L.L. & Parham, P. (1997). Human diversity in killer cell inhibitory receptor genes. Immunity, Vol.7, No.6, (December 1997), pp.753-763, ISSN 1074-7613

Venstrom, J.M., Ted, A. Gooley, T.A.; Spellman, S.; Pring, J.; Malkki, M.; Dupont, B.; Petersdorf, E. & Hsu, K.C. (2010). Donor activating KIR3DS1 is associated with decreased acute GVHD in unrelated allogeneic hematopoietic stem cell transplantation. Blood, Vol.115, No.15, (April 2010), pp.3162-3165, ISSN 0006-4971

Viel, D.O.; Tsuneto, L.T.; Sossai, C.R.; Lieber, S.R.; Marques, S.B.; Vigorito, A.C.; Aranha, F.J.; De Brito Eid, K.A.; Oliveira, G.B.; Miranda, E.C.; De Souza, C.A. & Visentainer, J.E. (2007). IL2 and TNFA gene polymorphisms and the risk of graft-versus-host disease after allogeneic stem cell transplantation. *Scandinavian Journal of Immunology*, Vol.66, No.6, (December 2007), pp.703-710, ISSN 0300-9475

Visentainer, J.E.; Lieber, S.R.; Persoli, L.B.; Vigorito, A.C.; Aranha, F.J.; Eid, K.A.; Oliveira, G.B.; Miranda, E.C. & de Souza, C.A. (2003). Serum cytokine levels and acute graft-versus-host disease after HLA-identical hematopoietic stem cell transplantation. *Experimental Hematology*, Vol.31, No.11, (November 2003), pp. 1044-1050, ISSN 0301-472X

Wilson, A.G.; Symons, J.A.; Mcdowell, T.L.; Mcdevitt, H.O. & Duff, G.W. (1997). Effects of a polymorphism in the human tumor necrosis factor alpha promoter on transcriptional activation. *Proceedings of the National Academy of Sciences of the United States of America*, Vol.94, No.7, (April 1997), pp.3195-319, ISSN 1091-6490

Witt, C.; Sayer, D.; Trimboli, F.; Saw, M.; Herrmann, R.; Cannell, P.; Baker, D. & Christiansen, F. (2000). Unrelated donors selected prospectively by block-matching have superior bone marrow transplant outcome. *Human Immunology*, Vol. 61, No.2, (February 2000), pp.85-91, ISSN 0198-8859

Witt, C.S. & Christiansen, F.T. (2006). The relevance of natural killer cell human leukocyte antigen epitopes and killer cell immunoglobulinlike receptors in bone marrow transplantation. *Vox Sanguinis*, Vol.90, No.1, (January 2006), pp.10-20, ISSN 0042-9007

Yi, T.; Zhao, D.; Lin, C.L.; Zhang, C.; Chen, Y.; Todorov, I.; LeBon, T.; Kandeel, F.; Forman, S. & Zeng, D. (2008). Absence of donor Th17 leads to augmented Th1 differentiation and exacerbated acute graft-versus-host disease. *Blood*, Vol.112, No.5, (September 2008), pp.2101–2110, ISSN 0006-4971

Yokoyama, W.M. & Kim, S. (2006). Licensing of natural killer cells by self major histocompatibility complex class I. *Immunological Reviews*, Vol.214, No.1, (December 2006), pp.143-154, ISSN 1529-2908

Zhang, C.; Todorov, I.; Zhang, Z.; Liu, Y.; Kandeel, F.; Forman, S.; Strober, S. & Zeng, D. (2006). Donor CD4+ T and B cells in transplants induce chronic graft-versus-host disease with autoimmune manifestations. *Blood*, Vol.107, No.7, (April 2006), pp.2993-3001, ISSN 0006-4971

Zhang, Y. & Stastny, P. (2006). MICA antigens stimulate T cell proliferation and cell-mediated cytotoxicity. *Human Immunology*, Vol.67, No.3, (March 2006), pp.215–222, ISSN 0198-8859

Zou, Y.; Stastny, P.; Susal, C.; Dohler, B. & Opelz G. (2007). Antibodies against MICA antigens and kidneytransplant rejection. *The New England Journal of Medicine*, Vol.357, No.13, (September 2007), pp. 1293-1300, ISSN 0028-4793

Zwirner, N.W.; Dole, K. & Stastny, P. (1999). Differential surface expression of MICA by endothelial cells, fibroblasts, keratinocytes, and monocytes. *Human Immunology*, Vol.60, No.4, (April 1999), pp.323–330, ISSN 0198-8859

4

Determination of Th1/Th2/Th17 Cytokines in Patients Undergoing Allogeneic Hematopoietic Stem Cell Transplantation

Adriana Gutiérrez-Hoya[1], Rubén López-Santiago[1],
Jorge Vela-Ojeda[2], Laura Montiel-Cervantes[2],
Octavio Rodríguez-Cortes[1] and Martha Moreno-Lafont[1]
*[1]Departamento de Inmunología, Escuela Nacional de
Ciencias Biológicas – Instituto Politécnico Nacional
[2]Unidad Médica de Alta Especialidad, Centro Médico
Nacional La Raza, Instituto Mexicano del Seguro Social
México*

1. Introduction

Allogeneic hematopoietic cell transplantation emerges as a therapy option to treat the sequels of exposure to radiation, a great concern at the beginning of the atomic age and cold war (Welniak et al., 2007). Hematopoietic cell transplantation emerged as a rescue strategy since there were already antecedents, like the study of Lorenz et al. in 1952 (as cited by Welniak et al., 2007), who showed that infusion of the bone marrow after lethal irradiation healed radiation disease in mice. This lay the foundations for the current consideration of allogeneic hematopoietic cell transplantation as the first-line therapy for many life-threatening oncological and hematological diseases. Today, it is primarily used to treat patients with hereditary anemias or immunological deficiencies through replacement of the hematopoietic system with cells from a healthy individual. It also allows cancer patients to be treated with myeloablative radiation and/or chemotherapy (known as myeloablative conditioning) in an attempt to eliminate tumoral cells, and although this strategy brings loss of bone marrow function, the latter can be recovered with infusion of normal hematopoietic cells (Jenq & Van den Brink, 2010).

2. Hematopoietic stem cell transplantation

Hematopoietic stem cell transplantation is today a simple procedure involving infusion of these cells intravenously. Once in the bloodstream, stem cells are able to migrate to the bone marrow in order to thus restore hematopoiesis during the first two weeks following transplantation (Léger & Nevill, 2004).

Stem cells giving rise to hematopoietic cells are known as hematopoietic stem cells due to their capacity for self-renewal, division and differentiation into a variety of specialized hematopoietic cells. This is the principle underlying hematopoietic stem cell transplantation (Hows, 2005).

One of the major difficulties in using hematopoietic stem cells has been their identification, since they are morphologically very similar to lymphocytes. This problem was solved with the use of biomarkers such as CD34, a transmembrane glycoprotein expressed by hematopoietic stem cells which is currently the main biomarker used to identify these cells. Hematopoietic cell transplantations are classified as isotransplantation, allotransplantation or autotransplantation. These are not the only types of transplantation, but they are the most commonly used in medical practice. It calls allotransplantation when donor and recipient are the same species but are not identical twins. The advantages of this type of transplantation compared to the allogeneic type are that the cells infused are normal cells and therefore the incidence of relapse is lower, as well as the fact that the graft cell is infused with immunocompetent cells that are able to induce a graft-versus-leukemia effect. The major concern with this type of transplantation is development of graft-versus-host disease (GVHD) or infections caused by opportunistic microorganisms, since patients are treated with immunosuppressant drugs (Léger & Neville, 2004; Vela-Ojeda et al., 2005).

2.1 Hematopoietic stem cell mobilization by G-CSF

At present peripheral blood hematopoietic stem cells are preferably used since grafting (particularly of blood platelets) is faster. This procedure is not excessively invasive – as is bone marrow procurement – and better results are obtained when mobilized peripheral blood is used as the hematopoietic stem cells source (Jaime et al., 2004). Normally, peripheral blood contains only a small amount of hematopoietic stem cells (<0.1% of nucleated cells). Different methods are therefore used to induce their egress from the bone marrow into the bloodstream in order to be able to collect them by apheresis for subsequent infusion in the patient. Hematopoietic stem cells mobilization was an innovative development in the 1990s, in particular after it was seen that the number of stem cells obtained from mobilized peripheral blood contained 1-log more lymphocytes than the number obtained from bone marrow (Champlin, 2000). The established, widely-used method of mobilization involves the use of G-CSF, which induces mobilization by initiating a stress process through neutrophil and osteoclast activation. This results in dissociation of the cell membrane unions between stem cells and the stroma cells as well as stem cell proliferation and activation and/or adhesion molecule degradation. Hematopoietic stem cells mobilization is also seen when chemotherapy is exclusively used (Devetten & Armitage, 2007).

The mechanism through which G-CSF mobilizes CD34+ hematopoietic stem cells from the bone marrow into the peripheral blood involves a series of steps. First of all, there is increased hematopoietic stem cell proliferation followed by exit of these cells from the bone marrow. Increased proliferation has been shown to occur with cytokines such as GM-CSF that temporarily increase the cell adhesion of CD34+ hematopoietic stem cells to the bone marrow stroma, a process that in turn increases cell proliferation. The mobilization of hematopoietic stem cells from the bone marrow to peripheral blood comprises several mechanisms. One hypothesis is modification of the cellular interactions occurring between hematopoietic stem cells and the bone marrow stroma. Analyses of peripheral blood mononuclear cells mobilized by G-CSF reveal a decrease in the expression of VLA-4 (*Very late antigen 4* [CD49d/CD29]) integrin which normally binds firmly to its ligand VCAM-1 (*Vascular cell adhesion molecule-1*) as well as to an extracellular-matrix fibronectine fragment. Other molecules in which a marked decrease occurs are LFA-1 (*Leucocyte functional antigen 1*

[CD11aCD18]) and c-kit. These molecules are expressed in most hematopoietic stem cells and are involved in binding of these cells to bone marrow stroma, a process that is expressed by the ligands of cells of the latter VCAM-1, ICAM-1 (*Intercellular adhesion molecule-1*) and ICAM-2 for LFA-1 and c-kitL. G-CSF can also initiate mobilization through neutrophils, by secretion of gelatinase B, breaking extracellular matrix molecules and

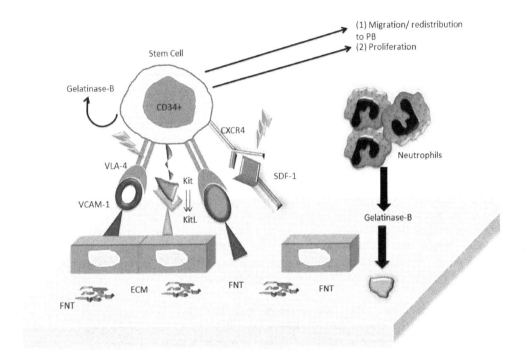

Fig. 1. Mechanism of hematopoietic stem cell mobilization from bone marrow to peripheral blood by stimulation with G-CSF. This process involves several steps, including modification of interactions occurring between stem cells and the stroma. Affected interactions include decreased expression of VLA-4 integrin, which normally binds to its ligand VCAM-1 and to FNT. Another molecule in which expression is decreased is c-kit; this process reduces the bond between this molecule and its ligand kit-L-. Decreased expression of these molecules reduces the bond between stem cells and the stromal cells. Another means by which G-CSF promotes stem cell mobilization is through neutrophils, by releasing gelatinase B, breaking extracellular matrix molecules and weakening adhesive interactions between stem cells and stroma cells. Yet another mechanism is stem cell secretion of gelatinase B, promoting faster migration of these cells to peripheral blood. A further mechanism involves indirect interaction of G-CSF with ligands, receptors/factors and stimulation of stem cell proliferation. PB: peripheral blood. G-CSF: granulocytic-colony stimulating factor. VCAM-1: vascular cell adhesion molecule-1, VLA-4: very late antigen 4 [CD49d/CD29] FNT: fibronectina (Modified from Gyger et al., 2000)

weakening adhesive interactions between stem cells and stroma cells. Stem cells have also been shown to secrete gelatinase B, a mechanism which may improve migration of these cells to peripheral blood (Figure 1). Finally, experimental evidence indicates that G-CSF may interact indirectly with a stem cell ligand to stimulate proliferation of these cells (Cashen et al., 2007; Cottler-Fox et al., 2003; Gyger et al., 2000).

In recent years, it has been demonstrated that G-CSF is also able to break one of the most important interactions between stem cells and stromal cells, which is formed by CXCL12 (formerly called SDF-1) and CXCR4 (Cashen et al., 2007).

2.1.1 Which stem cell source is best: bone marrow or mobilized peripheral blood?

This is one of the most commonly asked questions, since using mobilized peripheral blood rather than bone marrow in allogeneic transplantation is increasingly frequent. A retrospective study by Champlin et al. in 2000 examined the evolution of 288 allogeneic transplants in which mobilized peripheral blood was used and 536 in which bone marrow was used. They were followed-up during one year. The study found that in patients who had received mobilized peripheral blood, neutrophil engraftment was faster (14 days vs. 19) as was also platelet engraftment (19 days vs. 25). No significant differences were observed in development of acute GVHD. Chronic GVHD development was significantly higher in patients receiving mobilized blood, with a mean of 65% vs. 53%. The incidence of relapse did not differ significantly. Treatment-related mortality and leukemia-free survival were higher with mobilized blood transplants and hospitalization time was shorter. Additional studies similar to this one examining the benefits and drawbacks of allogeneic hematopoietic cell transplantation set the basis for mobilized peripheral blood being currently the most commonly used source in hematopoietic stem cell transplantation.

2.2 Points to consider before hematopoietic stem cell transplantation

When considering transplantation in patients in remission, two important aspects should be taken into account: whether medical evidence indicates that hematopoietic stem cells transplantation is more likely to heal the disease than other therapy forms and whether a suitable donor is available as a stem cell source. Although these are the major aspects to consider they are not the only ones. Other factors requiring consideration include biological characteristics at diagnosis, the specific disease that is being treated, presence of comorbidities that may complicate transplantation, and patient age (Deeg, 2010; Léger & Nevill, 2004).

2.3 Immunological typing of human leukocyte antigens

One reason for the progress that has taken place in hematopoietic cell transplantation is human leukocyte antigen (HLA) immunotyping. This is one of the major points to consider in allogeneic hematopoietic cell transplantation since, as already stated, it is important to have a suitable donor.

HLA proteins were first identified in 1950 by Jean Dausset upon observing that in many individuals, particularly those who previously received multiple blood transfusions or who were multiparous women, blood serum contained antibodies that reacted against a new kind of glycoprotein present on the outer surface of leukocytes of other members of the population; these glycoproteins were named human leukocyte antigens (HLAs). The latter behave as immunogenic markers making a person's cells distinct and are the major barrier to histocompatibility; they are therefore also called major histocompatibility complex (MHC) molecules. The importance of HLA molecules is not limited to the histocompatibility barrier, they are also essential in T-cell activation since HLA-molecules bind peptides to be presented to T cells. HLA class I molecules present peptides primarily to CD8+ T cells while CD4+ T cells recognize mainly peptides presented by class II molecules (Appelbaum, 2001; Bleakley & Riddell, 2004).

MHC genes are encoded on the short arm of chromosome 6 at locus p21. There are three different groups of genes called HLA-A, HLA-B and HLA-C, which individually code for the α chain of MHC class I. Similarly, there are three loci for the genes of class II MHC molecules known as HLA-DP, HLA-DQ and HLA-DR. Each of these includes genes coding for the α polypeptide chain and at least one β polypeptide chain. A person normally inherits two copies of the locus of each gene, one from each parent. Statistical data provided by the European Bioinformatics Institute (EBI) and the International Immunogenetics Organization Database (IMGT) suggest that the number of HLA class I and class II alleles discovered is on the increase. These data indicate that in human population there are 4,946 different class I alleles and 1,457 class II alleles, of which 1,601 are known alleles for HLA-A, 2,125 for HLA-B, 1,102 for HLA-C and 1,027 for HLA-DRβ of which 928 are HLA-DRβ1 alleles (these are the ones most commonly used to determine histocompatibility due to their high polymorphism) (Table 1).

Numbers of HLA Alleles	
HLA Class I Alleles	4,946
HLA Class II Alleles	1,457
HLA Alleles	6,403

HLA Class I					
Gene	A	B	C	E	F	G
Alleles	1,601	2,125	1,102	10	22	47
Proteins	1,176	1,641	808	3	4	15

HLA Class II									
Gene	DRA	DRB	DQA1	DQB1	DPA1	DPB1	DMA	DMB	DOA	DOB
Alleles	7	1,027	44	153	32	149	7	13	12	13
Proteins	2	774	27	106	16	129	4	7	3	5

HLA Class II- DRB Alleles								
Gene	DRB1	DRB2	DRB3	DRB4	DRB5	DRB6	DRB7	DRB8	DRB9
Alleles	928	1	57	15	19	3	2	1	1
Proteins	704	0	46	8	16	0	0	0	0

(Modified from http://www.ebi.ac.uk/imgt/hla/stats.html)

Table 1. Statistical data from the European Bioinformatics Institute (EBI) and the International Immunogenetics Organization database (IMGT) showing the number of each of the HLA alleles.

Historically, HLA immunotyping was performed by serological methods but now, with the advent of polymerase chain reaction (PCR), molecular immunotyping of the donor and recipient is possible. A study by Petersdorf et al. in 2001 examined patients who had previously undergone transplantation and were compatible by serological methods. When reexamined by molecular immunotyping, about 30%of these individuals were found to be incompatible in one or more alleles. These differences were correlated with increased GVHD and poor survival, indicating that a compatible donor and reliable HLA immunotyping are extremely important. The number of class I and class II HLA antigens is relatively large and therefore the probability of HLA matching between the recipient and an unrelated donor is extremely small.

2.4 Graft-versus-host disease and Th1/Th2/Th17 cytokines

Graft-versus-host disease (GVHD) may develop after hematopoietic stem cell transplantation. It is a reaction of immune cells from the donor against tissues of the host. Damage induced on epithelial cells of the host by activated T cells occurs after an inflammatory cascade that is unleashed by the conditioning regimen. Approximately 35-50%of allogenic hematopoietic cell transplantation recipients develop GVHD. The risk of developing the disease depends on several factors, primarily the stem cell source and donor cytokines, patient age, existing conditions and GVHD prophylaxis. GVHD involves mainly the skin, liver and gastrointestinal tract. Despite GVHD-related morbidity and mortality, its development is often desirable since it has been found to be associated with a lower recurrence of malignant disease, in other words, it is important for establishment of the graft-versus-tumor effect (Ferrara & Levine, 2008; Léger & Nevill, 2004; Saliba et al., 2007; Weisdorf 2007).

The physiopathology of acute GVHD described by Ferrara & Levine (2008) is a three-stage phenomenon. The initial stage involves damage to tissues of the host due to inflammation derived from chemo- and/or radiotherapy during the recipient conditioning. In the second stage, antigen-presenting cells (APC) of both donor and recipient as well as inflammatory cytokines unleash the activation of donor-derived T cells, with expansion and differentiation of the latter into effector cells. Antigens (Ag) of the minor histocompatibility complex have a central role in this activation. The pathway of T-cell activation results in activation of genes coding for cytokines such as IL-2 and interferon gamma (IFNγ). Cells that produce these cytokines are considered to be Th1 profile, as opposed to cells producing predominantly IL-4, IL-5, IL-10 and IL-13 which are considered to be Th2 phenotype and are assumed to be the ones that modulate GVHD. During the third stage, also known as the effector stage, donor-derived activated T cells mediate cytotoxicity against target cells of the recipient through FasL-Fas, perforin and granzyme B interactions as well as additional production of tumor necrosis factor α (TNFα). This cytokine is produced by monocytes and macrophages, and secondarily by T lymphocytes and natural killer (NK) cells (Figure 2). (Ferrara & Levine, 2008; Jacobsohn & Vogelsang, 2007; Socie & Blazar 2009).

TNFα is firmly involved in GVHD physiopathology at several steps of the process including induction of apoptosis in target tissues through the TNFα receptor. It also induces the activation of macrophages, neutrophils, eosinophils, and B and T cells; stimulates production of inflammatory cytokines such as IL-1, IL-6, IL-12 and TNFα itself; increases the expression of HLA molecules; and promotes lysis by T lymphocytes. High levels of TNFα are associated with a higher incidence of GVHD in bone marrow transplant recipients. This allogeneic dysregulation, in addition to dysregulation of cytokines, leads to the acute tissue damage produced by GVHD.

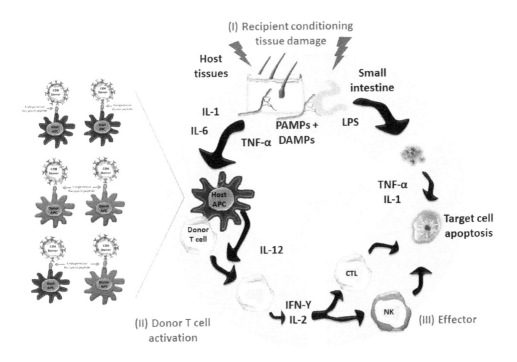

Fig. 2. Physiopathology of graft-versus-host disease. (I) Damage to host tissues by inflammation derived from the chemotherapy and/or radiotherapy conditioning regimen. (II) Antigen-presenting cells (APC) of both donor and recipient as well as inflammatory cytokines unleash the activation of donor-derived T cells, with expansion and differentiation of the latter into effector cells. The pathway of T-cell activation results in activation of the genes coding for cytokines such as IL-2 and IFNγ. (III) Effector stage: donor-derived activated T cells mediate cytotoxicity against target cells of the recipient through FasL-Fas, perforin and granzyme B interactions as well as additional production of tumor necrosis factor α (TNFα) (Modified from Ferrara & Levine, 2008).

In our laboratory, we have studied patients who underwent allogenic hematopoietic cell transplantation and developed GVHD, finding a correlation between these patients and an increased of CD14+ TNFα+ cells. Up to 32% of CD14+ cells secreting TNFα were found in a patient with stage II GVHD, increasing to 47% when the patient progressed to stage III, while in patients who did not develop GVHD this behavior was not observed. In patients with GVHD development, TNFα may promote increased expression of adhesion molecules such as VCAM-1, ICAM-1 and E-selectin in endothelium, therefore also promoting diapedesis of leukocytes in affected areas and degranulation of these cells with subsequent damage to tissues in which they are infiltrated (Aggarwal et al., 2000). On the other hand, activation of endothelium, release of nitric oxide, vasodilation and increased vascular permeability, and blood platelet activation are also promoted and, most importantly, increased expression of MHC-I and MHC-II molecules as well as co-stimulatory molecules such as CD40, CD80 and CD86 in dendritic cells, thus also activating T lymphocytes and giving rise to more effective antigen presentation, and along with this, more effective allorecognition (Steinman et al., 1998).

In addition to this, TNFα has a major role in the promotion of apoptosis (De Freitas et al., 2004) and due to the previously mentioned properties, TNFα overexpression contributes to GVHD emergence and severity (Figure 3). Recent studies reveal an increase not only in TNFα levels but also in TNF receptors (TNFR1 and TNFR2), and the latter are more stable and easier to quantify (Choi et al., 2009; Kitko et al., 2008).

The role of other cytokines such as those of the Th1 profile is worth noting. Diverse research groups initially correlated this profile with GVHD emergence, since large quantities of cytokines such as IFNγ, IL-2 and IL-12 were found in patients with GVHD development and this is correlated with GVHD severity (Das et al., 2001; Ju et al., 2005). However, these cytokines have a controversial role as they are necessary for development of both GVHD and the graft-versus-leukemia effect. We have found that mononuclear cells from patients with GVHD development in co-culture secrete large amounts of IFNγ and IL-2, but we have also observed that the capacity of these cells to secrete these cytokines is correlated with graft success unaccompanied by relapse or development of infections by opportunistic microorganisms, which tells us these cytokines have a dual role. Regarding the significance of the Th2 cytokine profile in GVHD control, some study teams point to the overexpression of IL-4, IL-5 and IL-10 as a positive prognostic factor (Das et al., 2001; Ju et al., 2005). In our laboratory, however, a correlation has been observed only between the overexpression of IL-10 by mononuclear cells of patients and control of GVHD.

There are new lymphocyte subsets to which great significance has been ascribed in inflammatory processes as well as in many pathologies previously thought to be associated with the Th1 profile. The subpopulation of Th17 cells discovered in 2005 is now known to have a controversial role as they are implicated in rejection of solid organ grafts (Kappel et al., 2008; Carlson 2009; Coghill et al., 2010).

In murine models, differences in GVHD development have been found between mice that were transferred CD4+ IL-17-/- T cells and mice that were transferred normal CD4+ cells. In the former, GVHD development took longer. However, no significant differences were noted between these groups in relation to mortality due to GVHD or in graft-versus-tumor activity. Another major finding was the fact that mice that were transferred CD4+ IL17-/- cells had fewer Th1 cells during early stages of GVHD. Also, a reduction occurred in the number of IFNγ-secreting macrophages and granulocytes as well as a decrease in the amount of pro-inflammatory cytokines. IL-17 is therefore believed to be essential for GVHD development and graft-versus-leukemia activity as it promotes pro-inflammatory cytokine production – all this in murine models (Kappel et al., 2008). These data and others showing the importance of the Th17 profile in inflammatory processes made several researchers think that this profile might be involved in GVHD development and severity in humans (Coghill, 2011). Our study team recently found that the Th17 profile is not relevant for GVHD development. We conducted a pilot study on the importance of this profile in six patients who underwent allogenic hematopoietic cell transplantation, following them for six months. This group was divided into patients with GVHD development and patients without GVHD. Peripheral blood and mononuclear cell cultures were analyzed at 30, 60, 100 and 180

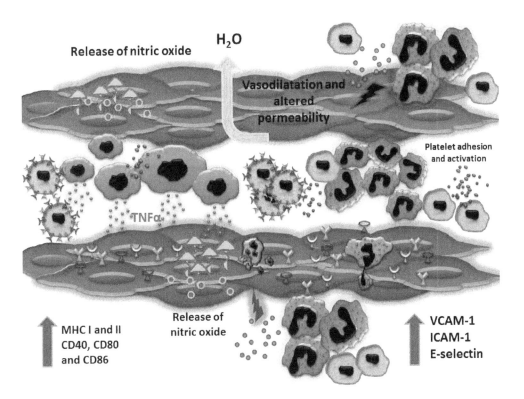

Fig. 3. The role of TNFα in GVHD emergence and exacerbation.

days after transplantation. Overproduction of Th17 profile was not observed neither in patients with GVHD nor in individuals without GVHD, as opposed to its production in healthy volunteers and in a patient who received a syngeneic transplant. Few months after concluding our study, Broady et al. (2010) published a similar study on patients who underwent allogenic hematopoietic cell transplantation, in which they evaluated Th1 and Th17 cells in tissue and peripheral blood in a cohort of 34 patients, of which 20 developed acute GVHD and 14 did not develop GVHD. The authors did not find an increase in the number of Th17 cells in patients with acute cutaneous GVHD as compared to healthy donors, but they did detect increased production of IFNγ-secreting cells (Broady, 2010).

GVHD diagnosis is suspected when the recipient develops all or some of the signs and symptoms that are characteristic of this disease such as dermatitis (rash), epidermal blistering, stomach cramps, abdominal pain with or without diarrhea which may be accompanied by passage of blood, nausea, persistent vomiting, and hepatitis (elevated bilirubins and/or liver enzymes). Typically, these signs and symptoms occur 100 days after allogenic hematopoietic cell transplantation but may also appear later. Because many of them are not specific of this complication, diagnosis must be supported with suitable biopsies, particularly if the symptoms are atypical or involve only the liver or gastrointestinal tract, since histological confirmation is extremely useful. A further reason for biopsy-taking is to help differentiate GVHD from other diseases with similar symptoms, such as viral infections or reactions to pharmaceutical agents (Ferrara & Levine 2008; Jacobsohn & Vogelsang, 2007).

In GVHD, mature T cells of the donor that accompany the graft attack host tissues, particularly the skin, liver and gastrointestinal tract. This explains the signs and symptoms that characterize this disease. To prevent GVHD development, all patients receive some type of prophylaxis with immunosuppressors and in some cases T cell depletion , being one of the most commonly used methods although its effectiveness has not been fully proven since T-cell elimination contributes to absence of GVHD development but patients die from relapse because lack of GVT effect. Another prophylactic method involves pharmacological treatment with agents that affect T-cell function. These types of prophylaxis elicit adverse effects since mature T cells of the donor have a major role in mediating the reconstitution of the adaptive immune system, particularly in adults with low thymus function (Jacobsohn & Vogelsang, 2007).

GVHD is classified according to the number and extent of the organs involved (Table 2). In the current classification system, established in 1994, GVHD is divided into four groups (I – IV). Skin damage is evaluated by the percentage of the body surface area involved, liver damage by elevated bilirubins, and gastrointestinal tract damage by the amount of diarrhea (Jacobsohn & Vogelsang, 2007; Vela-Ojeda et al., 2008).

Stage	Skin	Liver (bilirubin)	Gut (stool output/day)
0	No GVHD rash	< 2 mg/dl	< 500 ml/day or persistent nausea
1	Maculopapular rash < 25% BSA	2-3 mg/dl	500-999 ml/day
2	Maculopapular rash < 25 - 50% BSA	3.1-6 mg/dl	1000-1500 ml/day
3	Maculopapular rash > 50% BSA	6.1-15 mg/dl	Adult: >1500 ml/day
4	Generalized erythroderma plus bullous formation	>15 mg/dl	Severe abdominal pain with or without ileus
Grade			
I	Stage 1-2	None	None
II	Stage 3 or	Stage 1 or	Stage 1
III	-	Stage 2-3 or	Stage 2-4
IV	Stage 4 or	Stage 4	-

(Modified from Jacobsohn & Volgelsang 2007).

Table 2. Classification of acute graft-versus-host disease.

Chronic GVHD (cGVHD) is one of the most common and significant problems affecting recipients of allogenic hematopoietic cell transplantation at long term. It appears approximately 100 days after allogenic hematopoietic cell transplantation, which is the critical time at which close to 50% of patients develop some degree of cGVHD. Increased use of hematopoietic stem cells obtained from peripheral blood rather than bone marrow, increased age of recipients, and the use of busulfan in the conditioning regimen have led to a higher incidence of cGVHD. Other clinical risk factors for cGVHD development include previous acute graft-versus-host disease (aGVHD) and a second transplant. cGVHD most commonly affects the skin, liver, eyes and mouth, although other sites may also be affected. Death from severe cGVHD is generally a result of infectious complications. The standard treatment for severe cGVHD is a combination of cyclosporine and prednisone. An alternating daily regimen of these two agents prolongs survival and reduces drug-related adverse effects. Topical therapy in affected areas is recommended for patients with grade 1-2 cutaneous disease. Survival at 10 years in patients who develop light aGVHD is approximately 80%, but it is drastically reduced in patients with severe cGVHD, in whom this rate is reported to be 5% (Horwitz & Sullivan 2006; Lee 2005; Vela-Ojeda et al., 2008).

Alloreactivity is the basis for cGVHD pathogenesis. However, the exact phenotype and the origin of alloreactive cells remain somewhat ambiguous. Donor-derived alloreactive T-cells transplanted with hematopoietic stem cells play a key role in acute and chronic GVHD. Current animal models of cGVHD implicate Th2 cells as the first cell type to induce damage. However, in humans with cGVHD, Th1/Th2-polarized CD4+ cells have alloreactive properties. The formation of antibodies has been observed in experimental models and clinical studies of cGVHD. This suggests that B cells are implicated in the physiopathology of cGVHD as shown by antibody production in allogenic hematopoietic cell transplantation patients with donor of different sex, since antibodies against minor histocompatibility antigens are encoded in the Y chromosome. The presence of anti-nuclear, anti-double strand DNA and anti-smooth muscle antibodies in a frequency range of 11-62% has also been detected in patients with cGVHD as well as the presence of anti-cytoskeletal and anti-nucleolar antibodies. However, despite these findings, the role of antibodies in cGVHD remains unclear (Horwitz & Sullivan 2006; Lee 2005; Vela-Ojeda et al., 2008).

cGVHD can be classified according to type of clinical manifestations or extent of the disease. Most patients with cGVHD have previously had aGVHD. cGVHD may also be observed after achieving control of aGVHD. Similarly, patients may develop cGVHD without a previous history of aGVHD (*de novo* cGVHD). Classification according to the type and extent of clinical manifestations is shown in Table 3.

The International Center for Research on Bone Marrow and Blood Cell Transplantation estimates that 50,000 – 60,000 hematopoietic cell transplantations are performed each year throughout the world. Bone marrow is the main source of grafts for transplantation in children, although peripheral and umbilical cord blood are being increasingly used. Between 2004 and 2008 peripheral blood accounted for 27% and umbilical cord blood for 32% of transplants in patients fewer than 20 years in age. In patients over 20 years the most common source for allogenic hematopoietic cell transplantation is peripheral blood. Currently, very few adults receive grafts of umbilical cord blood but its use, although infrequent, increased 2-4% between 2004 and 2008. Mobilized peripheral blood is the main source for autologous transplantation, representing 91% of autotransplantations in children and 98% in adults. In recent years the number of hematopoietic cell transplantations, both allogeneic and autologous, in patients over 50 years old has increased. Approximately 40% of allogeneic transplants are unrelated donor transplantations. There has been a change lately: before 2002 the most commonly used source of hematopoietic stem cells was bone marrow but its use has declined since 2003 and peripheral and umbilical cord blood have been increasingly used.

Classification of GVHD	
Limited chronic GVHD	
Either or both:	
1	Localized skin involvement
2	Hepatic dysfunction due to chronic GVHD
Extensive chronic GVHD	
Either:	
1	Generalized skin involvement, or
2	Localized skin involvement and/or hepatic dysfunction due to chronic GVHD
Plus:	
3a	Liver histology showing chronic aggressive hepatitis, bridging necrosis, or cirrhosis, or
b	Involvement of eye (Schirmer test with <5-mm wetting), or
c	Involvement of minor salivary glands or oral mucosa demonstrated on labial biopsy, or
d	Involvement of any other target organ

Table 3. Classification of chronic graft-versus-host disease (Horwitz & Sullivan, 2006)

The most common cause of death after allogenic hematopoietic cell transplantation is relapse, although in unrelated donor transplants it is followed by GVHD and in HLA-matched sibling transplants by death from infections. Another major cause of death is interstitial pneumonitis (Pasquini & Wang, 2007).

2.5 Graft-versus-tumor effect
Existence of the graft-versus-tumor effect was first suggested in 1956 by Barnes et al., upon noting eradication of leukemia in irradiated mice receiving allogeneic bone marrow transplants, but not in those that after irradiation received syngeneic bone marrow transplants. The first evidence of this also occurring in humans came from studies reporting that the incidence of relapse was markedly lower in patients who developed GVHD than in those who did not (as cited in Appelbaum, 2001), and that just as in murine models, human allogenic hematopoietic cell transplantation recipients were at lower risk of relapse than recipients of syngeneic stem cell transplantations or allogenic hematopoietic cell transplantations in which T cells are previously depleted. Male patients receiving allogenic hematopoietic cell transplantation grafts from female donors are also seen to be a special group in that donor-derived T cells specific for receptors of minor histocompatibility antigens may contribute to development of the graft-versus-tumor or the graft-versus-leukemia effect as well as GVHD since the graft-versus-leukemia effect is associated with presence of GVHD. The potential impact of the graft-versus-leukemia effect can be observed

when the patient is administered infusions of donor-derived lymphocytes. Graft versus tumor effect formed the basis of the so-called non-myeloablative transplants in which intensive chemotherapy regimen are substituted by the antitumoral effect of lymphocytes (Jacobsohn & Vogelsang, 2007).

Factors inducing GVHD or the graft-versus-leukemia effect are not well defined and may to some extent be considered speculative. Minor histocompatibility antigens have been suggested to play a key role since some of them have limited expression in hematopoietic cells, including leukemic cells. These antigens are perhaps targeted by the selective effect of the graft-versus-leukemia effect while minor histocompatibility antigens that are expressed in general may be targeted by GVHD, but this is still not firmly established (Jacobsohn & Vogelsang 2007; Kolb, 2008; Riddell & Appelbaum, 2007).

Various minor histocompatibility antigens are encoded in Y-chromosome genes that exhibit significant polymorphism with their homologues genes of the X chromosome. The former genes are responsible for the immune reactions occurring between men and women. Differential expression of the genes encoding for minor histocompatibility antigens in tissues has been proposed for potential use as a basis to separate the graft-versus-leukemia effect from GVHD. Cells that recognize minor histocompatibility antigens which are expressed only in hematopoietic cell receptors, including leukemic cells, may have a major role in the elimination of the latter without GVHD development. Several minor histocompatibility antigens such as HA-1, HA-2, HB-1 and BCL2A1 are expressed by hematopoietic cells and are therefore being examined as potential targets in order to promote the graft-versus-leukemia effect (Randolph et al., 2004; Kolb, 2008).

2.6 Clinical relevance of regulation and induction of tolerance after allogenic hematopoietic cell transplantation

The potential benefits of allogenic hematopoietic cell transplantation are offset by the moderate survival rate of the graft at long term. This is to a large extent due to immunosuppressant agents that unspecifically inhibit immune response in order to prevent rejection, but bring multiple adverse effects which are responsible for chronic rejection. Therefore, one of the major goals of allogenic hematopoietic cell transplantation is to achieve absence of immune response in the face of donor-derived alloantigens without requiring prolonged administration of immunosuppressants and to promote the graft-versus-leukemia effect. To this end, research has focused on the study of regulatory T cells (Treg), particularly those of the CD4+CD25highFoxP3+ phenotype (natural Treg, nTreg) as they have been shown to be able to control immune response in the face of donor-derived alloantigens and therefore possess great potential to establish in vivo tolerance to the transplant. These cells have been studied the most but are not the only ones described as having a regulatory role since regulatory functions have also been observed in other subpopulations of CD4+ cells, in T CD8+ cells, Tγδ cells, NK cells and CD3+CD4-CD8-CD16+56+ cells, also known as NKT cells. The latter have been shown to have a powerful anti-tumoral effect and are important in the maintenance of tolerance. This is why many studies are focusing on transfer of these cells. The strategy that is being sought for use in the near future is ex vivo stimulation of Treg purified with alloantigens of the donor or even FoxP3-mediated transfection of alloreactive CD4+CD25⁻ cells (Bryceson & Ljunggren, 2007; Fehérvari & Sakaguchi, 2005).

Natural regulatory T cells (nTreg) express from the time of their differentiation in the thymus, CD4+, CD25+ and FoxP3 (*forkhead box P3 transcription factor*) expression patterns. They were identified by Sakaguchi et al. (1995) as a natural subset of CD4+ T lymphocytes (approximately 5-10% of the T lymphocytes present in peripheral blood) that constitutively express the CD25 molecule and suppress the response of effector T lymphocytes (CD4+ and CD8+) *in vivo*. Another lymphocyte subpopulation in peripheral blood are CD4+CD25− cells, which through the action of TGF-β and IL-2 may come to express CD25 and FoxP3, and are known as induced Treg (iTreg). Treg lymphocytes are also associated with low expression of CD127 which is positively correlated with regulatory function acquisition and negatively correlated with expression of FoxP3 (Curiel et al., 2004, Horwitz et al., 2008; Korn 2009; Liu et al., 2006; Seddiki et al., 2006).

CD4+CD25+FoxP3+ Treg cells have a key role in the maintenance of peripheral tolerance, and Treg deficiencies give rise to progressive autoimmune disorders. Similarly, improved Treg function can prevent graft rejection and suppress tumor immunity. In other words, an adequate balance between Treg and effector T cells is essential for maintenance of tolerance. In the context of allogenic hematopoietic cell transplantation, Treg have also been shown to have a major role in the establishment of tolerance between tissues of the recipient and donor-derived immunity. This was initially shown to occur in murine models where Treg depletion in the stem cell graft produced increased in GVHD and increased Treg numbers resulted in suppression of GVHD after transplantation (Lee 2005). In humans, patients with active cGVHD are reported to have a lower frequency of Treg than patients without cGVHD. These findings suggest that robust reconstitution of Treg post-allogenic hematopoietic cell transplantation is required to establish immune balance in order to be able to maintain adequate levels of peripheral tolerance. However, the mechanisms responsible for Treg reconstitution post-allogenic hematopoietic cell transplantation have not been adequately characterized and the factors contributing to inadequate recovery of Treg in patients who develop cGVHD are unknown (Matsuoka 2010).

Based on data obtained by Matsuoka et al. (2010) in patients examined during the first year after allogenic hematopoietic cell transplantation, thymus-dependent generation of Treg was considerably affected, but this subpopulation maintained high levels of cell proliferation in comparison to constitutive T cells. Such *in vivo* proliferation is apparently driven mainly by lymphopenia of CD4 cells. Among other findings, this study team has also shown that high levels of Treg proliferation were offset by higher susceptibility to apoptosis. Depletion of Treg in periphery in these patients was associated with development of extensive cGVHD.

On the other hand and in reference to lymphocyte populations that may take part in development of tolerance to alloantigens, the subpopulation of CD8+ Treg has been recently characterized. These lymphocytes, despite a long history in the field of immunology as described by Gershon & Kondo in 1970, have been difficult to characterize, and this factor combined with the discovery of CD4 Treg by Hall et al. (1990) and Sakaguchi et al. (1995) have considerably limited this area. The importance of CD8 Treg lies in the regulatory role observed in experimental autoimmune encephalitis (Lu & Cantor, 2008; Wang & Alexander 2009; Zheng et al., 2004).

The latter subpopulation has been said to be increased in peripheral blood analyses and infiltrated tissue of patients with colorectal cancer. Increased expression of TGF-β has also been found in these lymphocytes as compared to samples from healthy donors. These cells were able to suppress CD4+CD25- cell proliferation and cytokine Th1 production. The paper mentions the significance of immunological vigilance and the fact that CD8 Treg may promote tumoral growth. It also describes this cell subpopulation in patients with multiple sclerosis in whom lower numbers of these cells were correlated with relapse, a fact that may evidence their immunosuppressant role in the control of autoimmune diseases (Giovanni Frisullo, 2010; Chaput, 2009; Kiniwa, 2007).

Recently described populations of CD8+ Treg include CD8+ IL-10+ cells present in ovarian carcinoma, which are induced by plasmocytoid dendritic cells infiltrating the tumor. This differentiation towards CD8+ Treg was shown to be independent of CD4+ Treg. All these antecedents combined with the generation of CD8+ Treg through continuous antigen stimulation may indicate the importance of the latter in GVHD control.

3. Conclusions

TNFα levels have a major role in development and severity of graft-versus-host disease and can be used as a negative prognostic factor.

Th1 response is essential and required in post-transplant patients to prevent relapse, graft loss and appearance of infections caused by opportunistic microorganisms.

The Th17 profile has no essential role in development or severity of GVHD and is therefore not a target for therapy in these patients.

4. Acknowledgments

The present study was financially supported through grants from Consejo Nacional de Ciencia y Tecnología (CONACyT), number 82559; and Secretaría de Investigación y Posgrado, Instituto Politécnico Nacional, numbers SIP-20100710 and SIP-20110504.

5. References

[1] Welniak LA, Blazar BR & Murphy WJ. (2007). Immunobiology of allogeneic hematopoietic stem cell transplantation. *Annu Rev Immunol*. Vol. 25, pp. (139-17), ISSN:0732-0582

[2] Jenq RR & van den Brink MR. (2010). Allogeneic haematopoietic stem cell transplantation: individualized stem cell and immune therapy of cancer. *Nat Rev Cancer*. Vol. 10, No. 3, (March 2010), pp. (213-221), ISSN 1474-1768

[3] Léger CS & Nevill TJ. (2004). Hematopoietic stem cell transplantation: a primer for the primary care physician. *CMAJ*. Vol. 170, No. 10, (May 2004), pp. (1569-1577), ISSN 1488-2329

[4] Hows J. (2005). Adult stem cell therapy beyond haematopoietic stem cell transplantation? An update. *Transpl Immunol*. Vol. 14, No. 3-4, (August 2005), pp. (221-223), ISSN 0966-3274

[5] Vela-Ojeda J & Ruiz-Esparza MA. (2005). Hematopoietic stem cell transplantation in multiple myeloma. *Rev Invest Clin.* Vol. 57, No. 2, (March-April 2005), pp. (305-313), ISSN 0034-9887

[6] Jaime Fagundo JC, Dorticós Balea E, Pavón Morán V & Cortina Rosales L. (2004). Trasplante de células progenitoras hematopoyéticas: tipos, fuentes e indicaciones. *Rev Cubana Hematol Inmunol Hemoter.* Vol. 20, No. 2. ISSN 0864-0289

[7] Champlin RE, Schmitz N, Horowitz MM, Chapuis B, Chopra R, Cornelissen JJ, Gale RP, Goldman JM, Loberiza FR Jr, Hertenstein B, Klein JP, Montserrat E, Zhang MJ, Ringdén O, Tomany SC, Rowlings PA, Van Hoef ME & Gratwohl A. (2000). Blood stem cells compared with bone marrow as a source of hematopoietic cells for allogeneic transplantation. IBMTR Histocompatibility and Stem Cell Sources Working Committee and the European Group for Blood and Marrow Transplantation (EBMT). *Blood.* Vol. 95, No. 12, (June 2000), pp. (3702-3709), ISSN 1528-0020

[8] Devetten M & Armitage JO. (2007). Hematopoietic cell transplantation: progress and obstacles. *Ann Oncol.* Vol. 18, No. 9, (September 2007), pp. (1450-1456), ISSN 1569-8041

[9] Cashen AF, Lazarus HM & Devine SM. (2007). Mobilizing stem cells from normal donors: is it possible to improve upon G-CSF? *Bone Marrow Transplant.* Vol. 39, No. 10, (May 2007), pp. (577-588), ISSN 0006-4971

[10] Cottler-Fox MH, Lapidot T, Petit I, Kollet O, DiPersio J & Link. (2003). Stem cell mobilization. *Ame Soc Hematol.* Vol. 1, pp. (419-437), ISSN 0001-2001

[11] Gyger M, Stuart RK & Perreault C. (2000). Immunobiology of allogeneic peripheral blood mononuclear cells mobilized with granulocyte-colony stimulating factor. *Bone Marrow Transplant.* Vol. 26, No. 1, (July 2000), pp. (1-16), ISSN 0268-3369

[12] Champlin RE, Schmitz N, Horowitz MM, Chapuis B, Chopra R, Cornelissen JJ, Gale RP, Goldman JM, Loberiza FR Jr, Hertenstein B, Klein JP, Montserrat E, Zhang MJ, Ringdén O, Tomany SC, Rowlings PA, Van Hoef ME & Gratwohl A. (2000). Blood stem cells compared with bone marrow as a source of hematopoietic cells for allogeneic transplantation. IBMTR Histocompatibility and Stem Cell Sources Working Committee and the European Group for Blood and Marrow Transplantation (EBMT). *Blood,* Vol. 15, No. 95, (June 2000), pp. (3702-3709), ISSN 1528-0020

[13] Deeg HJ & Sandmaier BM. (2010). Who is fit for allogeneic transplantation? *Blood.* Vol. 116, No. 23, (Dec 2010), pp. (4762-4770), ISSN 1528-0020

[14] Appelbaum FR. (2001). Haematopoietic cell transplantation as immunotherapy. *Nature.* Vol. 411, No. 6835, (May 2001), pp. (385-389), ISSN 0028-0836

[15] Bleakley M & Riddell SR. (2004). Molecules and mechanisms of the graft-versus-leukaemia effect. *Nat Rev Cancer.* Vol. 4, No. 5, (May 2004), pp. (371-380), ISSN 1474-1768

[16] Petersdorf EW, Hansen JA, Martin PJ, Woolfrey A, Malkki M, Gooley T, Storer B, Mickelson E, Smith A & Anasetti C. (2001). Major-histocompatibility-complex class I alleles and antigens in hematopoietic-cell transplantation. *N Engl J Med.* Vol. 345, No. 25, (December 2001), pp. (1794-1800), ISSN 0028-4793

[17] Ferrara J & Levine J. (2008). A new approach to therapy for acute GVHD. *Cell Ther Transplant*. Vol. 1, No. 1, (May 2008), pp. (25-27), ISSN 1866-8836

[18] Saliba RM, de Lima M, Giralt S, Andersson B, Khouri IF, Hosing C, Ghosh S, Neumann J, Hsu Y, De Jesus J, Qazilbash MH, Champlin RE & Couriel DR. (2007). Hyperacute GVHD: risk factors, outcomes, and clinical implications. *Blood*. Vol. 109, No. 7, (Apr 2007), pp. (2751-2758), ISSN 1528-0020

[19] Weisdorf D. (2007). GVHD- The nuts and bolts. *Hematology Am Soc Hematol Educ Program*, Vol. 1, No. 1, (January 2007), pp. (62-67), ISSN 1520-4391

[20] Jacobsohn DA & Vogelsang GB. (2007). Acute graft versus host disease. *Orphanet J Rare Dis*. Vol. 2, No. 35, (Sep 2007), ISSN 0212-1611

[21] Socié G & Blazar BR. (2009). Acute graft-versus-host disease: from the bench to the bedside. *Blood*. Vol. 114, No. 20, (Nov 2009), pp. (4327-4336), ISSN 1528-0020

[22] Aggarwal BB, Samanta A & Feldmann M. (2000). TNFα. *Cytokine ref*. DOI:1006/RWEY/150001.200. pp. (414-434).

[23] Steinman RM. (1988). Cytokines amplify the function of accessory cells. *Immunol Lett*. Vol. 17, No. 3, (March 1988), pp. (197-202), ISSN 0165-2478

[24] De Freitas I, Fernández-Somoza M, Essenfeld-Sekler E & Cardier JE. (2004). Serum levels of the apoptosis-associated molecules, tumor necrosis factor-alpha/tumor necrosis factor type-I receptor and Fas/FasL, in sepsis. *Chest*. Vol. 125, No. 6, (June 2004), pp. (2238-2246), ISSN 1931-3543

[25] Choi SW, Kitko CL, Braun T, Paczesny S, Yanik G, Mineishi S, Krijanovski O, Jones D, Whitfield J, Cooke K, Hutchinson RJ, Ferrara JL& Levine JE. (2008). Change in plasma tumor necrosis factor receptor 1 levels in the first week after myeloablative allogeneic transplantation correlates with severity and incidence of GVHD and survival. *Blood*. Vol. 112, No. 4, (August 2008), pp. (1539-1542), ISSN 1528-0020

[26] Kitko CL, Paczesny S, Yanik G, Braun T, Jones D, Whitfield J, Choi SW, Hutchinson RJ, Ferrara JL & Levine JE. (2008). Plasma elevations of tumor necrosis factor-receptor-1 at day 7 postallogeneic transplant correlate with graft-versus-host disease severity and overall survival in pediatric patients. *Biol Blood Marrow Transplant*. Vol. 14, No. 7, (July 2008), pp. (759-765), ISSN 1083-8791

[27] Das H, Imoto S, Murayama T, Mizuno I, Sugimoto T, Taniguchi R, Toda K, Isobe T, Nakagawa T, Nishimura R & Koizumi T. (2001). Kinetic analysis of cytokine gene expression in patients with GVHD after donor lymphocyte infusion. *Bone Marrow Transplant*. Vol. 27, No. 4, (February 2001), pp. (373-380), ISSN 0006-4971

[28] Ju XP, Xu B, Xiao ZP, Li JY, Chen L, Lu SQ & Huang ZX. (2005). Cytokine expression during acute graft-versus-host disease after allogeneic peripheral stem cell transplantation. *Bone Marrow Transplant*. Vol. 35, No. 12, (June 2005), pp. (1179-1186), ISSN 0006-4971

[29] Kappel LW, Goldberg GL, King CG, Suh DY, Smith OM, Ligh C, Holland AM, Grubin J, Mark NM, Liu C, Iwakura Y, Heller G & van den Brink MR. (2009). IL-17 contributes to CD4-mediated graft-versus-host disease. *Blood*. Vol. 113, No. 4, (January 2009), pp. (945-952), ISSN 1528-0020

[30] Carlson MJ, West ML, Coghill JM, Panoskaltsis-Mortari A, Blazar BR & Serody JS. (2009). *In vitro*-differentiated TH17 cells mediate lethal acute graft-versus-host disease with severe cutaneous and pulmonary pathologic manifestations. *Blood*. Vol. 113, No. 6, (February 2009), pp. (1365-1374), ISSN 1528-0020

[31] Coghill JM, Sarantopoulos S, Moran TP, Murphy WJ, Blazar BR & Serody JS. (2011). Effector CD4+ T cells, the cytokines they generate, and GVHD: something old and something new. *Blood*. Vol. 117, No. 12, (March 2011), pp. (3268-3276), ISSN 1528-0020

[32] Broady R, Yu J, Chow V, Tantiworawit A, Kang C, Berg K, Martinka M, Ghoreishi M, Dutz J & Levings MK. (2010). Cutaneous GVHD is associated with the expansion of tissue-localized Th1 and not Th17 cells. *Blood*. Vol. 116, No. 25, (December 2010), pp. (5748-5751), ISSN 1528-0020

[33] Vela-Ojeda J, Ruiz-Esparza MA & Borbolla-Escoboza JR. (2008). *Trasplante de células progenitoras hematopoyéticas*. 1a. Ed, Ed. Prado, pp. (73-123, 485-515). México.

[34] Horwitz ME & Sullivan KM. (2006). Chronic graft-versus-host disease. *Blood Rev*. Vol. 20, No. 1, (January 2006), pp. (15-27), ISSN 1528-0020

[35] Lee SJ. (2005). New approaches for preventing and treating chronic graft-versus-host disease. *Blood*. Vol. 105, No. 11, (June 2005), pp. (4200-4206), ISSN 1528-0020

[36] Pasquini M & Wang Z. (2007). CIBMTR Newsletter. *Medical College of Wisconsin*. Vol. 14, pp. (1-16).

[37] Kolb HJ. (2008). Graft-versus-leukemia effects of transplantation and donor lymphocytes. *Blood*. Vol. 112, No. 12, (December 2008), pp. (4371-4383), ISSN 1528-0020

[38] Riddell SR & Appelbaum FR. (2007). Graft-versus-host disease: a surge of developments. *PLoS Med*. Vol. 4, No. 7, (July 2007), pp. (e198), ISSN 1549-1676

[39] Randolph SS, Gooley TA, Warren EH, Appelbaum FR & Riddell SR. (2004). Female donors contribute to a selective graft-versus-leukemia effect in male recipients of HLA-matched, related hematopoietic stem cell transplants. *Blood*. Vol. 103, No. 1, (January 2004), pp. (347-352), ISSN 1528-0020

[40] Bryceson YT & Ljunggren HG. (2007). Lymphocyte effector functions: armed for destruction? *Curr Opin Immunol*. Vol. 19, No. 3, (June 2007), pp. (337-338), ISSN 0952-7915

[41] Fehérvari Z & Sakaguchi S. (2005). CD4+ regulatory cells as a potential immunotherapy. *Philos Trans R Soc London B Biol Sci*. Vol. 360, No. 1461, (September 2005), pp. (1647-1661), ISSN 1471-2970

[42] Sakaguchi S, Sakaguchi N, Asano M, Itoh M & Toda M. (1995). Immunologic self-tolerance maintained by activated T cells expressing IL-2 receptor alpha-chains (CD25). Breakdown of a single mechanism of self-tolerance causes various autoimmune diseases. *J Immunol*. Vol. 155, No. 3, (August 1995), pp. (1151-1164), ISSN 1550-6606

[43] Curiel TJ, Coukos G, Zou L, Alvarez X, Cheng P, Mottram P, Evdemon-Hogan M, Conejo-Garcia JR, Zhang L, Burow M, Zhu Y, Wei S, Kryczek I, Daniel B, Gordon A, Myers L, Lackner A, Disis ML, Knutson KL, Chen L & Zou W. (2004). Specific recruitment of regulatory T cells in ovarian carcinoma fosters immune privilege

and predicts reduced survival. Nat Med. Vol. 10, No. 9 (September 2004), pp. (942-949), ISSN 1078-8956

[44] Horwitz DA, Zheng SG & Gray JD. (2003). The role of the combination of IL-2 and TGF-beta or IL-10 in the generation and function of CD4+ CD25+ and CD8+ regulatory T cell subsets. *J Leukoc Biol.* Vol. 74, No. 4, (October 2003), pp. (471-478), ISSN 1938-3673

[45] Korn T, Bettelli E, Oukka M & Kuchroo VK. (2009). IL-17 and Th17 cells. *Annu Rev Immunol.* Vol. 27, pp. (485-517), ISSN 0732-0582

[46] Liu W, Putnam AL, Xu-Yu Z, Szot GL, Lee MR, Zhu S, Gottlieb PA, Kapranov P, Gingeras TR, Fazekas de St Groth B, Clayberger C, Soper DM, Ziegler SF & Bluestone JA. (2006). CD127 expression inversely correlates with FoxP3 and suppressive function of human CD4+ T reg cells. *J Exp Med.* Vol. 203, No. 7, (July 2006), pp. (1701-1711), ISSN 1940-5901

[47] Seddiki N, Santner-Nanan B, Martinson J, Zaunders J, Sasson S, Landay A, Solomon M, Selby W, Alexander SI, Nanan R, Kelleher A & Fazekas de St Groth B. (2006). Expression of interleukin (IL)-2 and IL-7 receptors discriminates between human regulatory and activated T cells. *J Exp Med.* Vol. 203, No. 7, (July 2006), pp. (1693-1700), ISSN 1940-5901

[48] Matsuoka K, Kim HT, McDonough S, Bascug G, Warshauer B, Koreth J, Cutler C, Ho VT, Alyea EP, Antin JH, Soiffer RJ & Ritz J. (2010). Altered regulatory T cell homeostasis in patients with CD4+ lymphopenia following allogeneic hematopoietic stem cell transplantation. *J Clin Invest.* Vol. 120, No. 5, (May 2010), pp. (1479-1493), ISSN 0021-9738

[49] Gershon RK & Kondo K. (1970). Cell interactions in the induction of tolerance: The role of thymic lymphocytes. *Immunology.* Vol. 18, No. 5 (May 1970), pp. (723-737), ISSN 0019-2805

[50] Hall BM, Pearce NW, Gurley KE & Dorsch SE. (1990). Specific unresponsiveness in rats with prolonged cardiac allograft survival after treatment with cyclosporine. III. Further characterization of the CD4+ suppressor cell and its mechanisms of action. *J Exp Med.* Vol. 171, No. 1, (January 1990), pp. (141-157), ISSN 1940-5901

[51] Lu L & Cantor H. (2008). Generation and regulation of CD8(+) regulatory T cells. *Cell Mol Immunol.* Vol. 5, No. 6, (December 2008), pp. (401-406), ISSN 1672-7681

[52] Wang YM & Alexander SI. (2009). CD8 regulatory T cells: what's old is now new. *Immunol Cell Biol,* Vol.87, No.3, (March 2009) pp. (192-193), ISSN 0818-9641

[53] Zheng SG, Wang JH, Koss MN, Quismorio F Jr, Gray JD & Horwitz DA. (2004). CD4+ and CD8+ regulatory T cells generated ex vivo with IL-2 and TGF-beta suppress a stimulatory graft-versus-host disease with a lupus-like syndrome. *J Immunol.* Vol. 172, No. 3, (February 2004), pp. (1531-1539), ISSN 1550-6606

[54] Frisullo G, Nociti V, Iorio R, Plantone D, Patanella AK, Tonali PA & Batocchi AP. (2010). CD8(+)Foxp3(+) T cells in peripheral blood of relapsing-remitting multiple sclerosis patients. *Hum Immunol.* Vol. 71, No. 5, (May 2010), pp. (437-441), ISSN 0198-8859

[55] Chaput N, Louafi S, Bardier A, Charlotte F, Vaillant JC, Ménégaux F, Rosenzwajg M, Lemoine F, Klatzmann D & Taieb J. (2009). Identification of CD8+CD25+Foxp3+ suppressive T cells in colorectal cancer tissue. *Gut*. Vol. 58, No. 4, (April 2009), pp. (520-529), ISSN 1468-3288

[56] Kiniwa Y, Miyahara Y, Wang HY, Peng W, Peng G, Wheeler TM, Thompson TC, Old LJ & Wang RF. (2007). CD8+ Foxp3+ regulatory T cells mediate immunosuppression in prostate cancer. *Clin Cancer Res*. Vol. 13, No. 23, (December 2007), pp. (6947-6958), ISSN 1557-3265

5

The T-Cells' Role in Antileukemic Reactions - Perspectives for Future Therapies

Helga Maria Schmetzer[1] and Christoph Schmid[2]
*[1]Department of Medicine III, José Carreras Unit for Hematopoietic Stem Cell
Transplantation, Ludwig Maximilian University of Munich
[2]Stem Cell Transplantation Unit, Klinikum Augsburg,
Ludwig Maximilian University of Munich
Germany*

1. Introduction

1.1 Background (Schmid, Schmetzer)

Highly specialized and sensitive defence against infections as well as tumors is provided in great part by the adaptive, T-cell-mediated part of our immune system. Those T-cell specialists arise out of a cell pool of 25-100 million distinct naïve T-cell clones, after a very efficient priming phase by dendritic cells (DC), that present antigens in the context of major histocompatibility complexes (MHC), T-cell receptors (TCR) and costimulatory signals. It is well known, that T-cells are most important effectors of cellular tumor immunity and carry long lasting memory. Therefore recent tumor research has focused on the development and improvement of T-cell based immunotherapies (Barrett & Le Blanc, 2010; Smits et al., 2011).

The T-lymphocyte pool includes naïve (T_{naive}), effector (T_{eff}), effector memory (T_{em}) and central memory (T_{cm}), either CD8 or CD4 T-cells. After an antigen driven TCR engagement T_{naive} proliferate and give rise to large numbers of T_{eff}. Most of them die after depleting target cells. Some 'memory T-cells' of either T_{cm} or T_{em} phenotype remain, persist and can differentiate to T_{eff} after a re-challenge with antigens. It has been demonstrated that memory T-cells are able to self-renewal and differentiation (Sallusto et al., 2005). However antitumor immunity is limited by regulatory T-cells (T_{reg}) that are in general responsible for the prevention of autoimmunity, regulation of inflammatory antimicrobial or antitumor reactions and are regarded as the mediators of tolerance (Vignali et al., 2008). T_{reg} reactions can be either mediated by inhibitory cytokines (IL-10, IL-35, TGF-ß), Granzyme A/B dependent cytolysis, CD25 dependent IL-2 deprivation-mediated apoptosis, adenosine receptor mediated immunosuppression of DCs' maturation (Vignali et al., 2008). T_{reg} subtypes can be identified by their expression profiles and be subdivided in resting or activated T_{regs} of either CD4 or CD8 subtype (Miyora et al., 2009; Jordanova et al., 2008; Schick et al., 2011). Resting T_{regs} can convert to activated T_{regs} after proliferation. The functional repertoire of T-cells depends on their survival and their cooperation via cellular contact and the secretion of humoral factors. Improved knowledge of these properties should contribute to detect or select T-cells with defined markers or functional profiles for adoptive therapy.

In the past the potential of adoptively transferred T-cells to eradicate tumor cells has been intensively studied in patients with melanoma, EBV-associated tumors and especially in the context of a transplantation of allogeneic hematopoietic stem cells including immunocompetent cells in patients with lymphoid- or myeloid-derived malignant diseases (Kahl et al., 2007; Kolb et al., 2004; Schmid et al., 2011; Parmar et al., 2011; Moosmann et al., 2010).

In patients with acute myeloid leukemia (AML), a malignant clonal disease of the hematopoietic stem cells, conventional chemotherapy induces remission in 60- 80% of patients. However, relapse occurs in the majority of patients in the following two years (Buechner et al., 2003). Allogeneic stem cell transplantation (SCT) is considered as a curative therapy for patients with AML: Following engraftment of donor cells, the established hematopoietic chimerism persists even after discontinuation of immunsuppressive therapy, reflecting tolerance both in Graft-versus-Host and Host-versus-Graft direction (Kolb et al., 2004; Schmid et al., 2011). T-cells of the healthy donor mediate the 'graft versus leukemia' (GvL), effect which was perceived in principle as early as in the 1960ies. Clinical evidence for the efficacy of GvL reactions in AML came from the observation, that leukemia relapse after allogeneic SCT, the most frequent reason of treatment failure in AML, occurred most frequently in patients who had either been transplanted from a syngeneic twin, or had received a graft which had been depleted from donor T-cells prior to transfusion. In contrast, relapse incidence was lowest in patients developing acute or chronic Graft-versus-Host Disease (GvHD), which represents the second clinical manifestation of the allogeneic immune reaction mediated by donor T-cells (Hemmati et al., 2011; Schmid et al., 2007; Schmid et al., 2011; van den Brink et al., 2010). Based on these observations, the infusion of donor lymphocytes (DLI) was developed as a form of immunotherapy for relapsed disease after allogeneic SCT. However, up to now, not every patient, in particular those with rapidly proliferating AML, responds to or permanently benefits from those T-cell based immunotherapy.

1.2 Aims (Schmetzer)

The ability of T-cells to eliminate tumor cells and even to cure tumors has been demonstrated in experimental animal models. In man the development of effective T-cell therapies to treat human tumors remains still a challenge. Tumor antigens that elicit curative responses have been identified in animal models; in man tumor associated antigens are also known, but their use is limited due to HLA-restriction and limited duration of responses. This applies also to hematological malignancies as AML. In the last years several approaches have been made to further characterize T-cells and to explore the role of soluble and cellular factors on the regulation and mediation of antitumor reactions in AML-patients. Known tumor antigens may help to identify specific T-cells and their subtypes. This could be monitored in the course of treatment and they could be prepared for further treatment. However the majority of potential tumor antigens is unknown. Their presence may be deduced from T-cell reactions initiated and mediated by leukemia-derived dendritic cells (DC), presenting the whole antigenic repertoire of the leukemic cell. In analogy to T-cell reactions against known tumor antigens DC-stimulated T-cells reacting against unknown tumor antigens may be analysed against healthy cells before further use. In addition the identification of possible immune escape phenomena in cases without successful SCT or DLI or without antileukemic functions *ex vivo* could contribute to develop strategies to overcome those immunological barriers.

In this chapter we want to present experimental and clinical results of our group with a special focus on the following topics and discuss perspectives for future therapies:

- T-cells addressing known (leukemia-) specific antigens
- T-cells addressing unknown leukemia-specific antigens
- T-cell profiles to predict antileukemic reactions and prognosis
- Clinical use of donor T-cells for prevention and treatment of AML relapse after allogeneic SCT
- Perspectives for future therapies: adoptive transfer or *in vivo* activation of antileukemic T-cells?

2. Research methods (Schmetzer)

Cellular characterizations (especially of T-cells, leukemic blasts and dendritic cells) were performed by Flow Cytometric Analyses applying a panel of marker-specific, fluorochrome labelled monoclonal antibodies: **T-cells**: Naïve T-cells (T_{naive}) CD45RO-CCR7+; non-naïve T-cells ($T_{non-naïve}$) CD45RO+; central memory T-cells (T_{cm}) CD45RO+CCR7+CD8+; Effector memory T-cells (T_{em}) CD45RO+CCR7-CD27+; Effector T-cells (T_{eff}) CD45RO+CCR7-CD27-; Regulatory T-cells (CD8+T_{reg}) CD8+CD25+CD127$_{low}$; (CD4+T_{reg}) CD4+CD25+CD127$_{low}$; (T_{naive} $_{reg}$) CD25+CD127$_{low}$CCR7+CD45RO-; ($T_{cm\ reg}$) CD25+CD127$_{low}$CCR7+CD45RO+; ($T_{eff/em\ reg}$) CD25+CD127$_{low}$CCR7-CD45RO+ (Liepert et al., 2010; Vogt et al., 2011; Schick et al., 2011). **Blasts**: Myeloid cells co-expressing patient-specific markers (e.g. CD34, CD117, CD56, CD65); **DC:** DC co-expressing DC-antigens; Mature DC: DC coexpressing CD83; DC$_{leu}$: DC coexpressing DC-antigens (e.g. CD80, CD86, CD40) with blast-markers; (Schmetzer et al., 2007; Kremser et al., 2010). Untouched or touched CD4+, CD8+ or CD3+ T-cells were isolated by Magnetic labelled cell sorting (MACS) (Schick et al., 2011; Vogt et al., 2011; Grabrucker et al., 2010), leukemia-antigen specific T-cells by Interferon gamma (IFN-γ) capture assay (Neudorfer et al., 2007) or by MHC-multimer (Streptamers) staining for several described leukemia associated antigens (Knabel et al., 2002). In some cases spectratyping analyses were performed to observe clonal restriction among T-cells characterized by defined T-cell receptor-Vß chains (Schuster et al., 2008). The expression of leukemia-associated antigens (LAA; e.g. WT1, PRAME, PR1) was evaluated by PCR-technology (Steger et al., 2011). 'Taq man low density arrays' were used to study expressions of most of the known protein-coding Y-chromosome genes (Liu et al., 2005). To predict the HLA-A0201 binding potential of selected peptides a HLA-A0201 peptide binding assay was performed by using the HLA-A0201 positive TAP-deficient T2 cell line system (Nijman et al., 1993; Saller et al., 1985). Leukemic blasts were cultured in 'DC-media' containing a cocktail of immune-modulators and cytokines, (thereby converting blasts to leukemia-derived DC (DC$_{leu}$), theoretically presenting the whole leukemic antigen spectrum (Kremser et al., 2010; Schmetzer et al., 2007).

Alternatively LAA/HA1 or 'male specific' antigens were loaded as peptides or full length proteins on either unmanipulated or irradiated antigen presenting cells (APC; e.g. MNCs or CD4 cell depleted cell fraction (Adhikary et al., 2008), EBV-transformed B-cells 'mini-LCL' or DC (Moosmann et al., 2002) were irradiated with 45/80 Gray and used for T-cell stimulations as given in figure 3.1.3-1 (Steger et al., 2012; Bund et al., 2011). Antileukemic reactivity of T-effector cells was measured by chromium release-, IFN-γ ELISPOT assays or non-radioactive Fluorolysis assays (Bund et al., 2011; Kremser et al., 2010). Intracellular cytokine staining (ICS) and cytokine release profiles were performed by FACS (Cytometric Bead arrays (CBA)), ELISA or ELISPOT (Elbaz & Shaltout 2001; Schmittel 2000; Fischbacher et al., 2011; Merle et al., 2011; Bund et al., 2011). In a dog model we performed in addition an *in vivo* immunisation with antigen positive cells (Bund et al., 2011).

Using these methods we could evaluate antigen expression profiles on T-cells, antigen presenting cells or blast cells as well as cytokine secretion profiles assigning these profiles to cellular subtypes and correlate them with antileukemic reaction profiles or the clinical response to immunotherapies. Moreover we could contribute and quantify reaction profiles of 'antigen stimulated' or '-unstimulated' as well as of (specifically) selected, enriched or cloned T-cells against blast targets. Statistical evaluations were performed with standard excel programmes or SPSS software.

3. Experimental key results

In the following chapter the most important experimental results generated by our group are summarized. Responsible co-workers and cooperation partners are given and their contributions listed below.

3.1 T-cells addressing known (leukemia-) specific antigens
3.1.1 Y-chromosome encoded proteins overexpressed in acute myeloid leukemia and CD8+ T-cell reactions (Groupleaders: Kolb, Adamski; Scientists: Bund, Gallo)

In haploidentical SCT we and others observed that female-donors (especially mothers) show a higher GvL reactivity against male-patients (particularly sons) compared to all other haploidentical donor-recipient combinations for AML patients (Stern et al., 2008). These effects could be due to Y-chromosome-encoded male minor histocompatibility antigens (minor-H-Ags, mHAs) recognized by female alloimmune effector (memory) T-cells, immunized during pregnancy, in the context of a GvL-reaction (Ofran et al., 2010). We studied the expression profiles of Y-chromosome genes in healthy male stem cell donors compared to male AML patients in order to possibly detect new AML-typical Y-restricted expression patterns. Blasts from male patients with acute (myelo) monocytic leukemia and monocytes from healthy male donors as the healthy control counterpart were used to determine and compare the expression profiles of Y-chromosome genes. We could detect several genes being up-regulated in male AML-cells. Among those, we focused on *PCDH11*, *VCY*, *TGIF2LY*, known to be expressed only in male tissues and its X-chromosome-encoded homolog *TGIF2LX* (Blanco-Arias et al., 2002; Skaletsky et al., 2003; Gallo et al., 2011). In a next step, we studied the immunological impact of the identified Y-encoded genes. We analyzed the proteins encoded by those four genes for the presence of nonameric peptides that could potentially bind HLA-A0201 molecules. Such analysis was performed with the help of publicly available peptide-motif scoring systems (*http://bimas.dcrt.nih.gov/molbio/ hla_bind/* and *http://www.syfpeithi.de*; Rammensee et al., 1995). High-scoring peptides were not found for *PCDH11*, whereas HLA-A0201-binding peptides could be identified *in silico* for the *VCY*, *TGIF2LY* and *TGIF2LX* genes. Their effective binding efficacy was determined in a standard HLA-A0201-T2 binding assay: Two peptides derived from VCY as well as from TGIF2LX and one derived from TGIF2LY were able to bind to the HLA-A0201-molecules of the T2 cells. Furthermore these peptides were tested for their ability to induce a CD8+ T-cell response: we selected CD3+ T-cells from female volunteers and cultured them in the presence of T2 cells loaded with the different Y-chromosome-encoded peptides for four weeks. We could show that the *VCY*-encoded peptide G54 stimulated female effector T-cells as shown by a specific lysis of G54-loaded T2 target cells in a chromium release assay

(Figure 3.1.1-1). Further research will focus on the immunogenic G54-peptid particularly with respect to our assumption that mothers (who had given birth to a son) bear CD8+ T-cells being reactive to male-specific antigens, leading to a strong GvL effect. Moreover, peptides restricted to other HLA-types will also be investigated.

In conclusion we identified three new potentially antileukemic, male-specific human genes being upregulated in blasts of male AML-patients. These might be valuable targets for T-cells. As a rule Y-chromosome coded antigens are expressed in all cells of the organism. However some data have been reported, that differentially spliced forms of the Y-linked UTY (ubiquitously-transcribed tetratricopeptide-repeat-gene, Skaletsky et al., 2003) may be restricted in a tissue restricted fashion (Warren et al., 2000). UTY is highly conserved in man and animal species. We worked out in a dog model *in vitro* and *in vivo* that the Y-chromosome coded mHA UTY might be a promising candidate target-structure to improve GvL immune reactions after SCT: female T-cells were stimulated with either autologous (female) DCs, loaded with three different UTY-derived (male) peptides or with allogeneic, donor-matched male cells (PBMCs) endogenously expressing UTY. We identified 3 out of 15 identified UTY-encoded peptides bearing immunological potential to stimulate 'antimale'- (i.e. anti-UTY-) directed immune reactions. Amongst those, W248 showed highest immunogenic potential in both *in vitro* and *in vivo* settings: *In vitro* expanded CTLs specifically recognized mainly bone-marrow (BM) from DLA-identical male littermates in an MHC-I-restricted manner (Figure 3.1.1-2; *in vitro*). *In vivo*, comparable W248-(UTY-) specific reactivity against BM was also obtained after stimulation and immunization of a female dog with DLA-identical male PBMCs (Table 3.1.1-1; *in vivo* (Bund et al., 2001)).

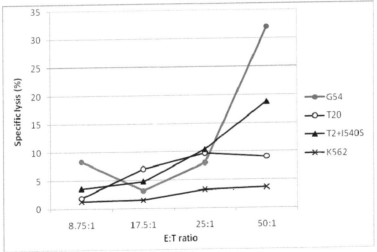

T2-cells were loaded with the VCY-derived G54-peptide and incubated with female HLA-A0201+ T-cells for 4 weeks. Cytotoxic activity of the generated G54-specific CTLs were tested in Chromium release assays (E:T = 8.75:1 to 50:1). T-cells specifically lysed T2-cells loaded with the cognate peptides G54 (G54, ● red). T2-cells alone (T20, ○), T2-cells loaded with I540S (non-HLA-A0201 binding; HFLLWKLIA; T2+I540S, ▲) and K562-cells (NK-cell target, ×) were not recognized or only to a low extent

Fig. 3.1.1-1. Female T-cells stimulated with the Y-chromosomally encoded G54-peptid can specifically lyse T2-cells loaded with G54 *in vitro*.

	E:T*	male DLA-identical target cells	W248-specific spots/100,000 T-cells*
In vitro	80:1	BM	85
		BM + <anti MHC-I antibody>	24
In vivo	20:1	BM	45
		BM + <anti MHC-I antibody>	25
		BM + W248-peptide	35
		BM + W248-peptide + <anti MHC-I antibody>	15

BM bone marrow; <MHC-I>=<MHC-I>-antibody.
* E:T= Effector-to-target-ratio
**number of UTY-specific spots per 100,000 T-cells

T-cells from female dog(s) were expanded using autologous DCs pulsed with the UTY-encoded peptide W248 (in vitro; n=3/6) or male DLA-identical PBMCs (in vivo; n=1). Female UTY-specific T-cell recognition was determined in IFN-γ-ELISPOT-assays (day 21-28 (E:T = 80:1) and day 49 (E:T = 20:1), respectively). Female T-cells mainly recognized male DLA-identical BM in vitro and in vivo verifying the male-specific UTY-presentation. T-cells` MHC-I-restriction was shown by an anti-MHC-class-I-mAb.

Table 3.1.1-1 Female dog T-cells stimulated with UTY (W248)-peptides loaded on autologous DC *in vitro* or male DLA-identical PBMC *in vivo* specifically recognized 'male' target cells

Taken together we could demonstrate, that female dog effector T-cells could be specifically stimulated against male, *UTY*-gene product specific cells meaning in turns, that UTY seems to be a promising candidate antigen to improve GvL reactions after SCT.

3.1.2 LAA-specific CD8+ T-cells (Groupleaders: Busch, Borkhardt, Kolb; scientists: Doessinger, Steger, Schuster)

Between 60-90% of AML cases overexpress leukemia-associated antigens (LAA), that means antigens that are absent or only weakly expressed in normal tissues (e.g. WT1, PR1 or PRAME (Greiner et al., 2006; Steger et al., 2011)). Therefore T-cell based immunotherapeutic strategies addressing those LAA-expressing cells could be promising. Alternatively mHAs, preferentially expressed on hematopoietic cells, could qualify as T-cell targets in a GvL reaction (Mutis & Goulmy, 2002). Principally T-cell based strategies could be based on a vaccination with LAA/mHAs or by identification, selection and transfer of LAA/mHAs specific T-cells already present in the donor. LAA/mHAs specific T-cells can be found at a low frequency in normal persons implying a low level of immunity. Vice versa a long lasting immunity against leukemic cells overexpressing LAA or mHAs should imply the presence of specific T-cells. Therefore our experimental approach was to detect LAA-specific T-cells by MHC-multimer technology in AML patients after SCT. We constructed human HLA-A2 peptide multimers (Knabel et al., 2002) and tested CD8+ T-cells in 5 AML- and 2 MDS-patients after SCT for antigen specificity, as given in table 3.1.2-1

Patients (pt)	Dgn.	stage of the disease at T-cell aquisition	Cytogen. Marker at first dgn.	Blasts in PB at sample aquisition	IC blast phenotype (CD) in acute phases	IC monocytes (%)	IC B-cells (%)	IC T-cells (%)	IC NK-cells (%)	performed analyses
pt 1147	AML-M2	CR2 after SCT and DLI	+21,+21, +21	0	7,33,34,117	nd	nd	nd	nd	MHC-multimer staining
pt 1148	AML-M2	CR after 3rd SCT	inv (3qq)	0	13,33,34,117	nd	nd	nd	nd	MHC-multimer staining, ICS
pt 1149	AML-M4	CR after SCT and DLI	46, XX	0	13,15,33,34, 117	7	6	14	6	MHC-multimer staining, ICS
pt 1150	MDS-RAEB I	CR after SCT and DLI	-5, +1 (at relapse)	0	13,33,34,117	11	6	13	7	MHC-multimer staining, ICS
pt 1151	AML-M4	CR after SCT	46, XX	5	15,33,7,65,64,4	nd	nd	28	12	MHC-multimer staining, ICS
pt 1152	AML-M5	CR after SCT	46, XX	0	nd	nd	nd	nd	nd	MHC-multimer staining, Spectratyping
pt 1153	MDS-CMML	Pers after SCT and DLI	46, XX	8	nd	nd	nd	nd	nd	MHC-multimer staining, ICS, LAA, CD4+ exp.
pt 1154	MDS-RAEB II	CR after SCT and DLI	46, XY	0	nd	10	3	34	8	ICS, LAA, CD4+ exp.
pt 1155	MPS-atyp. CML	CR after SCT and DLI	t (8;22)	0	nd	nd	nd	nd	nd	ICS, LAA, CD4+ exp.

nd not done; CR complete remission; Rel. relapse; MDS myelodysplastic syndrome; RAEB Refractory Anaemia with Excess Blasts; AML-M3 acute myeloid leukemia FAB M2; CMML Chronic Myelomonocytic Leukemia; LAA leukemia associated antigen, overexpression analyses compared to healthy controls, detected by the RQ= $2^{-\Delta\Delta ct}$ method in MNCs; dgn. diagnosis; ICS intracellular staining; CD4+ exp. CD4+ experiments

Table 3.1.2-1 Patients'characteristics I:

In all of these 7 cases we could detect LAA-specific CD8+ T-cells (that means more than 0.1% T-cells with LAA specificity) –although not directed against all given LAA, suggesting the persistence of T-cells with antileukemic potential (table 3.1.2-1 and fig 3.1.2-2). Four of five cases with two different types of LAA- specific CD8+ T-cells (pt 1149, 1151, 1152, 1153) were characterized by long-lasting clinical remissions for more than 2 years. One patient with two different types of LAA-specific CD8+ T-cells relapsed after 9 months (pt 1151) and in addition the patient with only one type of LAA-specific T-cells, who relapsed after one year (pt 1147). One patient could not be analysed under a clinical point of view since he died one month after sample acquisition of an infect (pt 1148, table 3.1.2-2, Steger et al., 2012).

Patients (pt)	LAA over-expression in MNCs (at sample preparation)	Peak response MHC-Multimer staining (% of specific CD8+ T-cells)	Cytokine profile (IFN-γ, IL-2) after LAA-stimulation CD 4+/C8+ T-cells	Time to relapse or last follow up
pt 1147	nd	A2/WT1 0.11 A2/PR1 0.13 A2/PRAME 0.034	NR/NR	04/07 local rel.; 08/09 systemic rel., 05/11 CR after 2nd SCT, DLI and 3th rel.
pt 1148	nd	A2/WT1 0.37 A2/PR1 0.4 A2/PRAME nd	NR/NR	03/06 death with infect in CR after SCT
pt 1149	nd	A2/WT1 0.61 A2/PR1 0.39 A2/PRAME 0.4	NR/NR	until 02/11 in CR after SCT
pt 1150	nd	A2/WT1 0.27 A2/PR1 0.13 A2/PRAME 0.081	NR/NR	until 03/11 in CR after SCT
pt 1151	nd	A2/WT1 0.16 A2/PR1 0.088 A2/PRAME 0.42	NR/NR	11/06 rel; 04/07 death after 3th DLI, rel. and 2nd SCT
pt 1152*	nd	A2/WT1 0.16 A2/PR1 0.074 A2/PRAME 0.38	NR/NR	until 04/11 in CR after SCT
pt 1153	WT1 (-), PRAME (+), PR1 (-)	A2/WT1 0.1 A2/PR1 0.14 A2/PRAME 0.13	*PRAME 0.32*/NR	until 02/11 in CR after SCT
pt 1154	WT1 (-), PRAME (-), PR1 (-)	nd	NR/NR	until 07/11 in CR after SCT
pt 1155	WT1 (-), PRAME (-), PR1 (-)	nd	NR/NR	until 07/11 in CR after SCT

No LAA overexpression (-), 1–10x LAA overexpression (+), compared to healthy controls, analysed by the RQ= $2^{-\Delta\Delta ct}$ method; nd not done

Bold: > 0.1% CD8+ T-cells defined as 'LAA-specific T-cells present'; * restricted T-cells by spectratyping in *PRAME*- MHC multimer selected T-cells detectable

Table 3.1.2-2 Anti-LAA-peptide reactive T-cells are detectable by MHC-Multimer staining in all given PB samples from AML/MDS patients after allogeneic SCT

In one case (pt 1152) we performed spectratyping in T-cells selected for PRAME-specificity and could demonstrate a highly restricted TCR-repertoire. This points to a specific clonal expansion of CD8+ cells after (*in vivo*) PRAME challenge by residual PRAME overexpressing blasts (Figure 3.1.2-1).

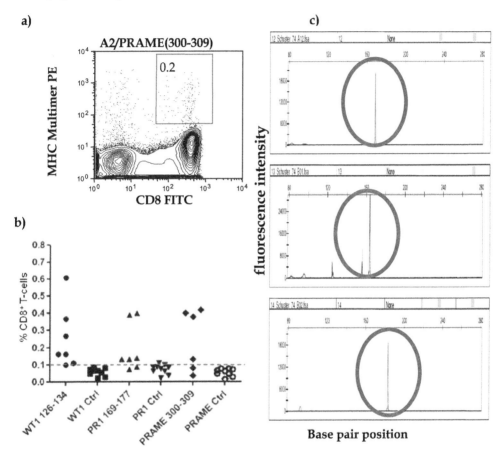

a) representative FACS-plot shows MHC-Multimer staining from peripheral blood of an AML-patient after SCT.
b) LAA-specific T-cells from PBMCs from AML-pts after SCT were labelled with MHC multimers binding T-cells, that recognize frequently overexpressed LAA antigens. PBMCs were analyzed by FACS. Healthy donors served as controls and multimer-staining revealed a threshold value of 0.11% multimer-positive cells in the CD8 cell fraction.
c) MHC-multimer positive CD8+ T-cells from peripheral blood of an AML-patient after SCT were enriched by FACS sorting. RNA was extracted and Spectratyping of the Vβ-composition reveals strong clonal restriction among TCR-species (1rd row: Vß3-Jß1.5; 2nd row: Vß3-Jß2.1; 3rd row: Vß3-Jß2.5)

Fig. 3.1.2-1. LAA-specific T-cells can be isolated from AML-patients after SCT by MHC multimer technique. Selected T-cells are highly Vß restricted

Upon in vitro peptide-challenge we could not detect secretion of IFN-γ or IL-2 in T-cells by intracellular cytokine staining in 7 out of 8 patients tested (table 3.1.2-2). This however does not exclude a cytokine-independent functionality of multimer positive T-cells. Interestingly we could detect an IFN-γ response in CD4+ T-cells in one case (pt 1153) with PRAME overexpressing leukemic blasts detectable during persisting relapse after SCT. This is very surprising as the peptide triggering this response is MHC class I restricted and could indicate a CD8 coreceptor independent binding of a MHC I directed TCR and an unusual involvement of CD4+ T-cells in the leukemia directed immune response.

In summary that means, that in general LAA-specific, HLA-A2-restricted CD8+ T-cells can be prepared by MHC multimer technology from most of the patients after SCT at various time points. Possibly the simultaneous detection of two different LAA-specific CD8+ T-cells correlates with a higher chance of longlasting remissions. Optimal time points have to be evaluated for the preparation of (sufficient) LAA-specific CD8+ T-cells that could be used for adoptive transfer and concerning minimal amounts needed for maintenance of remission.

3.1.3 LAA-specific CD4+ T-cells (Groupleaders: Buhmann, Milosevic, Kolb, Schmetzer; scientists: Steger)

CD8+ T-cells recognize HLA-class I restricted peptides, therefore they can mediate strong cytotoxic, antileukemic reactions, but also severe graft versus host (GvH) disease. In contrast CD4+ T-cells recognize HLA class II restricted peptides that are mainly expressed by cells of the haematopoetic system and absent from other organs. In order to further analyse the antileukemic function of CD4+ T-cells we prepared (untouched) CD4+ T-cells from 6 patients, as given in table 3.1.3-1, after SCT or DLI immunotherapies and stimulated them with LAA-proteins (WT1, PRAME, PR1 and the mHA HA-1), that were loaded on the CD4 depleted cell fraction (containing monocytes and DC as antigen presenting cells (APCs)) or on 'mini-LCL'.

During the stimulation phase the cells lost their naïve (and central memory) T-cell phenotype and gained an effector memory or effector cell phenotype (data not shown).

As already shown for CD8 selected T-cells cytokine release assays for IFN-γ (ELISPOT, ICS) or GM-CSF (ELISA) did not reveal clear and specific cytokine release profiles of LAA or HA-1 stimulated, expanded or cloned CD4+ T-cells (data not shown).

Therefore we performed a functional Fluorolysis assay in case pt 1158: *blast cells* of the patient, that were characterized by a overexpression of WT1, PRAME and PR1 at first diagnosis served as leukemic target and *fibroblasts, effector cells* or *non-blast cells* of the patient as negative controls. *Effector cells* (E) used for these assays were: unstimulated MNC, CD3+ or CD4+ T-cells obtained in different stages of the disease, LAA or HA-1 stimulated CD4+ T-cells in different stimulation phases, enriched proliferating and CD40L+ CD4+ cells before or after single cell cloning (table 3.1.3-2).

We could demonstrate that most of the CD4+ T- cell containing effector cell fractions (except MNCs before SCT, CD4+ T-cells after 16 stimulation rounds (E11) and two of the CD4+ T-cell clones (E13, E15)) were able to regularly and specifically lyse leukemic blasts, but not fibroblasts or non-blast-cells of the patient. Highest antileukemic activity was demonstrated for enriched proliferating and CD40L+CD4+ T-cells followed by one of the three tested clones. Unfortunately despite of provable (CD4+) immunity against leukemic cells the patient died two years after SCT in hematological CR from a myocardial chloroma.

Patients (pt)	Dgn.	T-cell source (stage of disease)	Blasts in PB at sample aquisition	Cell source	Analyses performed in addition to CD4+experiments
pt 1153	MDS-CMML	Pers after SCT	8	CD4+, CD8+, MNCs	ICS, IFN-γ ELISPOT, MHC-Multimer staining, LAA analyses
pt 1154	MDS-RAEB II	CR after SCT	0	CD4+, CD8+, MNCs	ICS, IFN-γ ELISPOT, LAA analyses
pt 1155a and 1155 b	MPS-atyp. CML	CR after SCT	0	CD4+, CD8+, MNCs	ICS, IFN-γ ELISPOT, GM-CSF ELISA, LAA analyses
pt 1156	Biphen. ALLL/ AML	CR after SCT	0	CD4+	IFN-γ ELISPOT
pt 1157	AML-M4	CR after SCT	0	CD4+	IFN-γ ELISPOT
pt 1158 a ('E1')	AML-M4	CR before SCT	0	MNCs	LAA analyses, Fluorolysis assay
pt 1158 b ('E2')	AML-M4	CR after 1st SCT and 1st DLI	0	CD4+	Fluorolysis assay
pt 1158 c ('E3') pt 1158 d ('E12': after P5) pt 1158 e ('E11': after P16) pt 1158 f ('E6': after P17,FACS-Sort, P14) pt 1158 g, h, i ('E13, 14, 15' clones, after FACS-Sort, P14)	AML-M4	CR after 1st SCT and 1st DLI	0	CD4+	ICS, IFN-γ ELISPOT, GM-CSF ELISA , Fluorolysis assay
pt 1158 p ('blast targets')	AML-M4	Rel. after 1st SCT and 2nd DLI	34	CD3 depleted blasts	Fluorolysis assay
pt 1158 j ('E4')	AML-M4	Rel. after 1st SCT and 2nd DLI	nd	CD4+	Fluorolysis assay
pt 1158 k ('E5')	AML-M4	CR after 2nd SCT and 4th DLI	0	CD4+	Fluorolysis assay
pt 1158 l ('E16')	AML-M4	CR after 2nd SCT and 4th DLI	0	CD4+	Fluorolysis assay
pt 1158 m, n, o ('E7, 8, 9')	AML-M4	CR after 2nd SCT and 4th DLI	0	MNCs, CD3+, CD4+	LAA analyses, Fluorolysis assay

Dgn. diagnosis; Pers persistant disease; Rel. relapse; CR complete remission; MDS myelodysplastic syndrome; RAEB Refractory Anaemia with Excess Blasts; AML-M3 acute myeloid leukemia FAB M3; CMML Chronic Myelomonocytic Leukemia; LAA leukemia associated antigen, overexpression analyses compared to healthy controls, detected by the RQ= $2^{-\Delta\Delta ct}$ method in MNCs; E effector cells prepared at different time points in the course of the disease or after stimulation with CD4 depleted LAA/HA1 protein loaded APCs; P passage after x stimulations with CD4 depleted LAA/HA1 protein loaded APCs; nd not done;

Table 3.1.3-1 Patients´ characteristics II:

A flow chart with the methodological strategy to create LAA-presenting nonCD4+ cells or mini-LCL is given in figure 3.1.3-1. We could demonstrate that in general it is possible to stimulate untouched CD4+ T-cells using the CD4 depleted fraction or 'mini-LCL' as stimulator fraction. Furthermore we enriched LAA-stimulated cells from these stimulation settings by either enrichment of proliferating, CD40L+CD4+ T-cells or by T-cell single-cell cloning after repeated stimulation with LAA- and HA-1- loaded stimulator cells. Resulting cells were characterized by proliferation, CD40L upregulation and cellular expansion.

I.

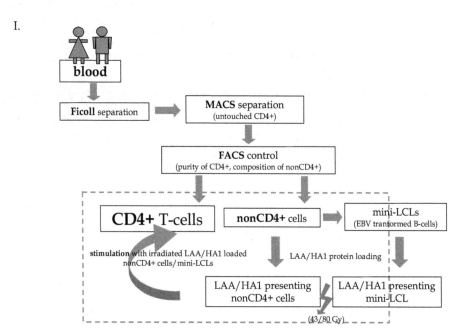

I. Untouched CD4+ T-cells prepared from AML patients' PBMNC after SCT were stimulated (6-16 stimulations with 20 U IL2 twice a month) with irradiated (43 Gy, 80 Gy by mini-LCLs), LAA/HA1 protein loaded nonCD4 cells (as APCs) for 24h. Alternative stimulation of the nonCD4+ cell fraction with EBV transformed B-cells as APCs.

II.

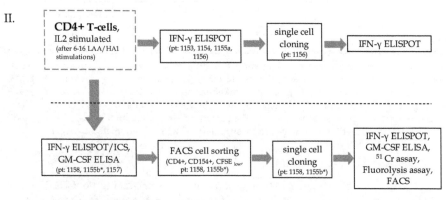

•* mini-LCLs stimulated;

• ⁵¹Cr Chromium-release assay

II. Stimulated CD4+ T-cells were characterized by ELISPOTS, ELISAS or ICS for secretion of IFN-γ or GM-CSF before or after single cell cloning or sorting of CD40L+ CFSE$_{low}$ cells. Moreover some cases were tested for antileukemic activity in a chromium-release or fluorolysis assay.

Fig. 3.1.3-1. Preparation, stimulation (I) and characterisation (II) of (untouched) CD4+T-cell

Patient 1158	T-cell source (stage of disease)	Cell source of the effectors	Proportion of blasts lysed by different effector cells (%)	Patient	T-cell source (stage of disease)	Cell source of the effectors	Proportion of blasts lysed by different effector cells (%)
pt 1158 a ('E1')	CR before SCT	MNCs	0	pt 1158 f ('E6')	CR after 1st SCT and 3 weeks after 1st DLI	CD4+ (after P17 and FACS Sort P14)	87
pt 1158 b ('E2')	CR after 1st SCT and 3 weeks after 1st DLI	CD4+	51	pt 1158 e ('E11')		CD4+ (after P16)	0
pt 1158 c ('E3')	CR after 1st SCT and 5 weeks after 1st DLI	CD4+	42	pt 1158 d ('E12')	CR after 1st SCT and 3 weeks after 1st DLI	CD4+ (after P5)	9
pt 1158 j ('E4')	Rel. after 1st SCT and 2nd DLI	CD4+	61	pt 1158 g ('E13')			0
pt 1158 k ('E5')	CR after 2nd SCT and 4th DLI	CD4+	60	pt 1158 h ('E14')		CD4+ T-cell clones (after FACS Sort P14)	16
pt 1158 m ('E7')		MNCs	22	pt 1158 i ('E15')			0
pt 1158 n ('E8')	CR after 2nd SCT and 4th DLI	CD3+	19 (38, 4h)	pt 1158 l ('E16')	CR after 2nd SCT and 4th DLI	CD4+	86
pt 1158 o ('E9')		CD4+	9	pt 1158 q	† Myocardial Chloroma		

E effector cells prepared at different time points in the course of the disease or after stimulation with CD4 depleted LAA/HA1 protein loaded APCs (table 3.1.3-1); P passage after x stimulations with CD4 depleted LAA/HA1 protein loaded APCs; † Exitus letalis

Table 3.1.3-2 Antileukemic functionality (demonstrated by fluorolysis assay) of different CD4+ effector cells prepared before or after specific stimulation, enrichment or sorting

In summary this means that the cytokine release of IFN-γ or GM-CSF is no reliable tool to detect specificity in T-cell fractions. We could demonstrate however, that CD4+ T-cells in general can mediate cytotoxic reactions and that certain enriched CD4+ subtypes might be even more promising candidates for GvL- without GvH reactions.

3.2 T-cells addressing unknown leukemia-specific antigens
3.2.1 Establishment and maintenance of protective immunity by dendritic cells derived from leukemic blasts (Groupleaders: Borkhardt, Buhmann, Schmetzer; Scientists: Fischbacher, Freudenreich, Grabrucker, Liepert, Merle, Reuther, Schick, Schuster, Vogt)

Although technically possible the preparation of LAA-specific T-cells is cumbersome, in case of MHC-Multimer technology HLA-A2 restricted and moreover restricted to defined LAAs. Therefore we wanted to study the antileukemic activity of T-cells stimulated with DC derived from leukemic blasts (DC_{leu}), as those DC bear the advantage of potentially presenting the whole (including as yet unknown) and patient-typical antigen pool of the leukemic cells. We have already established the methods to generate sufficient amounts of DC and especially of DC_{leu} in every given case with AML: in a minimalized assay we cultured DC in three different media and choose the DC generation method with the quantitatively highest DC/DC_{leu} counts (Kremser et al., 2010; Schmetzer et al., 2007). In a next step we study the functional profiles of DC/DC_{leu}-stimulated T-cells. We could demonstrate, that isolated *unstimulated* T-cells were able to lyse blasts in 47% of cases, whereas only 26% of those T-cells showed antileukemic activity after a 10 days culture with blasts – pointing to an establishment of a T-cell inhibitory microenvironment in the presence of blasts. However, stimulation of T-cells with blasts after their conversion to DC_{leu} resulted in a blast lytic activity in 58% of all cases. These data suggest, that the inhibitory (blast-induced) atmosphere could be abolished after blast-conversion to DC_{leu}, although not completely: even a DC/DC_{leu} stimulation of T-cells was not effective to induce antileukemic T-cells in every case (Schmetzer et al., 2011; Grabrucker et al., 2010). Therefore we analysed potential conditions and factors being responsible for these impaired immune reactions. We could demonstrate that the *quality of DC* – especially with respect to proportions of mature DC and DC_{leu} – is predictive for their activation capacity for antileukemic T-cells. Those DC/DC_{leu} induce an ‚antileukemically effective' T-cell composition of DC-stimulated T-cells, characterized by higher proportions of CD4+ and non-naive T-cells (Grabrucker et al., 2010; Liepert et al., 2010). A detailed analysis of T-cells' compositions in cases *with* compared to those *without* antileukemic activity revealed significantly higher proportions of naïve (T_{naive}) and central memory T-cells (T_{cm}) and lower proportions of effector memory regulatory ($T_{eff/em\ reg}$) as well as CD8+ regulatory T-cells (CD8+ T_{reg}) (Schick et al., 2011; Vogt et al., 2011). Moreover we could define soluble factors that are predictive for the mediation of antileukemic activity of DC/DC_{leu}-stimulated T-cells: A higher release of 'inflammatory' chemokines (CXCL8, CCL2) in DC culture supernatants or of 'T-cell-promoting' cytokines (IFN-γ, IL-6) in mixed lymphocyte culture (MLC) supernatants of T-cells with DC clearly correlated with antileukemic activity of DC-stimulated T-cells (Fischbacher et al., 2011; Merle et al., 2011; Schmetzer et al., 2011).

Detailed studies of T-cell subsets via spectratyping analysis could verify that especially after DC-stimulation CD4+ as well as CD8+ T-cells were characterized by a highly restricted Vβ T-cell-receptor (TCR) repertoire (Schuster et al., 2008). Interestingly, in one patient studied comprehensively *in vitro* stimulation with DC/DC_{leu} resulted into an identical TCR β chain restriction pattern which could be identified *in vivo* in the patient's T-cells 3 months after allo-SCT (Reuther et al., 2011).

In summary, DC_{leu} are promising candidates to stimulate and enrich antileukemic T-cells without knowledge of defined antigen targets which is attended with the creation of an 'antileukemic cellular microenvironment' and could contribute to develop strategies to overcome immunological resistances. With our experimental *in vitro* models combining culture methods and functional flow cytometry with spectratyping we can moreover provide explanations for clinical observations and might provide predictive information about T-cellular response patterns *in vivo*. Further studies of selected T-cells (e.g. by their Vß type) for their phenotype and function will allow to understand clinical responses and to prepare T-cells for treatment.

3.2.2 Antileukemic T-cell profiles to predict antileukemic reactions of DC/DC$_{leu}$ stimulated T-cells and prognosis of patients (Groupleaders: Schmetzer; Scientists: Fischbacher, Freudenreich, Grabrucker, Liepert, Merle, Schick, Vogt)

Since not every AML patient responds to immunotherapy (SCT, DLI) *in vivo* and since not every *ex vivo* T-cell stimulation with DC$_{leu}$ results in antileukemia effector T-cells we wanted to elucidate responsible cells or soluble factors. We could evaluate 'cut-off values' for DC- or T-cell subtypes in the cellular settings and in addition amounts of soluble factors that allow a *prediction of the antileukemic function of T-cells* in this cellular or microenvironmental context or a *prediction of the clinical response to immunotherapy*. We could demonstrate, that T-cells stimulated with DC$_{leu}$ in a 'favorable cellular and soluble chemokine/cytokine context' (with >45% mature DC and >65% DC$_{leu}$ with a release of >200pg CXCL8, >100pg CCL2, >10pg IFN-γ or >15pg IL-6, resulting in >65% CD4+, T$_{non-naive}$ and <60% CD8+ T-cells and especially >3% T$_{naive}$, >11% T$_{cm}$ and low proportions of CD8+ T$_{reg}$ after the DC stimulation) had a more than 75% chance to gain antileukemic *ex vivo* activity. In addition we could demonstrate, that clinical responders to immunotherapy were characterized by a higher *ex vivo* generability of DC$_{leu}$ and mature DC, a better *ex vivo* T-cell proliferation and CD4:CD8 and T$_{non-naive}$: T$_{naive}$ ratios>1 and in addition by a high release of CCL2, IFN-γ and IL-6 (Liepert et al., 2010; Schmetzer et al., 2011; Fischbacher et al., 2011; Merle et al., 2011; Grabrucker et al., 2010).

That means, that we can not only associate cellular subtypes of T-cells and DC or cytokine/chemokine release patterns with antileukemic functions of T-cells in *ex vivo* settings and in the context of a clinical response to immunotherapies, but in addition define predictive 'cut-off values' , that means proportions of cells with certain cellular subtypes or concentrations of soluble factors, that allow a correlation with cellular responses or the clinical course of the disease after immunotherapy.

4. Clinical key results

4.1 Clinical use of donor T-cells for prevention and treatment of AML relapse after allogeneic SCT (Schmetzer, Schmid)

Donor lymphocyte infusion (DLI) for treatment of leukemic relapse after allogeneic hematopoietic stem cell transplantation (SCT) has been introduced in the early nineties (Kolb et al., 1990). Being extremely effective in chronic myeloid leukemia, the procedure was less successful in AML, although remissions were observed in selected cases (Kolb et al., 1995; Collins et al., 1997). Therefore, on behalf of the Acute leukemia Working Party of the European Group of Blood and Marrow Transplantation (EBMT) our group performed a retrospective analysis of patients who had been transplanted for AML in complete remission, and had suffered from leukemia relapse post SCT (Schmid et al., 2007). The analysis was based on the EBMT transplant registry, and included 399 adult patients who had received (n=171) or not (n=228) DLI as part of their treatment. With a median follow up of 27 and 40 months in the both groups, overall survival (OS) at two years was 21±3% for patients receiving, and 9±2% for patients not receiving DLI. After adjustment for differences between the groups, better outcome was associated with younger age (p= 0.008), remission duration >5 months after SCT (p<0.0001), and use of DLI (p=0.04). Among DLI recipients, a lower tumour burden at relapse (<35% of bone marrow blasts; p=0.006), female gender (p=0.02), favorable cytogenetics (p=0.004) and remission at time of DLI (p<0.0001) were predictive for survival in a multivariate analysis. Two-year survival was 56±10%, if DLI was performed in remission or with favourable karyotype, and 15±3% if DLI was given in aplasia or with active disease. Therefore, an algorithm for the clinical use of DLI in the treatment of relapsed AML after allogeneic SCT was developed, comprising the sequence of cytoreductive chemotherapy for disease control or induction of complete remission, followed by DLI for long term control of the leukemia based on cellular immune effects (Schmid et al., 2011).

In an approach to increase the antileukemic efficacy of donor T-cells against myeloid leukemias, systemic application of GM-CSF was studied after DLI for relapse of AML or MDS after SCT (Schmid et al., 2004). GM-CSF was chosen due to its capacity to contribute *in vitro* to the generation of antigen-presenting cells (APC) from leukemic blasts (Woiciechowsky et al., 2001; Kufner et al., 2005; Kremser et al., 2010; Dreyssig et al., 2011). As described above, blasts from myeloid leukemias should have the full genetic repertoire for effective antigen presentation, but might be ineffective stimulators or even induce specific anergy, due to inferior or aberrant expression of co-stimulatory molecules, such as CD80 or CD86. GM-CSF has been shown to induce up-regulation of these molecules on the surface of leukemia blasts and to improve cytotoxic efficacy of autologous and allogeneic T-cells. In a clinical pilot trial for AML relapse after SCT, mild chemotherapy with low dose AraC, infusion of donor T-cells together with stem cells for reconstitution of haematopoiesis, and s.c. or i.v. application of GM-CSF, was studied. Overall response rate was 67% among evaluable patients', overall survival at 2 years was 29%. Long term survival was associated with longer remission post transplant, disease control by low dose AraC and development of chronic GvHD. These results confirm the proposed strategy of initial cytoreduction by chemotherapy and induction of a GvL reaction for long term disease control. Systemic application of GM-CSF was safe in this setting, however, its clinical efficacy remains to be evaluated in randomised studies. Nevertheless, in accompanying *ex vivo* experiments we could demonstrate, that cases in which DC could be generated *ex vivo* using GM-CSF-based protocols showed a more favourable outcome after *in vivo* immunotherapy (Freudenreich et al., 2011).

Since overall, the outcome of patients with AML who relapse after allogeneic SCT is poor, strategies to prevent occurrence of overt haematological relapse are of increasing interest. Intensive monitoring of minimal residual disease and donor chimerism in different cellular compartments (CD34+, CD3+) of bone marrow or peripherial blood has gained in importance by allowing early interventions (chemotherapy, DLI, second SCT) *before* haematological relapse has occurred (Bornhauser et al., 2009). Our group has developed a protocol for the use of prophylactic or preemptive DLI (pDLI) for patients with high-risk AML. Starting from day +120 after SCT, patients in haematologic remission, free of immunosuppression for at least 30 days without clinically evident GvHD, and free of infections receive up to 3 courses of DLI in 4 weeks' intervals, using an escalating cell dose schedule. Patients receiving prophylactic DLI have been compared to a control group of high-risk AML patients, who were treated according to the same transplant protocol, would have fulfilled the criteria for pDLI, but did not receive the cells since their transplant centres did not take part at this part of the study (Schmid et al., 2005; Schleuning et al., unpublished results). Hence, patients receiving pDLI showed a significantly lower incidence of relapse and achieved a longer overall survival as compared to controls without pDLI. The treatment was also safe and induction of severe GvHD was a rare event in this setting.

In summary, although less effective as in CML, the clinical use of DLI for AML patients after SCT is an effective therapeutic tool for prevention or as part of treatment of relapses after SCT in AML.

5. Perspectives for future therapies: Adoptive transfer or *in vivo* activation of antileukemic T-cells? (Schmetzer, Schmid)

We could clearly demonstrate, that it is possible to *detect and monitor* leukemia specific T-cells by LAA-peptid specific (HLA-A2 restricted) MHC-Multimer analyses or LAA-protein specific CD4+ T-cells, especially if combined with spectratyping and cellular subtype analyses. Concerning 'known' (leukemia-) specific antigens we can conclude from our data, that LAA-peptide specific CD8+ T-cells can be prepared by MHC multimer-technology, LAA-protein specific CD4+ T-cells by preparation of (enriched) proliferating CD40L+ or cloned CD4+ cells and both cell types could be used for adoptive therapies. Moreover we could work out *in vitro* as well as in a dog model, that male specific antigens might be promising candidate antigens for immunotherapies. In addition we could show, that (enriched) T-cells addressing known as well as unknown leukemia-associated antigens, as demonstrated after DC/DC$_{leu}$-stimulation, can mediate cytotoxic reactions. Those cells could be promising candidates for *adoptive immunotherapies* in selected patients.

Since the manipulation and selection of antigen-specific T-cells is not only an oncological challenge, but has to be approved by special committees before a clinical application another strategy circumventing T-cell manipulations could be more promising: *applicating immune-modulators* and cytokines like GM-CSF or IFN-α *in vivo* could possibly induce the conversion of (residual) blasts in patients to DC$_{leu}$. In a small patients' cohort we could already show, that patients receiving GM-CSF in the context of a DLI-relapse therapy had a better chance to respond to this relapse therapy compared to patients without additionally applicated GM-CSF (Freudenreich et al., 2011). Moreover we could show, that the convertibility of blasts to DC$_{leu}$ in *ex vivo* settings correlated with the clinical response and outcome to immunotherapies, what can be interpreted by an '*ex vivo* simulation' of the DC-generating potential out of blasts. We could even demonstrate, that cases, in that higher proportions of DC$_{leu}$ could be generated *ex vivo* had a longer overall survival compared to cases with lower DC$_{leu}$ proportions.

Our *ex vivo* focus in the future will therefore be to thoroughly investigate and optimize *in vivo* strategies with allo SCT applying different donor transplants or *ex vivo* 'manipulated' grafts. We further want to develop and test different 'immune modulating cocktails' (Ansprenger et al., 2011; Deen et al., 2011) that can be applicated to patients with the aim to induce leukemia-derived DC *in vivo* and in consequence to stimulate the generation of leukemia-specific T-cells *in vivo*. In parallel we want to further enlighten the role of different (enriched, selected) effector cells – e.g. CD4+, CD8+, NK, NK-T- cells) in the mediation of antileukemic reactions in order to find promising candidates for adoptive T-cell transfer.

6. Acknowledgements

This book chapter was written by Helga Schmetzer (experimental parts) and Christoph Schmid (clinical part) in cooperation with groupleaders and scientists as listed below. The chapter summarizes, among others, the main results worked out in the course of SFB TR project 36 (supported by the DFG; applicants Prof. Borkhardt, Prof. Busch, Prof. Kolb), Deutsche Jose Carreras Stiftung, DLR-grant 01GU 0516 (Prof. Kolb) and TRANSNET project MRTN-CT-2004-512253 (EC Marie Curie grant, Prof. Kolb).

All authors thank technicians, nurses and physicians for skilful work and data contribution. Many of the data presented were worked out in the course of theses (MD, PhD).

6.1 Groupleaders and responsibilities

Adamski   Jerzi (Prof., PhD, Helmholtz Research Center for Environmental Health, responsible for male specific antigens)

Borkhardt Arndt (Prof., MD, Director of the Department for Pediatric Oncology and Hematology, University of Duesseldorf, responsible for spectratyping)

Buhmann Raymund (MD, Helmholtz Research Center for Environmental Health, responsible for LAA analyses, CD4 characterization)

Busch Dirk (Prof., MD, Director of the Department for Immunology, Technical University of Munich, responsible for MHC-Multimer analyses)

Kolb Hans-Jochem (Prof., MD, former head of the Stem Cell Transplantation Unit of the Med Dept III, University of Munich, responsible for clinical development and application of stem cell transplantation protocols , initiation and discussions of T-cell projects)

Milosevic Slavoljub (PhD, Helmholtz Research Center for Environmental Health, responsible for the LAA-specific CD4+ T-cells)

Schmetzer Helga (PhD, PD, Prof., Med Dept 3, dept for stem cell transplantations, University of Munich, responsible for DC-projects, CD4 project, author of this book chapter)

Schmid Christoph (PD, MD, head of the Stem Cell Transplantation unit at Klinikum Augsburg, responsible for clinical development and application of stem cell transplantation protocols, main coauthor of this book chaper)

6.2 Scientists and responsibilities

Ansprenger Christian (MD student; thesis student, Med Dept 3, working group Schmetzer, responsible for characterization of immunomodulatory DC culture additives)

Bund Dagmar (PhD student, Helmholtz Research Center for Environmental Health, working group Buhmann/Kolb; responsible for male specific antigens/T-cell reactions)

Deen Diana (MD student, thesis student, Med Dept 3, working group Schmetzer, responsible for characterization of immunomodulatory DC culture additives)

Doessinger Georg (PhD student, Department for Immunology, Technical University of Munich, working group Busch, responsible for MHC-Multimer analyses)

Fischbacher Dorothea (MD, thesis student, Med Dept 3, working group Schmetzer, responsible for cytokine analyses in DC project)

Freudenreich Markus (MD, thesis student, Med Dept 3, working group Schmetzer, responsible for *in vivo* correlations in DC project)

Gallo Antonio (PhD, formerly Helmholtz Research Center for Environmental Health, working group Kolb/Adamsky, responsible for male specific antigens/T-cell reactions)

Grabrucker Christine (MD, Med Dept 3, working group Schmetzer, responsible for DC- or blast-stimulations of T-cells in DC project)
Liepert Anja (MD, thesis student, Med Dept 3, working group Schmetzer, responsible for characterization of DC-stimulated T-cells in DC project)
Merle Marion (MD, thesis student, Med Dept 3, working group Schmetzer, responsible for chemokine analyses in DC project)
Reuther Susanne (PhD student, Department for Pediatric Oncology and Hematology, University of Duesseldorf, working group Borkhardt, responsible for spectratyping)
Schick Julia (MD student, thesis student, Med Dept 3, working group Schmetzer, responsible for characterization of regulatory T-cells in DC project)
Schuster Friedhelm (MD, Department for Pediatric Oncology and Hematology, University of Duesseldorf, working group Borkhardt, responsible for spectratyping)
Steger Brigitte (PhD student, Helmholtz Research Center for Environmental Health, working group Kolb/ Buhmann/ Schmetzer, responsible for LAA analyses and LAA-specific CD4+ T-cell project)
Vogt Valentin (MD student, thesis student, Med Dept 3, working group Schmetzer, responsible for characterization of T-cell differentiation subtypes)

7. References

Adhikary, D.; Behrends, U.; Feederle, R.; Delecluse, H.J.; Mautner, J. (2008). Standardized and highly efficient expansion of Epstein-Barr virus-specific CD4+ T-cells by using virus-like particles. *Journal of virology.*,Vol.82(8), pp. 3903-3911.

Ansprenger, C.; Grabrucker, C.; Kroell, T.; Schmetzer, H. (2011). Modulation of blasts using paraimmunity- inducing factors (PINDS) to improve leukemic antigen presenting function. Manuscript in preparation.

Barrett, AJ & Le Blanc, K. (2010). Immunotherapy prospects for acute myeloid leukemia. *Clin. Exp. Immunol.*;161(2), pp.223-32.

Blanco-Arias, P.; Sargent, C.A. & Affara N.A. (2002). The human-specific Yp11.2/Xq21.3 homology block encodes a potentially functional testis-specific TGIF-like retroposon. *Mamm Genome* 13, pp. 463-468.

Bornhauser,M., Oelschlaegel,U., Platzbecker,U., Bug,G.; Lutterbeck,K.; Kiehl,M.G.; Schetelig,J.; Kiani,A.; Illmer,T.; Schaich,M.; Theuser,C.; Mohr,B.; Brendel,C.; Fauser,A.A.; Klein,S.; Martin,H.; Ehninger,G.; Thiede,C. (2009). Monitoring of donor chimerism in sorted CD34+ peripheral blood cells allows the sensitive detection of imminent relapse after allogeneic stem cell transplantation. *Haematologica*, 94, pp. 1613-1617.

Buechner, T.; Hiddemann, W.; Berdel, W.E.; Wörmann, B.; Schoch, C.; Fonatsch, C.; Löffler, H.; Haferlach, T.; Ludwig, W.D.; Maschenmeyer, G.; Staib, P.; Aul, C.; Gruneisen, A.; Lengfelder, E.; Frickhofen, N.; Kern, W.; Serve, H.L.; Mesters, R.M.; Sauerland, M.C.; Heinecke, A.(2003). 6-Thioguanine, cytarabine and daunorubicin (TAD) and high-dose cytarabine and mitoxantrone (HAM) for induction, TAD for consolidation and either prolonged maintenance by reduced monthly TAD or TAD-HAM-TAD and one course of intensive consolidation by sequential HAM in adult patients at all ages with de novo acute myeloid leukemia (AML): a randomized trial of the German AML Cooperative Group. *J Clin Oncol* 21; pp. 4496-504.

Bund, D.; Schmetzer, H.; Buhmann, R.; Zorn, J.; Gökmen, F.; Kolb, H.J. (2011). UTY encoded minor-histocompatibility antigens as targets for a graft-versus-haematopoiesis (GvHm) and graft versus leukemia (GvL) in the canine model. Submitted for publication.

Collins, R.H., Jr.; Shpilberg, O.; Drobyski, W.R.; Porter, D.L.; Giralt, S.; Champlin, R.; Goodman, S.A.; Wolff, S.N.; Hu, W.; Verfaillie, C.; List, A.; Dalton, W.; Ognoskie, N.; Chetrit, A.; Antin, J.H.; Nemunaitis, J. (1997). Donor leukocyte infusions in 140 patients with relapsed malignancy after allogeneic bone marrow transplantation. *J Clin Oncol.* 15, pp. 433-444.

Deen, D.; Ansprenger, C.; Grabrucker, C.; Kroell, T.; Schmetzer, H. (2011). Modulation of blasts by a combination of immunomodulatory factors and cytokines to stimulate the generation of DC *in vivo*. Manuscript in preparation

Dreyßig, J.; Kremser, A.; Liepert, A.; Grabrucker, C.; Freudenreich, M.; Schmid, C.; Kroell, T.; Scholl, N.; Tischer, J.; Kufner, S.; Salih, H.; Kolb, H.J.; Schmetzer, H. (2011). Various 'Dendritic Cell Antigens' (DCA) are already expressed on uncultured blasts in acute myeloid Leukemia (AML) and myelodysplastic Syndromes (MDS). *J. Immunotherapy* 3(9), pp. 1113-1124.

Elbaz, O. & Shaltout, A. (2001). Implication of granulocyte-macrophage colony stimulating factor (GM-CSF) and interleukin-3 (IL-3) in children with acute myeloid leukaemia (AML). *Hematology* 5(5), pp. 383-388.

Fischbacher, D.; Merle, M.; Liepert, A.; Grabrucker, C.; Kremser, A.; Loibl, J.; Schmid, C.; Kroell, T.; Kolb, H.J.; Schmetzer, H. (2011). CXCL8 and CCL2 secretion by dendritic cells generated from AML-blasts (DCleu) as well as IFN-γ or IL-6 release in mixed lymphocyte cultures (MLC) from T-cells after DC-priming are predictive for antileukemic T-cell reactions. Manuscript in preparation

Freudenreich, M.; Schmid, C.; Kremser, A.; Dreyßig, J., Kroell, T.; Tischer, J.; Kolb, H.J.; Schmetzer, H. (2011). Clinical relevance of in vitro generation of Dendritic cells in patients with AML or MDS. Manuscript in preparation.

Gallo, A.; Bund, D.; Moeller, G.; Schmetzer, H.; Mindnich, R.; Buhmann, R.;, Kolb, H.J., Adamski, J. (2011) Characterization of TGIF2LY, a human Y chromosome encoded gene which is up-regulated in acute myelomonocytic leukemia. Submitted

Grabrucker, C.; Liepert, A.; Dreyssig, J.; Kremser, A.; Kroell, T.; Freudenreich, M.; Schmid, C.; Schweiger, C.; Tischer, J.; Kolb, H.J, Schmetzer, H. (2010). The quality and quantity of leukaemia-derived dendritic cells (DC) from patirnts with acute myeloid leukaemia and myelodysplastic syndrome are a predictive factor for the lytic potential of DC-primed leukaemia-specific T-cells. *J. Immunotherapy* 33,5, pp. 523-537.

Greiner, J.; Döhner, H.; Schmitt, M. (2006). Cancer vaccines for patients with acute myeloid leukaemia-definition of leukaemia-associated antigens and current clinical protocols targeting these antigens. *Haematologica* 91(12), pp. 1653-61.

Hemmati, P.G.; Terwey, T.H.; le Coutre, P.; Vuong, L.G.; Massenkeil, G.; Dörken, B.; Arnold, R. (2011). A modified EBMT risk score predicts the outcome of patients with acute myeloid leukaemia receiving allogeneic stem cell transplants. *Eur.J. Haematol.* ;86(4), pp. 305-16.

Jordanova, E.S.; Gorter, A.; Ayachi, O.; Prins, F.; Durrant, L.G.; Kenter, G.G.; van der Burg, S.H.; Fleuren, G.J. (2008). Human leukocyte antigen class I, MHC class I chain-related molecule A, and CD8+/ regulatory T-cell ratio: which variable determines survival of cer vical cancer patients?. *Clin. Cancer Res.* 14(7), pp. 2028-2035.

Kahl, C.; Storer, B.E.; Sandmaier, B.M.; Mielcarek, M.; Maris, M.B.; Blume, K.G.; Niederwieser, D.; Chauncey, T.R.; Forman, S.J.; Agura, E.; Leis, J.F.; Bruno, B.; Langston, A.; Pulsipher, M.A.; McSweeney, P.A.; Wade, J.C.; Epner, E.; Bo Petersen, F.; Bethge, W.A.; Maloney, D.G.; Storb R. (2007). Relapse risk in patients with malignant diseases given allogeneic hematopoetic cell transplantation after nonmyeloablative conditioning. *Blood.* 110(7) pp. 2744-8.

Knabel, M.; Franz, T.J.; Schiemann, M.; Wulf, A.; Villmow, B.; Schmidt, B.; Bernhard, H.; Wagner, H.; Busch, D.H.(2002). Reversible MHC multimer staining for functional isolation of T-cell populations and effective adoptive transfer. *Nat. Med.* 8(6), pp. 631-7.

Kolb, H.J.; Mittermüller, J.; Clemm, C.; Holler, E.; Ledderose, G.; Brehm, G.; Heim, M.; Wilmanns, W.(1990). Donor leukocyte transfusions for treatment of recurrent chronic myelogenous leukemia in marrow transplant patients. *Blood*, 76(12), pp. 2462-2465.

Kolb, H.J.; Schattenberg, A.; Goldman, .JM.; Hertenstein, B.; Jacobsen, N.; Arcese, W.; Ljungman, P.; Ferrant, A.; Niederwieser, D.; van Rhee, F.; Mittermüller, J.; de Witte, T.; Holler, E.; Ansari, H. Graft-versus-leukemia effect of donor lymphocyte transfusions in marrow grafted patients. European Group for Blood and Marrow Transplantation Working Party Chronic Leukemia. *Blood.* ; 86, pp. 2041-2050.

Kolb, H.J.; Simoes, B.; Schmid, C. (2004). Cellular immunotherapy after allogeneic stem cell transplantation in hematologic malignancies. *Current Opinions in Oncology* 16, pp. 167-173.

Kremser, A.; Kufner, S.; Konheuser, E.; Kroell, T.; Doehner, C.; Schoch, C.; Kolb, H.J.; Zitzelsberger, H.; Schmetzer, H. (2011). Combined immunophenotyping and FISH ('FISH-IPA') with chromosome-specific DNA-probes allows the quantification and differentiation of *ex vivo* generated dendritic cells (DC), leukaemia-derived DC and clonal leukemic cells in patients with AML. Manuscript in preparation

Kufner, S.; Kroell, T.; Pelka-Fleischer, R.; Schmid, C.; Zitzelsberger, H.; de Valle, F; Zirpel, I; Schmetzer, H.(2005). Serum-free generation and quantification of functionally active leukemia-derived dendritic cells is possible from malignant blasts in acute myeloid leukemia (AML) and myelodysplastic syndromes (MDS). *Cancer Immunol. Immunother.* 54, pp. 953-970.

Liepert, A.; Grabrucker, C.; Kremser, A.; Dreyssig, J.; Ansprenger, C.; Freudenreich, M.; Kroell, T.; Reibke, R.; Tischer, J.; Schweiger, C.; Schmid. C.; Kolb, H.J; Schmetzer, H. (2010). Quality of T-cells after stimulation with leukaemia-derived dendritic cells (DC) from patients with acute myeloid leukaemia (AML) or myeloid dysplastic syndrome (MDS) is predictive for their leukaemia cytotoxic potential. *Cellular Immunity* 265, pp. 23-30.

Liu, D.W., Chen, S.T. & Liu, H.P. (2005). Choice of endogenours control for gene expression in nonsmall cell lung cancer. *Eur Respir J,*. 26, pp. 1002-1008.

Merle, M.; Fischbacher, D.; Liepert, A.; Kroell, T.; Grabrucker, C.; Kremser, A.; Dreyssig, J.; Freudenreich, M.; Schmid, C.; Kolb, H.J; Schmetzer, H. (2011). Chemokines secreted by dendritic cells (DC) from patients with acute myeloid leukaemia (AML)

are a predictive factor for the lytic potential of DC-stimulated leukaemia specific T-cells. Manuscript in preparation

Miryara, M. ; Yoshioka, Y. ; Kitoh, A. ;Shima, T. ; Wing, K. ; Niwa, A. ; Parizot, C. ; Taflin, C. ; Heike, T. ; Valeyre, D. ; Mathian, A. ; Nakahata, T. ; Yamaguchi, T. ; Nomura, T. ; Ono, M. ; Amoura Z. ; Gorochov, G. ; Sakaguchi, S. (2009). Functional delineation and differentiation dynamics of human CD4+ T-cells expressing the FoxP3 transcription factor. *Immunity* 30, pp. 899-911.

Moosmann , A.; Khan, N.; Cobbold, M.; Zentz, C.; Delecluse, H.J.; Hollweck, G.; Hislop, A.D.; Blake, N.W.; Croom-Carter, D.; Wollenberg, B.; Moss, P.A.; Zeidler, R.; Rickinson, A.B.; Hammerschmidt, W. (2002). B cells immortalized by a mini-Epstein-Barr virus encoding a foreign antigen efficiently reactivate specific cytotoxic T cells.*Blood,* 100(5), pp.1755-1764.

Moosmann,A.; Bigalke,I.; Tischer,J.; Schirrmann,L.; Kasten,J.; Tippmer,S.; Leeping,M.; Prevalsek,D.; Jaeger,G., Ledderose,G.; Mautner,J.; Hammerschmidt,W.; Schendel,D.J.; Kolb,H.J. (2010) Effective and long-term control of EBV PTLD after transfer of peptide-selected T cells. *Blood,* 115, pp. 2960-2970.

Mutis, T. & Goulmy, E. (2002). Hematopoietic system specific antigens as targets for cellular immunotherapy of hematological malignancies. *Semin Hematol.* ;39, pp. 23–31.

Neudorfer, J.; Schmidt, B.; Huster, K.M; Anderl, F.; Schiemann, M.; Holzapfel, G.; Schmidt, T.; Germeroth, L.; Wagner, H.; Peschel, C.; Busch, D.H; Bernhard, H. (2007). Reversible HLA multimers (Streptamers) for the isolation of human cytotoxic T lymphocytes functionally active against tumor-and virus-derived antigens. *J. of Immunol. Meth.* 320, pp. 119-131.

Nijman, H.W.; Houbiers, J.G.; Vierboom MP.; van der Burg, S.H.; Drijfhout, J.W.; D'Amaro, J.; Kenemans, P.; Melief, C.J.; Kast, W.M.(1993). Identification of peptide sequences that potentially trigger HLA- A2.1-restricted cytotoxic T lymphocytes. *Eur J Immunol.* 23, pp. 1215–1219.

Ofran, Y.; Kim, H.T.; Brusic, V.; Blake, L.; Mandrell, M.; Wu, C.J.; Sarantopoulos, S.; Bellucci, R.; Keskin, D.B.; Soiffer, R.J.; Antin, J.H.; Ritz, J. (2010). Diverse patterns of T-cell response against multiple newly identified human Y chromosome-encoded minor histocompatibility epitopes. *Clin Cancer Res.*16, pp. 1642–1651.

Parmar, S.; Fernandez-Vina, M; de Lima, M. (2011). Novel transplant strategies for generating graft-versus-leukemia effect in acute myeloid leukaemia. *Curr. Opin. Hematol.* 18(2), pp. 98-104.

Rammensee, H.G.; Friede, Stevanovic, S. (1995). MHC ligands and peptide motifs: 1st listing. *Immunogenetics.* 41, pp. 178-228.

Reuther, S.; Schuster, F.; Hubner, B.; Grabrucker, C.; Liepert, A.; Reibke, R.; Lichtner, P.; Yang, T.; Kroell, T.; Kolb, H.J.; Borkhardt, A.; Schmetzer, H.; Buhmann, R.(2011). *In vitro* induced response patterns of antileukemic T cells- characterization by spectratyping and immunophenotyping. Submitted for publication

Saller, R.D.; Howell, D.N.; Cresswell, P.(1985). Genes regulating HLA class I antigen expression in T-B lymphoblast hybrid. *Immunogenetics.* 1985;21, pp. 235–46.

Sallusto, F.; Geginat, J.; Lanzavecchia, A.(2004). Central memory and effector memory T cell subsets: function, generation and maintenance. *Annu. Rev. Immunol.* 22, pp. 745-763.

Schick, J.; Vogt, V.; Zerwes, M.; Kroell, T.; Schweiger, C.; Köhne H, Kolb H.J, Buhmann R, Schmetzer H. (2011). Antileukemic T-cell responses after dendritic cell (DC)

stimulation can be predicted by compositions of regulatory T-cell subpopulations, especially with respect to regulatory central memory and regulatory CD8 cells. *Bone Marrow Transplantation* 46, supp 1, abstr. 1048.

Schleuning, M.; Schmid, C.; Koenecke, C.; Hertenstein, B.; Baurmann, H.; Schwerdtfeger, R.; Kolb, H.J.(2008). Long term follow-up and matched pair analysis of adjuvant donor lymphocyte transfusions following allogeneic stem cell transplantation after reduced intensity conditioning for high-risk AML. ASH 2008; *Blood* supplement, abstract No 2142.

Schmetzer, H.; Kremser, A.; Loibl, J.; Kröll, T.; Kolb, H.J.(2007). Quantification of *ex vivo* generated dendritic cells (DC) and leukaemia-derived DC ('DCleu') contributes to estimate the quality of DC, to detect optimal DC-generating methods or to optimize DC-mediated T-cell-activation-procedures *ex vivo* or *in vivo*. *Leukemia* 21, pp. 1338-41.

Schmetzer, H. (2011). Antileukemic T-cell-mediated immune reactions: limitations and perspectives for future therapies. Editorial, *Immunotherapy* 3(7), pp. 809-811.

Schmid,C.; Schleuning,M; Aschan,J.; Ringden,O.; Hahn,J.; Holler,E.; Hegenbart,U.; Niederwieser,D.; Dugas,M.; Ledderose,G.; Kolb,H.J. (2004) Low-dose ARAC, donor cells, and GM-CSF for treatment of recurrent acute myeloid leukemia after allogeneic stem cell transplantation. *Leukemia*, 18, pp. 1430-1433.

Schmid, C.; Schleuning, M.; Ledderose, G.; Tischer, J.; Kolb, H.J.(2005). Sequential regimen of chemotherapy, reduced-intensity conditioning for allogeneic stem-cell transplantation, and prophylactic donor lymphocyte transfusion in high-risk acute myeloid leukemia and myelodysplastic syndrome. *J Clin Oncol.* 23, pp. 5675-5687.

Schmid, C.; Labopin,M.; Nagler,A.; Bornhauser,M.; Finke,J.; Fassas,A.; Volin,L.; Gurman,G.; Maertens,J.; Bordigoni,P.; Holler E.; Ehninger,G.; Polge,E.; Gorin,N.; Kolb,H.-J.; Rocha,V. (2007) Donor lymphocyte infusion in the treatment of first hematological relapse after allogeneic stem cell transplantation in adults with acute myeloid leukaemia: A retrospective risk factors analysis and comparison with other strategies by the EBMT Acute Leukemia Working Party Journal of Clinical Oncology, 2007, 25 (31); 4938-4945. *J Clin Oncol.*, 25, pp. 4938-4945.

Schmid, C., Labopin, M., Nagler, A., Niederwieser, D., Castagna, L., Tabrizi, R., Stadler, M., Kuball, J., Cornelissen, J., Vorlicek, J., Socié, G., Falda, M., Vindeløv, L., Ljungman, P., Jackson, G., Kröger, N., Rank, A., Polge, E., Rocha, V., Mohty, M. (2011) Treatment, risk factors, and outcome of adults with relapsed AML after reduced intensity conditioning for allogeneic stem cell transplantation. *Blood.* 2011 Dec 13. [Epub ahead of print]

Schmittel, A.; Keilholz, U.; Thiel, E.; Scheibenbogen, C. (2000). Quantification of tumor-specific T lymphocytes with the ELISPOT assay. *Journ. of Immunother,*23(3), pp.289-295.

Schuster, F.; Buhmann, R.; Reuther, S.; Hubner, B.; Grabrucker, C.; Liepert, A.; Reibke, R.; Lichtner, P.; Yang, T.; Kroell, T.; Kolb, H.J.; Borkhardt, A.; Schmetzer, H.(2008). Improved effector functions of leukaemia-specific T-lymphocyte clones trained with AML-derived dendritic cells. *Cancer Genomics Proteomics* 5, pp. 275-286.

Skaletsky,H; Kuroda-Kawaguchi, T; Minx, P.J.; Cordum, H.S.; Hillier, L.; Brown, L.G.; Repping, S.; Pyntikova, T.; Ali, J.; Bieri, T.; Chinwalla, A.; Delehaunty, A.; Delehaunty, K.; Du, H.; Fewell, G., Fulton, L.; Fulton, R.; Graves, T., Hou, S.F.;

Latrielle, P.; Leonard, S.; Mardis, E., Maupin, R., McPherson, J., Miner, T., Nash, W.; Nguyen, C.; Ozersky, P.; Pepin, K.; Rock, S.; Rohlfing, T.; Scott, K.; Schultz, B.; Strong, C.; Tin-Wollam, A.; Yang, S.P.; Waterston, R.H.; Wilson, R.K.; Rozen, S., Page, D.C.(2003). The male-specific region of the human Y chromosome is a mosaic of discrete sequence classes. *Nature*. 423, pp. 825–837.

Smits, EL.; Lee, C.; Hardwick, N.; Brooks, S.; Van Tendeloo, V.F.; Orchard, K.; Guinn, B.A. (2011). Clinical evalution of cellular immunotherapy in acute myeloid leukaemia. *Cancer Immunol. Immunother.* 60(6), pp.757-69.

Steger, B.; Schmetzer, H.; Floro, L.; Kroell, T.; Tischer, J.; Kolb, H.J.; Buhmann, R. (2011). Clinical relevance of mRNA overexpressions of the leukaemia associated antigens (LAA) WT1, PRAME and PR1 in patients (pts) with Acute Myeloid Leukaemia (AML): an analysis of (co)expressions in different cellular compartments, subtypes or stages. Submitted for publication.

Steger, B.; Milosevic, S.; Doessinger, G.; Reuther, S.; Liepert, A.; Zerwes, M.; Schick, J.; Vogt, V.; Schuster, F.; Kroell, T.; Busch D.; Borkhardt, A.; Kolb, H.J. ; Tischer, J.; Buhmann, R.; Schmetzer, H. (2012). CD4+ as well as CD8+ T-cells addressing leukaemia-associated antigens (LAA: WT1, PRAME, PR1) or minor histocompatibility antigens (mHags: HA1) can be identified and mobilized to recognize and kill leukemic cells expressing from patients (pts) with acute myeloid leukaemia (AML). Submitted for publication

Stern, M.; Loredana, R.; Mancusi, A.; Bernardo, M.E.; de Angelis, C.; Bucher, C.; Locatelli, F.; Aversa, F.; Velardi, A. (2008). Survival after T cell-depleted haploidentical stem cell transplantation is improved using the mother as donor. *Blood*, Vol 112(7), pp. 2990-2995.

van den Brink,M.R.; Porter,D.L.; Giralt,S.; Lu,S.X.; Jenq,R.R.; Hanash,A.; Bishop,M.R. (2010) Relapse after allogeneic hematopoietic cell therapy. *Biol.Blood Marrow Transplant.*, 16, pp. S138-S145.

Vignali, D.A.; Collison, L.W.; Workman, C.J.(2008). How regulatory T cells work. *Nat. Rev. Immunol.* 8(7), pp. 523-32.

Vogt, V.; Schick, J.; Zerwes, M.; Kroell, T.; Schweiger, C.; Koehne, C.; Buhmann, R.; Kolb, H.J.; Schmetzer, H. (2011). Antileukemic T cell responses after DC-stimulation can be predicted by composition of regulatory T-cell subpopulations, especially with respect to regulatory central memory and regulatory CD8 cells. Bone Marrow Transplantation 46, supp 1, abstr. 1047

Warren, E.H.; Gavin, M.A.; Simpson, E.; Chandler, P.; Page, D.C.; Disteche, C.; Stankey, K.A.; Greenberg, P.D.; Riddell, S.R. (2000). The human UTY gene encodes a novel HLA-B8-restricted H-Y antigen. J. Immunol.164(5), pp. 2807-2814

Woiciechowsky, A.; Regn, S.; Kolb, H.J.; Roskrow, M.(2001). Leukemic dendritic cells generated in the presence of FLT3 ligand have the capacity to stimulate an autologous leukemia-specific cytotoxicT cell response from patients with acute myeloid leukemia.*Leukemia*. 15, pp. 246–255.

6

Licensed to Kill: Towards Natural Killer Cell Immunotherapy

Diana N. Eissens, Arnold van der Meer and Irma Joosten
Radboud University Nijmegen Medical Centre
The Netherlands

1. Introduction

Allogeneic stem cell transplantation (SCT) is often the final treatment modality for patients with leukemia or other hematological malignancies (Schaap et al., 1997; Thomas & Blume, 1999). However, relapse of the underlying malignancy is still a major complication post SCT. To prevent the occurrence of relapse post SCT, patients are treated with pre-emptive donor lymphocyte infusions (DLI) consisting of donor-derived T cells from the same donor used for allogeneic SCT in order to boost the donor-derived immune system to terminally eradicate residual tumour cells (Barge et al., 2003; Peggs et al., 2004; Schaap et al., 2001). Unfortunately, DLI treatment using donor-derived T cells does not only provoke graft-versus-leukemia (GVL) reactivity, but also increases the risk for the development of graft-versus-host disease (GVHD). Thus, post allogeneic SCT, long-term remission is still greatly dependent on effective GVL reactivity, while strictly controlling GVHD. Therefore, the development of treatment strategies augmenting GVL reactivity while reducing GVHD is of clinical importance.

In allogeneic SCT, natural killer (NK) cells have shown to play an important role in GVL reactivity within the first months after transplantation (Cook et al., 2004; Giebel et al., 2006; Ruggeri et al., 2002; van der Meer et al., 2008). Ruggeri *et al.* showed that alloreactive donor NK cells were able to lyse recipient tumour cells *in vitro*, implying that these NK cells may be able to provide immune reactivity by targeting residual tumour cells still present in the recipient (Ruggeri et al., 1999). Moreover, fast recovery of NK cells and predicted GVL reactivity towards host tumour cells has been associated with reduced GVHD, decreased relapse rates, and better overall survival of the patient (Kim et al., 2005a; Kim et al., 2006; Ruggeri et al., 2007; Savani et al., 2007). Altogether, this makes NK cells important candidates for immunotherapeutic use in the treatment of leukemia and other malignancies.

2. Natural Killer cells

NK cells are members of the innate immune system. They are important in the initial phase of defense against infections and play an important role in tumour surveillance. Their name was based on their ability to kill target cells without prior sensitization (Kiessling et al., 1975a; Kiessling et al., 1975b). As they are morphologically recognized as relatively large lymphocytes containing azurophilic granules, they have also been known as large granular lymphocytes (LGL) (Herberman, 1986). NK cells comprise approximately 5-15% of the peripheral blood lymphocyte (PBL) population and are also found in lymph nodes, spleen, bone marrow, lung, liver, intestine, omentum and placenta (Vivier, 2006). NK cells are believed to originate from the same common lymphoid progenitor lineage as T and B cells in bone marrow (Spits et al., 1995). However, they do not rearrange T cell receptor genes or immunoglobulin (Ig) like, respectively, T and B cells do.

Resting NK cells can be recognized based on their expression of CD56 (neural cell adhesion molecule; NCAM). Since CD56 is also expressed by other immune cells, NK cells are identified by the expression of CD56 combined with the lack of CD3, which are both present on NKT cells. NK cells can be further characterized based on their expression of CD56 in combination with CD16, a low affinity Fc receptor (Figure 1) (Cooper et al., 2001).

In peripheral blood, approximately 90% of NK cells shows low expression of CD56 and high expression of CD16 on the cell surface. These cells are collectively referred to as the CD56dimCD16+ or CD56dim NK cell subset. The other 10% of NK cells shows a high level of CD56 expression and almost no expression of CD16 on the cell surface. Together, these cells are known as the CD56brightCD16+/- or CD56bright NK cell subset. The CD56dim NK cell subset is characterized by a highly cytolytic behaviour towards target cells, whereas CD56bright NK cells abundantly produce cytokines, such as IFN-γ and TNF-α, upon activation. The production of cytokines by NK cells influences the T_H1/T_H2 bias of the adaptive immune response by activating T_H1 cells. Thereby, NK cells form a bridge between innate and adaptive immunity (Seaman, 2000).

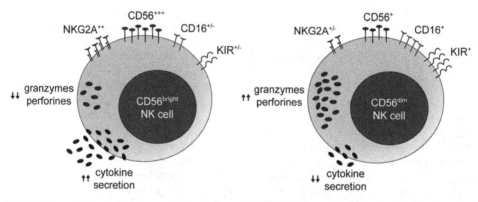

Fig. 1. Natural Killer cell subsets. NK cells can be divided in two major subsets based on their expression of CD56 and CD16. CD56bright NK cells have a high CD56 and low CD16 expression profile, and are specialized in cytokine secretion (e.g. TNF-α, IFN-γ). In addition they highly express inhibitory receptor NKG2A. CD56dim NK cells have a low CD56 and high CD16 expression profile, and are highly cytolytic. Their function is predominantly inhibited through KIR.

NK cells lyse susceptible target cells (e.g. virus infected cells, malignant transformed cells) by one of two mechanisms: "natural killing" (no prior sensitization) or antibody dependent cellular cytotoxicity (ADCC). Natural killing is initiated by activating signals from a variety of stimulatory receptors that can be inhibited by a variety of inhibitory receptors. In ADCC, the activating receptor FcRγIII (CD16) binds to the Fc piece of antibodies bound to target cells. In both mechanisms, target cells are lysed by the release of cytolytic proteins (i.e. granzymes and perforines) or by the induction of apoptosis (Bossi & Griffiths, 1999).

2.1 NK cell receptors
The NK cell receptor repertoire forms the basis for NK cell immune surveillance and NK cell activity. NK cell immune surveillance is regulated through the recognition of HLA class I molecules by inhibitory receptors. Subsequent activation of NK cells is triggered through the recognition of activating ligands by stimulatory receptors.

2.1.1 Inhibitory receptors
NK cells survey potential target cells for the absence or loss of expression of classical HLA class I molecules or non-classical HLA class I specific signals through inhibitory killer cell immunoglobulin-like receptors (KIRs) and lectin-like receptors (Farag & Caligiuri, 2006; Papamichail et al., 2004). The cytoplasmic domains of all inhibitory NK cell receptors contain an immunoreceptor tyrosine-based inhibitory motif (ITIM) (Burshtyn et al., 1996; Fry et al., 1996; Vivier & Daeron, 1997). These domains recruit intracellular tyrosine phosphatases SHP-1 or SHP-2 that mediate the inhibition of cytotoxicity and cytokine release (Burshtyn et al., 1996; Fry et al., 1996; Le et al., 1998; Olcese et al., 1996).
The lectin-like receptor complex CD94:NKG2A forms an inhibitory receptor that recognizes non-classical HLA-E molecules (Braud et al., 1998). As the expression of HLA-E is promoted by the binding of signal sequence-derived peptides from HLA class I molecules, it is thought that HLA-E expression serves as a barometer of classical HLA class I expression (Braud et al., 1997). The purpose of the inhibitory CD94:NKG2A receptor complex may, therefore, be to monitor the overall HLA class I expression. KIRs, on the other hand, allow for a more subtle immune surveillance as these receptors scan the presence of specific classical HLA class I molecules.
KIRs are encoded by a family of polymorphic and highly homologous genes, and recognize polymorphic epitopes present on HLA-A, -B, or -C molecules; HLA-A3 and -A11 are recognized by KIR3DL2, HLA-Bw4 is recognized by KIR3DL1 and receptors KIR2DL1, KIR2DL2, and KIR2DL3 are able to distinguish HLA-C into HLA group C1 and HLA group C2 molecules (Parham, 2005). The various KIRs are classified by the number of immunoglobulin-like (Ig) extracellular domains as 2-domain (2D) or 3-domain (3D). They are further subdivided on the basis of the length of their cytoplasmic tail L (long) or S (short) (Vilches & Parham, 2002). Different KIRs sharing the same number of Ig domains and length of the cytoplasmic tail are distinguished by number at the end of their name, e.g. KIR2DL2 or KIR2DL3. KIRs are clonally distributed among NK cells within each individual, which creates a complex combinatorial repertoire of NK cell specificities for HLA class I molecules (Vilches & Parham, 2002).

2.1.2 Stimulatory receptors
Some members of the CD94:NKG2 receptor and KIR family have stimulatory properties. NKG2C is a stimulatory member of the CD94:NKG2 family and competes with CD94:NKG2A for the recognition of HLA-E (Braud et al., 1998; Houchins et al., 1997). KIR2DS and KIR3DS are stimulatory members of the KIR family (Biassoni et al., 1996; Bottino et al., 1996; Moretta et al., 1995). Instead of ITIM, these stimulatory receptors contain

a positively charged amino acid residue in their transmembrane domain that associates with the negatively charged DAP-12 molecule. DAP-12 contains an immunoreceptor tyrosine-based activating motif (ITAM) (Lanier et al., 1998). There is evidence that the stimulatory KIRs bind self-HLA class I molecules with lower affinity as compared with the inhibitory receptors (Vales-Gomez et al., 1998a; Vales-Gomez et al., 1998b). Thus autoimmunity can be prevented by a balance towards negative NK cell regulation. Similar to the inhibitory receptors, the HLA class I-specific stimulatory receptors are expressed in a variegated and predominantly stochastic fashion by NK cells (Raulet et al., 2001).

Besides stimulatory members of the CD94:NKG2 receptor and KIR family, NK cells also express a variety of other stimulatory receptors. The biological roles of many of these receptors are not well understood, primarily because the ligands for these receptors have not been fully identified. The main triggering receptors for NK cell activity are the natural cytotoxicity receptors (NCR) and NKG2D (Arnon et al., 2001; Bauer et al., 1999; Mandelboim et al., 2001; Sivori et al., 1997). Their stimulation causes direct killing of target cells and their stimulatory signals can even override the inhibition of NK cells.

NCR consist of three members; NKp30, NKp44, and NKp46. NCR belong to the immunoglobulin superfamily and molecular cloning of NCR confirmed that they are structurally distinct (Bottino et al., 2000; Pende et al., 1999). The ligands for NCR remain controversial. Some groups have proposed viral antigens as being the ligands for NCR based on their role in the lysis of virus infected cells (Arnon et al., 2001; Arnon et al., 2005; Mandelboim et al., 2001). NCR have also been shown to mediate lysis of tumour cells and that NK cells with a NCR[dull] phenotype are unable to kill tumour cells, suggesting that their ligands may be upregulated or induced upon malignant transformation of cells (Bottino et al., 2005; Fauriat et al., 2005; Fauriat et al., 2007). NKp30 and NKp46 are both uniquely expressed on resting and activated NK cells, whereas NKp44 is only present on IL-2 activated NK cells (Cantoni et al., 1999).

Unlike NKG2A, NKG2D is not associated with CD94, but is a homodimer that needs association to the adaptor molecule DAP10 for stable cell surface expression (Wu et al., 1999). NKG2D recognizes HLA class I-like molecules, such as MIC A and MIC B. It has been shown that the expression of NKG2D ligands, i.e. MIC A/B, ULPB1, ULPB2, and ULPB3, are upregulated by cells in times of stress, virus infection, and malignant transformation (Bauer et al., 1999; Cosman et al., 2001; Farrell et al., 2000). NKG2D is constitutively expressed on all human NK cells and can be upregulated through stimulation by IL-15, IL-12 and IFN-α (Diefenbach et al., 2000; Sutherland et al., 2006). Stimulation of NKG2D complements NCR activation in mediating NK cell lysis of tumour cells (Pende et al., 2001). Similarly, cooperation between NKG2D and stimulatory KIRs has been shown for both cytolytic activity and IFN-γ secretion (Wu et al., 2000). Therefore, it is possible that NKG2D may serve both as a primary stimulatory receptor, whose engagement triggers cytotoxicity, and also as a co-stimulatory receptor, which cooperates with other activating receptors (e.g. activating KIR or NCR) for cytokine secretion. A similar phenomenon is seen on cytomegalovirus-specific T cells, where NKG2D acts as a co-stimulatory receptor for TCR-dependent signals (Das et al., 2001; Groh et al., 2001; Ugolini & Vivier, 2001).

Other stimulatory receptors that are involved in NK cell activation are co-stimulatory receptors NKp80 and 2B4 (CD244) (Biassoni et al., 2001). NKp80 and 2B4 both function synergistically with NCR (Sivori et al., 2000; Vitale et al., 2001). In addition, CD16, CD69 and DNAM-1 have been shown to trigger NK cell-mediated lysis in redirected cytotoxicity assays (Lanier et al., 1988; Moretta et al., 1991; Shibuya et al., 1996).

2.2 NK cell allorecognition
2.2.1 The "missing self" hypothesis

In 1976, Snell *et al.* observed a correlation between the susceptibility of target cells to NK cell lysis and the absence or loss of expression of HLA class I molecules on the target cells (Snell, 1976). Absent or low expression of HLA class I molecules is common in virus infected and malignant transformed cells, which are the usual targets for NK cell lysis. Therefore, they proposed that NK cell receptors may not only interact with HLA class I molecules, but that these receptors are also able to detect a decrease in HLA class I expression.

It was not until 10 years later that Kärre and Ljunggren demonstrated the regulation of NK cell activity (Kärre et al., 1986a). They showed that murine lymphoma cells with low, or absent, MHC class I expression were less malignant than wild-type cells after low dose inoculation in syngeneic mice, and that the rejection of these cells was regulated through innate immunity, preferably through NK cell-mediated lysis (Kärre et al., 1986b). Resistance to NK cell-mediated lysis of tumours with low MHC class I expression could be restored by reintroduction of MHC class I molecules (Franksson et al., 1993; Ljunggren et al., 1990). Based on these data, they proposed the "missing self" hypothesis, which is nowadays still appreciated as the basic model for NK cell activation (Figure 2) (Ljunggren & Kärre, 1990).

2.2.2 Licensed to kill

As the KIR repertoire of NK cells is encoded by a set of highly polymorphic genes and segregates independently from HLA class I genes during NK cell development, it is essential that the KIR repertoire of NK cells properly corresponds with the HLA environment to provide self-tolerance and prevent autoimmunity. There have been several hypotheses on the acquisition of self-tolerance by NK cells. Raulet *et al.* proposed that an individual NK cell can simultaneously express multiple inhibitory KIRs in a stochastic fashion (Raulet et al., 2001). The only rule appears to be that every NK cell has at least one inhibitory KIR specific for self-HLA class I in order to avoid autoreactivity. This is referred to as the "at least one receptor" model (Raulet et al., 2001). Others have suggested a "receptor calibration" model in which the acquisition of the KIR repertoire may be related to changes in the HLA class I environment and is dependent on the HLA class I haplotype (Salcedo et al., 1997; Sentman et al., 1995; Valiante et al., 1997). However, these studies involved *in vitro* cultures that could alter the intrinsic features of NK cells that may be different from the *in vivo* situation.

Recently, the acquisition of self-tolerance was demonstrated in an *in vivo* murine study. Kim *et al.* showed that NK cells from MHC-deficient mice were functionally immature as they were defective in cytokine secretion upon *ex vivo* stimulation as compared with wild type NK cells, indicating that MHC-specific receptors are involved in the acquisition of functional competence (Kim et al., 2005b). They also found a correlation between the expression of an inhibitory receptor for self-MHC class I and the capacity of an individual naive NK cell to be activated to produce cytokines and lyse susceptible target cells. Based on their findings they proposed the "licensing" model, in which NK cells acquire functional competence through "licensing" by self-HLA class I molecules, resulting in two types of self-tolerant NK cells: licensed or unlicensed. This model was confirmed by others, both in mice and human, demonstrating that NK cells without expression of known self-receptors were found to be hyporesponsive (Cooley et al., 2007; Fernandez et al., 2005). Thus, in order for NK cells to get their "license to kill", they need to fulfil the requirement of HLA class I-specific receptor engagement by self-HLA. There appears to be one exception to this rule: Orr *et al.* showed in a mouse model that, contrary to the licensing hypothesis, unlicensed NK cells were the main mediators of NK cell-mediated control of mouse cytomegalovirus infection (MCMV) *in vivo* (Orr et al., 2010). It would be highly relevant to check whether such a cell population harbours increased allo- or tumour reactivity.

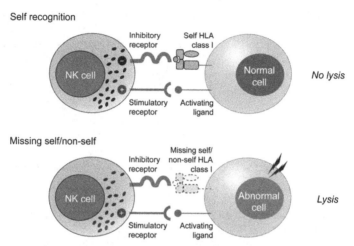

Fig. 2. "Missing self" hypothesis. NK cell activity depends on a balance between inhibitory (i.e. KIR, CD94/NKG2A) and stimulatory (e.g. NCR, NKG2D) signals. In steady state, NK cells are inhibited from activation by the recognition of self-HLA class I molecules, which overrules potential stimulatory signals (self recognition). In case of virus infection or malignant transformation, cells may downregulate self-HLA class I molecules, while upregulating activating ligands that trigger NK cells to respond resulting in lysis of the infected/transformed cells (missing self). After allogeneic SCT, donor NK cells may be triggered by host leukemic cells due to reduced HLA-matched class I molecules (HLA-matched SCT), or the presence of non-self HLA class I molecules (HLA-mismatched SCT), combined with strong stimulation by upregulated activating ligands.

3. NK cells and their therapeutic role in SCT

3.1 Evidence for GVL
Deficient HLA class I expression has been described for leukemic cells making them susceptible targets for NK cell-mediated lysis. However, this phenomenon was not ubiquitously observed in the autologous setting for patients with different forms of leukemia. In CML, NK cell numbers and NK cell function have been shown to decrease progressively during the spontaneous course of the disease, but could be recovered upon IFN-α treatment (Pawelec et al., 1995; Pierson & Miller, 1996). Moreover, activated autologous NK cells were shown to suppress the growth of primitive CML progenitors in long-term *in vitro* cultures (Cervantes et al., 1996). In AML, however, autologous NK cells were demonstrated to be impaired in their cytolytic function, which correlated with a low NCR cell surface density (NCR[dull]) (Fauriat et al., 2007). Moreover, these NK cells were impaired in regulating DC physiology (killing the surplus of immature DCs), which could

lead to specific T cell tolerization by expanded immature DCs expressing leukemia-derived antigens (Fauriat et al., 2005). Allogeneic SCT may overcome the impairment of NK cell-mediated lysis.

In different allogeneic SCT settings, NK cells have been shown to play an important role in the anti-tumour response within the first months after transplantation (Cook et al., 2004; Giebel et al., 2006; Ruggeri et al., 2002; van der Meer et al., 2008). In haploidentical SCT, Ruggeri *et al.* showed that donor alloreactive NK cells isolated from peripheral blood of the recipient were able to lyse tumour cells derived from the recipient, implying that within one month after SCT, NK cells may be able to provide some degree of immune reactivity by targeting residual tumour cells still present in the recipient (Ruggeri et al., 1999). Moreover, fast recovery of NK cells and predicted GVL reactivity towards host tumour cells has been associated with decreased relapse rates and better overall survival of the patient (Kim et al., 2006; Ruggeri et al., 2007; Savani et al., 2007). Altogether these data suggest that NK cells play an important role in the control and clearance of leukemic cells after allogeneic SCT.

3.2 Evidence for the prevention of GVHD

The haploidentical transplantations performed by Ruggeri *et al.* additionally suggested that NK cells may prevent the development of GVHD (Ruggeri et al., 2002). For patients, the prevalence of GVHD was significantly lower using grafts with potential NK cell alloreactivity in the GVL direction as compared with grafts without potential NK cell alloreactivity. In a murine model, they demonstrated that mice transplanted with non-T cell depleted grafts could be rescued from GVHD upon infusion of alloreactive NK cells. Mice infused with non-alloreactive NK cells died as they were not protected from GVHD. They also demonstrated that alloreactive NK cells are able to lyse recipient antigen presenting cells (APCs), thereby preventing interaction with donor T cells which otherwise would initiate GVHD. Recently, a novel mechanism for NK cell-mediated GVHD reduction was demonstrated, whereby alloreactive donor NK cells were able to inhibit and lyse alloreactive donor T cells during the initiation of GVHD (Olson et al., 2010). Overall, these studies demonstrate that alloreactive NK cells may, directly or indirectly, reduce or prevent the occurrence of GVHD while retaining GVL reactivity.

4. Exploitation of NK cell alloreactivity

4.1 Infusion of mature donor NK cells as part of the graft

Immediately after allogeneic SCT, alloreactive NK cells have been shown to be beneficial not only for boosting the anti-tumour response, but also for the prevention of GVHD as well as infections. In these cases, optimal functional activity of NK cells already in the early phase after SCT is essential, and therefore the presence of NK cells in the graft appears to be beneficial for transplant outcome (Bethge et al., 2006; Kim et al., 2005a).

As part of a prospective randomized phase III study, we directly compared the alloreactive potential of allogeneic donor NK cells between patients having either received a CD3$^+$/CD19$^+$ cell depleted graft (containing substantial NK cell numbers) or a conventional CD34$^+$ selected graft (devoid of NK cells) in the setting of HLA-matched SCT (Eissens et al., 2010a). Results demonstrate that patients having received a CD3$^+$/CD19$^+$ cell depleted graft, exhibited a faster recovery of NK cells and a functional NK cell receptor repertoire of inhibitory and stimulatory receptors as compared with patients having received a conventional CD34+ graft. Furthermore, transplantation with a CD3+/CD19+ cell depleted graft resulted in the development of a functionally different NK cell population that was more prone to activation via the CD94:NKG2C receptor complex and less sensitive to inhibition via the CD94:NKG2A receptor complex. Although it was demonstrated that human cytomegalovirus (CMV) infection may result in increased CD94:NKG2C expression levels and subsequent loss of CD94:NKG2A expression (Guma et al., 2004; Guma et al., 2006; van Stijn et al., 2008), this phenomenon remained present in the CD3/19 depletion group after exclusion of CMV positive patients from analysis. Unfortunately, later interim analysis on 25 patients per group showed that the primary objectives of this clinical study could not be reached resulting in early termination of the study. Thus, the alternative reconstitution of the NK cell receptor repertoire using CD3+/19+ depleted grafts, characterized by the change in balance of CD94:NKG2A+ NK cells to more CD94:NKG2C+ NK cells, and its impact on clinical outcomes after HLA-matched SCT remains a subject for further study.

Recently, the reconstitution of allogeneic donor NK cells was evaluated in haploidentical SCT after reduced intensity conditioning (RIC) using CD3+/19+ depleted grafts (Federmann et al., 2011). Data showed similar results as compared with our study, including fast recovery of NK cells and fast immune reconstitution of the NK cell receptor repertoire. In addition, a similar decrease of NKG2A+ NK cells was seen post SCT. However, the expression of NKG2C was not evaluated. Nevertheless, this study confirms our findings that different graft manipulation methods may trigger differential NK cell reconstitution, which may be beneficial for transplant outcome. Previously, Gentilini *et al.* even showed a significant faster and sustained recovery of NK cells in a group of patients after RIC allogeneic SCT with CD3+/CD19+ depleted grafts in comparison with patients with myeloablative allogeneic SCT with CD34+ selected grafts combined with adoptive NK cell infusion two days post SCT (Gentilini et al., 2007).

Overall, these studies suggest that the use of NK cell rich grafts is favourable for the facilitation of fast and sustained NK cell recovery and differential reconstitution of the NK cell receptor repertoire, which may lead to improved donor NK cell alloreactivity in the GVL direction (Eissens et al., 2010a). Further prospective comparisons of the different graft manipulation methods for allogeneic SCT in the HLA-matched or haploidentical setting are warranted for more detailed analysis of the impact of graft composition on immune reconstitution. Subsequently, the impact of adoptive NK cell infusions after allogeneic SCT for boosting GVL reactivity needs to be studied in further detail.

4.2 Skewing donor NK cell alloreactivity before SCT

In allogeneic SCT, donor NK cell alloreactivity can be facilitated by allowing mismatches for specific HLA molecules (e.g. HLA-C) between donor and recipient. This is referred to as the "ligand-ligand" model. The introduction of certain HLA mismatches has been shown to induce NK cell-mediated GVL reactivity, without inducing severe GVHD, and to contribute to decreased relapse, better engraftment and improved overall survival (Ruggeri et al., 1999; Ruggeri et al., 2004; Ruggeri et al., 2007). However, others state that the induction of NK cell alloreactivity is not dependent on HLA mismatching, but is rather induced by the presence of an inhibitory KIR in the donor's genotype with the absence of the corresponding KIR-ligand in the recipient's HLA repertoire ("receptor-ligand" model) (Hsu et al., 2005; Leung et al., 2004; Leung et al., 2005). This makes the exploitation of NK cell alloreactivity not only feasible for HLA-mismatched settings, but may also be promising for HLA-matched settings.

For further exploitation, however, the "licensing/education" model needs to be considered as well. Upon maturation, NK cells obtain their "license to kill" through interactions of inhibitory KIRs with self-HLA class I molecules (Parham, 2006; Raulet & Vance, 2006; Vivier et al., 2008). NK cells that fail to interact with self-HLA class I molecules remain functionally immature and will reside in a hyporesponsive state. Recently, it was shown that the strength of response by an individual NK cell is even quantitatively controlled by the extent of inhibitory signals that are received from HLA class I molecules during NK cell education (Brodin et al., 2009). Concerning adoptive transfer of mature NK cells for immunotherapeutic purposes, this suggests that the presence of inhibitory KIR on donor NK cells in absence of its cognate ligand in the recipient ("receptor-ligand" model) as well as the HLA-background of the donor NK cells ("licensing/education" model) are two key factors that need to be taken into account for the successful exploitation of alloreactive donor NK cell responses.

4.3 Interference by immunosuppressive drugs

For optimal NK cell-mediated GVL reactivity, NK cells need to be fully functional in the early phase after allogeneic SCT, despite that at this stage a high level of immunosuppressive treatment is given. Among the various immunosuppressive drugs (ISDs), cyclosporin A (CsA), rapamycin (Rapa) and mycophenolate mofetil (MMF) have successfully been applied for the prevention of GVHD (Cutler et al., 2007; Haentzschel et al., 2008; Neumann et al., 2005; Schleuning et al., 2008; Vogelsang & Arai, 2001). Therefore, we studied the influence of CsA, Rapa and mycophenolic acid (MPA; the active metabolite of MMF) on NK cell phenotype and function in an *in vitro* cytokine-based culture system (Eissens et al., 2010b). Results showed that the modulation of the NK cell receptor repertoire during culture was arrested by Rapa and MPA treatment. This was reflected in the cytolytic activity, as MPA- and Rapa-treated NK cells, in contrast to CsA-treated NK cells, lost their cytotoxicity against leukemic target cells. In contrast, IFN-γ production was not only impaired by MPA and Rapa, but also by CsA upon target encounter. A recent study, however, suggested that IFN-γ production upon target encounter may be limited to the CD56[dim] NK cell subset, whereas the CD56[bright] NK cell subset produces IFN-γ upon cytokine-stimulation (Fauriat et al., 2010). Thus, as CD56[bright] NK cells were still abundantly present in the CsA-treated cultures, in contrast to MPA- and Rapa-treated cultures, the IFN-γ production upon cytokine stimulation may largely be preserved after CsA treatment. This was confirmed in a study showing sustained IFN-γ production by CsA-treated NK cell cultures upon IL-12 and IL-18 stimulation (Wang et al., 2007), suggesting that IFN-γ-mediated GVL reactivity after allogeneic SCT should remain intact when using CsA as GVHD prophylaxis.

Our findings on the effect of CsA and MPA on the cytolytic response by *in vitro* cytokine-stimulated NK cells are in concert with previous findings on this subject (Ohata et al., 2011). Besides CsA and MPA, they also evaluated the effect of tacrolimus (TAC) and methotrexate (MTX), which are also successfully used as GVHD prophylaxis after allogeneic SCT (Alyea et al., 2008; Cutler et al., 2007; Ho et al., 2009). Both ISDs did not interfere with NK cell-mediated cytolytic activity against different leukemic cell lines. However, a dose range of each ISD is lacking in this study, which would be more appropriate when studying the effect of ISDs on NK cell functionality.

Overall, these *in vitro* studies clearly suggest that the choice of immunosuppressive treatment might affect the outcome of NK cell immunotherapy *in vivo* after transplantation. Additional studies on NK cell phenotype and function of patients after allogeneic SCT using different immunosuppressive strategies are warranted to survey the *in vivo* effect of the different immunosuppressive regimens in more detail.

4.4 Clinical grade NK cell products for adoptive cancer immunotherapy
4.4.1 Development of clinical grade NK cell products
The facilitation of donor NK cell alloreactivity is not restricted to HLA-matched/mismatched allogeneic SCT, but may also be exploited for adoptive immunotherapy in non-transplantation settings. Previously, several clinical studies have examined the feasibility of allogeneic NK cells for adoptive immunotherapy using allogeneic NK cells selected from leukapheresis products by immunomagnetic beads selection protocols (Iyengar et al., 2003; Klingemann & Martinson, 2004; Koehl et al., 2005; McKenna, Jr. et al., 2007; Meyer-Monard et al., 2009; Passweg et al., 2004). In all these studies, the adoptive transfer of allogeneic NK cells proved to be safe and well tolerated by patients. Nevertheless, for optimal exploitation of NK cell adoptive immunotherapy, the development of innovative strategies producing allogeneic NK cell products with high cell numbers, high purity and functionality are needed. In this respect, recent studies have developed culture systems for large scale *ex vivo* expansion of allogeneic NK cells using either hematopoietic progenitor cells from bone marrow or UCB (Carayol et al., 1998; Kao et al., 2007; Miller et al., 1992). However, most of these culture systems are unsuitable for clinical application due to the use of animal sera, animal-derived proteins, and/or supportive feeder cells.

Previously, in our centre a cytokine-based method for high log-scale *ex vivo* expansion of functional allogeneic NK cells from hematopoietic stem and progenitor cells from umbilical cord blood (UCB) using a novel clinical grade medium was developed (Spanholtz et al., 2010). The *ex vivo* generated NK cell products are of high purity and contain developmentally mature NK cell populations expressing inhibitory NKG2A and KIRs, and a variety of stimulatory receptors. Furthermore, these NK cell products show the ability to efficiently kill myeloid leukemia and melanoma tumour cell lines. The findings in this study provide an important advance for the clinical application of *ex vivo* generated NK cell products to be exploited for adoptive immunotherapy either following allogeneic SCT for boosting NK cell-mediated GVL reactivity or in the non-transplant setting following lymphodepleting immunosuppressive regimens. In addition, human *in vitro* studies and *in vivo* evidence in mice suggest that NK cell-based immunotherapy may also be beneficial for patients with melanoma or renal cell carcinoma when applied in the setting of the "receptor-ligand" model (Burke et al., 2010; Igarashi et al., 2004; Lakshmikanth et al., 2009). Overall, further exploitation of this culture system may provide a broad clinical application for NK cell-based immunotherapy against hematological and non-hematological malignancies.

4.4.2 Clinical feasibility of *ex vivo* generated NK cells: a phase I trial
Recently, the NK cell generation protocol described by Spanholtz et al. was transferred to clinical applicable conditions (Spanholtz et al., 2011) and medical ethical approval was given to study the feasibility of adoptive transfer of *ex vivo* generated NK cell products in elderly patients diagnosed with poor prognosis AML (Spanholtz et al., 2010). In the second quartile

of 2011, a phase I dose-escalating study has started for a group of 12 AML patients (age >65 years), not eligible for allogeneic SCT, who have achieved clinical remission after standard remission-induction chemotherapy and who have completed consolidation chemotherapy. Patients will receive allogeneic NK cells generated *ex vivo* from CD34⁺ UCB cells in a single escalating dose up to 10x10⁷ donor NK cells/kg body weight after completing standard chemotherapy and preparative immunosuppressive conditioning consisting of fludarabine and cyclophosphamide in order to prevent rejection. The primary goal is to evaluate the safety and dose-limiting toxicity of adoptive transfer of the allogeneic *ex vivo* generated NK cells. Secondly, the *in vivo* lifespan of the adoptively transferred allogeneic NK cells will be evaluated together with an assessment of NK cell-mediated GVL reactivity in study participants.

5. Towards NK cell immunotherapy

Within the last decade, different NK cell-based immunotherapy strategies have successfully been developed. They have either already been proved safe in clinical phase I/II trials or are currently under clinical evaluation. Today, applications for NK cell-based immunotherapy can generally be divided into three main categories: (1) the use of enriched NK cell grafts for allogeneic SCT; (2) administering NK-DLI after allogeneic SCT and; (3) adoptive NK cell transfer in non-transplantation settings (Figure 3).

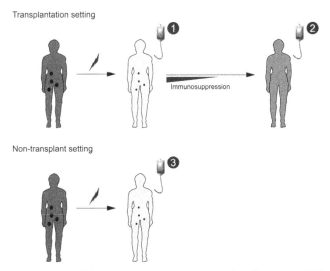

Fig. 3. Applications for NK cell-based immunotherapy. In the allogeneic SCT setting, patients are first treated with a conditioning regimen to eradicate healthy hematopoietic recipient cells and to minimize the tumour burden within the recipient. Subsequently, enriched NK cell grafts (1) and/or NK-DLI (2) may be applied in the further course of allogeneic SCT in order to facilitate alloreactive donor NK cell-mediated GVL reactivity. In the non-transplant setting (e.g. patients no longer eligible for allogeneic SCT or with solid tumours), adoptive NK cell transfer can be used as a NK cell-based immunotherapeutic strategy in patients after completing standard chemotherapy and preparative immunosuppressive conditioning in order to prevent rejection.

5.1 Allogeneic SCT setting

The use of enriched NK cell grafts for allogeneic SCT has shown to be beneficial for transplant outcome and provides enhanced GVL reactivity directly after transplantation as compared with conventional grafts that lack NK cells (Bethge et al., 2006; Eissens et al., 2010a; Kim et al., 2006). In addition, the head start in GVL reactivity may lead to better outcomes in terms of infectious events and overall survival after allogeneic SCT (Kim et al., 2005a). Altogether, this indicates the immunotherapeutic value of the exploitation of donor NK cells in the allogeneic SCT setting. In order to further increase the beneficial effects of such NK cell-based immunotherapy strategies in the setting of allogeneic SCT, donor NK cells can also be administered as part of the conditioning regimen prior to transplantation instead of, or in combination with, the use of enriched NK cell grafts. This can have three potential beneficial effects. First, NK cell-mediated GVL reactivity could provide anti-tumour activity prior to allogeneic SCT (Lundqvist et al., 2007; Ruggeri et al., 2002). Second, NK cell-mediated depletion of host dendritic cells before transplantation could prevent the development of acute GVHD allowing for a less stringent depletion of T cells in the graft (Lundqvist et al., 2007; Ruggeri et al., 2002). Third, NK cells may facilitate better engraftment through eradication of host T cells, thereby reducing the need for toxic myeloablative regimens and shortening the neutropenic period (Ruggeri et al., 2002). However, to be able to implement the combinatorial strategy of NK cell infusions as part of the conditioning regimen together with the use of enriched NK cell grafts in the clinic, the necessary amount of NK cells used for infusion prior to allogeneic SCT to provoke beneficial immunotherapeutic effects still needs to be established. Insufficient numbers may cause the necessity to choose between the use of NK cell infusions as part of the conditioning regimen and the use of enriched NK cell grafts. In this respect, also in case of the combinatorial strategy, it is important that more research is performed on the effects of conditioning and immunosuppressive regimens on NK cells in exploiting NK cell-mediated (GVL) reactivity in the allogeneic SCT setting.

The use donor T cells for DLI after allogeneic SCT has developed into an effective treatment of recurrent hematological malignancy as well as prophylactic treatment in high-risk leukemia and lymphoma (Kolb et al., 2004). Still, the main risk of T-DLI is the induction of life-threatening GVHD. To minimize the risk of GVHD, studies have been initiated to modify conventional DLI by using donor NK cells instead of donor T cells (Passweg et al., 2004; Passweg et al., 2005). Additionally, the administration of NK-DLI may facilitate engraftment and induce NK cell-mediated GVL reactivity (Passweg et al., 2004; Passweg et al., 2005). Although no firm conclusions can be drawn on the clinical efficacy of NK-DLI after allogeneic SCT at this point, data indicate that NK-DLI is safe and well tolerated, and can generate GVL reactivity and long-term remission in some patients after leukemia relapse. As non-malignant tissues generally do not overexpress ligands for activating NK cell receptors, NK-DLI should not cause GVHD (Bottino et al., 2005; Ruggeri et al., 2004; Ruggeri et al., 2006). Until now, NK-DLI has been tested in the haploidentical SCT setting. Thus, further research on the efficacy of NK-DLI in the HLA-matched SCT setting is warranted.

5.2 Non-transplant settings

In non-transplant settings, donor NK cells can be exploited for immunotherapeutic strategies for the treatment of hematological and non-hematological malignancies.

Previously, Miller et al. showed that haploidentical donor NK cell infusions after high-dose cyclophosphamide and fludarabine treatment resulted in long-term survival and *in vivo* expansion of donor NK cells in patients with metastatic melanoma (n=10), metastatic renal cell carcinoma (n=13), refractory non-Hodgkin's disease (n=1), and poor-prognosis AML (n=19) (Miller et al., 2005). The *in vivo* NK cell expansion was associated with increased levels of endogenous IL-15, which were possibly responsible for driving the survival and proliferation of donor NK cells. In general, the donor NK cell infusions were well tolerated without evidence for the induction of GVHD. Furthermore, 5 out of 19 patients with poor-prognosis AML achieved complete remission. Only 4 of the 19 AML patients were KIR-ligand (HLA) mismatched in the graft-versus-host direction. Interestingly, out of these 4 patients, 3 achieved complete remission. These findings indicate that haploidentical donor NK cells can persist and expand *in vivo* and may have a role in the treatment of (non-)hematological malignancies in non-transplant settings or in combination with allogeneic SCT. In addition, when using haploidentical donors the choice of a KIR-ligand mismatched donor, based on the "ligand-ligand" model, may be needed to obtain successful results in future clinical trials (Miller et al., 2005). In case of HLA-matched donors, the choice of a "receptor-ligand" mismatched donor is preferred.

In parallel, adoptive transfers are currently being performed with the NK cell line NK-92. This cell line can be cultured under good manufacturing practice (GMP) conditions and shows significant cytotoxicity against several tumour cell lines (Tam et al., 2003). Infusions of NK-92 cells have been administered to more than 20 patients with advanced renal-cell carcinoma and malignant melanoma. This proved to be safe and generated anti-tumor effects in some cases (Klingemann, 2005). Furthermore, NK-92 cells can easily be obtained in high numbers during GMP culture providing sufficient amounts of cells for adoptive immunotherapeutic strategies. However, to prevent that the success of NK cell adoptive immunotherapy is solely based on the use of one NK cell line and the use of donor NK cells are still preferred, recent studies have developed culture systems for large scale *ex vivo* expansion of allogeneic NK cells using either hematopoietic progenitor cells from bone marrow or UCB (Carayol et al., 1998; Kao et al., 2007; Miller et al., 1992; Spanholtz et al., 2010). After transferring these culture systems to GMP conditions, these allogeneic donor NK cells may also be proven safe for use in NK cell adoptive immunotherapy.

6. Conclusion

Several issues remain crucial for the development and implementation of successful NK cell-based immunotherapy in the future. In the non-transplant setting , these include issues relating to the type of NK cell preparation to be used (activation, degree of enrichment and possible selection or skewing of specific subpopulations), criteria for donor selection ("ligand-ligand" versus "receptor-ligand" model, KIR genotyping and phenotyping, and size of the alloreactive subset), conditioning of patients prior to immunotherapy, clinical context of therapy, criteria for patient selection, and strategies for the identification of susceptible tumours within patient groups. Besides these issues, the effects of immunosuppressive regimens given after allogeneic SCT are also important when implementing NK cell-based immunotherapy in the setting of allogeneic SCT.

7. References

Alyea, E.P.; Li, S.; Kim, H.T.; Cutler, C.; Ho, V.; Soiffer, R.J. & Antin, J.H. (2008). Sirolimus, Tacrolimus, and Low-Dose Methotrexate as Graft-versus-Host Disease Prophylaxis in Related and Unrelated Donor Reduced-Intensity Conditioning Allogeneic Peripheral Blood Stem Cell Transplantation. *Biology of Blood and Marrow Transplantation,* 14(8), 920-926.

Arnon, T.I.; Achdout, H.; Levi, O.; Markel, G.; Saleh, N.; Katz, G.; Gazit, R.; Gonen-Gross, T.; Hanna, J.; Nahari, E.; Porgador, A.; Honigman, A.; Plachter, B.; Mevorach, D.; Wolf, D.G. & Mandelboim, O. (2005). Inhibition of the NKp30 activating receptor by pp65 of human cytomegalovirus. *Nature Immunology,* 6(5), 515-523.

Arnon, T.I.; Lev, M.; Katz, G.; Chernobrov, Y.; Porgador, A. & Mandelboim, O. (2001). Recognition of viral hemagglutinins by NKp44 but not by NKp30. *European Journal of Immunology,* 31(9), 2680-2689.

Barge, R.M.; Osanto, S.; Marijt, W.A.; Starrenburg, C.W.; Fibbe, W.E.; Nortier, J.W.; Falkenburg, J.H. & Willemze, R. (2003). Minimal GVHD following in-vitro T cell-depleted allogeneic stem cell transplantation with reduced-intensity conditioning allowing subsequent infusions of donor lymphocytes in patients with hematological malignancies and solid tumors. *Experimental Hematology,* 31(10), 865-872.

Bauer, S.; Groh, V.; Wu, J.; Steinle, A.; Phillips, J.H.; Lanier, L.L. & Spies, T. (1999). Activation of NK cells and T cells by NKG2D, a receptor for stress-inducible MICA. *Science,* 285(5428), 727-729.

Bethge, W.A.; Haegele, M.; Faul, C.; Lang, P.; Schumm, M.; Bornhauser, M.; Handgretinger, R. & Kanz, L. (2006). Haploidentical allogeneic hematopoietic cell transplantation in adults with reduced-intensity conditioning and CD3/CD19 depletion: fast engraftment and low toxicity. *Experimental Hematology,* 34(12), 1746-1752.

Biassoni, R.; Cantoni, C.; Falco, M.; Verdiani, S.; Bottino, C.; Vitale, M.; Conte, R.; Poggi, A.; Moretta, A. & Moretta, L. (1996). The human leukocyte antigen (HLA)-C-specific "activatory" or "inhibitory" natural killer cell receptors display highly homologous extracellular domains but differ in their transmembrane and intracytoplasmic portions. *Journal of Experimental Medicine,* 183(2), 645-650.

Biassoni, R.; Cantoni, C.; Pende, D.; Sivori, S.; Parolini, S.; Vitale, M.; Bottino, C. & Moretta, A. (2001). Human natural killer cell receptors and co-receptors. *Immunological Reviews,* 181, 203-214.

Bossi, G. & Griffiths, G.M. (1999). Degranulation plays an essential part in regulating cell surface expression of Fas ligand in T cells and natural killer cells. *Nature Medicine,* 5(1), 90-96.

Bottino, C.; Biassoni, R.; Millo, R.; Moretta, L. & Moretta, A. (2000). The human natural cytotoxicity receptors (NCR) that induce HLA class I-independent NK cell triggering. *Human Immunology,* 61(1), 1-6.

Bottino, C.; Castriconi, R.; Moretta, L. & Moretta, A. (2005). Cellular ligands of activating NK receptors. *Trends in Immunology,* 26(4), 221-226.

Bottino, C.; Sivori, S.; Vitale, M.; Cantoni, C.; Falco, M.; Pende, D.; Morelli, L.; Augugliaro, R.; Semenzato, G.; Biassoni, R.; Moretta, L. & Moretta, A. (1996). A novel surface molecule homologous to the p58/p50 family of receptors is selectively expressed on a subset of human natural killer cells and induces both triggering of cell functions and proliferation. *European Journal of Immunology*, 26(8), 1816-1824.

Braud, V.M.; Allan, D.S.; O'Callaghan, C.A.; Soderstrom, K.; D'Andrea, A.; Ogg, G.S.; Lazetic, S.; Young, N.T.; Bell, J.I.; Phillips, J.H.; Lanier, L.L. & McMichael, A.J. (1998). HLA-E binds to natural killer cell receptors CD94/NKG2A, B and C. *Nature*, 391(6669), 795-799.

Braud, V.M.; Jones, E.Y. & McMichael, A. (1997). The human major histocompatibility complex class Ib molecule HLA- E binds signal sequence-derived peptides with primary anchor residues at positions 2 and 9. *European Journal of Immunology*, 27(5), 1164-1169.

Brodin, P.; Lakshmikanth, T.; Johansson, S.; Karre, K. & Hoglund, P. (2009). The strength of inhibitory input during education quantitatively tunes the functional responsiveness of individual natural killer cells. *Blood*, 113(11), 2434-2441.

Burke, S.; Lakshmikanth, T.; Colucci, F. & Carbone, E. (2010). New views on natural killer cell-based immunotherapy for melanoma treatment. *Trends in Immunology*, 31(9), 339-345.

Burshtyn, D.N.; Scharenberg, A.M.; Wagtmann, N.; Rajagopalan, S.; Berrada, K.; Yi, T.; Kinet, J.P. & Long, E.O. (1996). Recruitment of tyrosine phosphatase HCP by the killer cell inhibitor receptor. *Immunity*, 4(1), 77-85.

Cantoni, C.; Bottino, C.; Vitale, M.; Pessino, A.; Augugliaro, R.; Malaspina, A.; Parolini, S.; Moretta, L.; Moretta, A. & Biassoni, R. (1999). NKp44, a triggering receptor involved in tumor cell lysis by activated human natural killer cells, is a novel member of the immunoglobulin superfamily. *Journal of Experimental Medicine*, 189(5), 787-796.

Carayol, G.; Robin, C.; Bourhis, J.H.; naceur-Griscelli, A.; Chouaib, S.; Coulombel, L. & Caignard, A. (1998). NK cells differentiated from bone marrow, cord blood and peripheral blood stem cells exhibit similar phenotype and functions. *European Journal of Immunology*, 28(6), 1991-2002.

Cervantes, F.; Pierson, B.A.; McGlave, P.B.; Verfaillie, C.M. & Miller, J.S. (1996). Autologous activated natural killer cells suppress primitive chronic myelogenous leukemia progenitors in long-term culture. *Blood*, 87(6), 2476-2485.

Cook, M.A.; Milligan, D.W.; Fegan, C.D.; Darbyshire, P.J.; Mahendra, P.; Craddock, C.F.; Moss, P.A. & Briggs, D.C. (2004). The impact of donor KIR and patient HLA-C genotypes on outcome following HLA-identical sibling hematopoietic stem cell transplantation for myeloid leukemia. *Blood*, 103(4), 1521-1526.

Cooley, S.; Xiao, F.; Pitt, M.; Gleason, M.; McCullar, V.; Bergemann, T.; McQueen, K.L.; Guethlein, L.A.; Parham, P. & Miller, J.S. (2007). A subpopulation of human peripheral blood NK cells that lacks inhibitory receptors for self MHC is developmentally immature. *Blood*, 110(2), 578-586.

Cooper, M.A.; Fehniger, T.A. & Caligiuri, M.A. (2001). The biology of human natural killer-cell subsets. *Trends in Immunology*, 22(11), 633-640.

Cosman, D.; Mullberg, J.; Sutherland, C.L.; Chin, W.; Armitage, R.; Fanslow, W.; Kubin, M. & Chalupny, N.J. (2001). ULBPs, novel MHC class I-related molecules, bind to CMV glycoprotein UL16 and stimulate NK cytotoxicity through the NKG2D receptor. *Immunity*, 14(2), 123-133.

Cutler, C.; Li, S.; Ho, V.T.; Koreth, J.; Alyea, E.; Soiffer, R.J. & Antin, J.H. (2007). Extended follow-up of methotrexate-free immunosuppression using sirolimus and tacrolimus in related and unrelated donor peripheral blood stem cell transplantation. *Blood,* 109(7), 3108-3114.

Das, H.; Groh, V.; Kuijl, C.; Sugita, M.; Morita, C.T.; Spies, T. & Bukowski, J.F. (2001). MICA engagement by human Vgamma2Vdelta2 T cells enhances their antigen-dependent effector function. *Immunity,* 15(1), 83-93.

Diefenbach, A.; Jamieson, A.M.; Liu, S.D.; Shastri, N. & Raulet, D.H. (2000). Ligands for the murine NKG2D receptor: expression by tumor cells and activation of NK cells and macrophages. *Nature Immunology,* 1(2), 119-126.

Eissens, D.N.; Schaap, N.P.; Preijers, F.W.; Dolstra, H.; van, C.B.; Schattenberg, A.V.; Joosten, I. & van der, M.A. (2010a). CD3(+)/CD19(+)-depleted grafts in HLA-matched allogeneic peripheral blood stem cell transplantation lead to early NK cell cytolytic responses and reduced inhibitory activity of NKG2A. *Leukemia,* 24(3), 583-591.

Eissens, D.N.; van der, M.A.; van, C.B.; Preijers, F.W. & Joosten, I. (2010b). Rapamycin and MPA, but not CsA, impair human NK cell cytotoxicity due to differential effects on NK cell phenotype. *American Journal of Transplantation,* 10(9), 1981-1990.

Farag, S.S. & Caligiuri, M.A. (2006). Human natural killer cell development and biology. *Blood Reviews,* 20(3), 123-137.

Farrell, H.; gli-Esposti, M.; Densley, E.; Cretney, E.; Smyth, M. & vis-Poynter, N. (2000). Cytomegalovirus MHC class I homologues and natural killer cells: an overview. *Microbes and Infection,* 2(5), 521-532.

Fauriat, C.; Just-Landi, S.; Mallet, F.; Arnoulet, C.; Sainty, D.; Olive, D. & Costello, R.T. (2007). Deficient expression of NCR in NK cells from acute myeloid leukemia: evolution during leukemia treatment and impact of leukemic cells in NCRdull phenotype induction. *Blood,* 109(1), 323-330.

Fauriat, C.; Moretta, A.; Olive, D. & Costello, R.T. (2005). Defective killing of dendritic cells by autologous natural killer cells from acute myeloid leukemia patients. *Blood,* 106(6), 2186-2188.

Fauriat, C.; Long, E.O.; Ljunggren, H.G. & Bryceson, Y.T. (2010). Regulation of human NK cell cytokine and chemokine production by target cell recognition. *Blood,* 115(11), 2167-2176.

Federmann, B.; Hagele, M.; Pfeiffer, M.; Wirths, S.; Schumm, M.; Faul, C.; Vogel, W.; Handgretinger, R.; Kanz, L. & Bethge, W.A. (2011). Immune reconstitution after haploidentical hematopoietic cell transplantation: impact of reduced intensity conditioning and CD3/CD19 depleted grafts. *Leukemia,* 25(1), 121-129.

Fernandez, N.C.; Treiner, E.; Vance, R.E.; Jamieson, A.M.; Lemieux, S. & Raulet, D.H. (2005). A subset of natural killer cells achieves self-tolerance without expressing inhibitory receptors specific for self-MHC molecules. *Blood,* 105(11), 4416-4423.

Franksson, L.; George, E.; Powis, S.; Butcher, G.; Howard, J. & Karre, K. (1993). Tumorigenicity conferred to lymphoma mutant by major histocompatibility complex-encoded transporter gene. *Journal of Experimental Medicine,* 177(1), 201-205.

Fry, A.M.; Lanier, L.L. & Weiss, A. (1996). Phosphotyrosines in the killer cell inhibitory receptor motif of NKB1 are required for negative signaling and for association with protein tyrosine phosphatase 1C. *Journal of Experimental Medicine,* 184(1), 295-300.

Gentilini, C.; Hägele, M.; Meussig, A.; Nogai, A.; Kliem, C.; Bartsch, K.; Bazara, N.; Vogel, W.; Faul, C.; Kanz, L.; Thiel, E.; Niederwieser, D.W.; Uharek, L. & Bethge, W.A. (2007). NK cell recovery and immune reconstitution after haploidentical hematopoietic cell transplantation using either CD34 selected grafts and adoptive NK cell transfer or CD3/CD19 depleted grafts: comparison of two strategies for NK cell based immunotherapy. *Blood (ASH Annual Meeting Abstracts)*, 110, 2988.

Giebel, S.; Nowak, I.; Wojnar, J.; Markiewicz, M.; Dziaczkowska, J.; Wylezol, I.; Krawczyk-Kulis, M.; Bloch, R.; Kusnierczyk, P. & Holowiecki, J. (2006). Impact of activating killer immunoglobulin-like receptor genotype on outcome of unrelated donor-hematopoietic cell transplantation. *Transplantation Proceedings*, 38(1), 287-291.

Groh, V.; Rhinehart, R.; Randolph-Habecker, J.; Topp, M.S.; Riddell, S.R. & Spies, T. (2001). Costimulation of CD8alphabeta T cells by NKG2D via engagement by MIC induced on virus-infected cells. *Nature Immunology*, 2(3), 255-260.

Guma, M.; Angulo, A.; Vilches, C.; Gomez-Lozano, N.; Malats, N. & Lopez-Botet, M. (2004). Imprint of human cytomegalovirus infection on the NK cell receptor repertoire. *Blood*, 104(12), 3664-3671.

Guma, M.; Budt, M.; Saez, A.; Brckalo, T.; Hengel, H.; Angulo, A. & Lopez-Botet, M. (2006). Expansion of CD94/NKG2C+ NK cells in response to human cytomegalovirus-infected fibroblasts. *Blood*, 107(9), 3624-3631.

Haentzschel, I.; Freiberg-Richter, J.; Platzbecker, U.; Kiani, A.; Schetelig, J.; Illmer, T.; Ehninger, G.; Schleyer, E. & Bornhauser, M. (2008). Targeting mycophenolate mofetil for graft-versus-host disease prophylaxis after allogeneic blood stem cell transplantation. *Bone Marrow Transplantation*, 42(2), 113-120.

Herberman, R.B. (1986). Natural killer cells. *Annual Review of Medicine*, 37, 347-352.

Ho, V.T.; Aldridge, J.; Kim, H.T.; Cutler, C.; Koreth, J.; Armand, P.; Antin, J.H.; Soiffer, R.J. & Alyea, E.P. (2009). Comparison of Tacrolimus and Sirolimus (Tac/Sir) versus Tacrolimus, Sirolimus, and Mini-Methotrexate (Tac/Sir/MTX) as Acute Graft-versus-Host Disease Prophylaxis after Reduced-Intensity Conditioning Allogeneic Peripheral Blood Stem Cell Transplantation. *Biology of Blood and Marrow Transplantation*, 15(7), 844-850.

Houchins, J.P.; Lanier, L.L.; Niemi, E.C.; Phillips, J.H. & Ryan, J.C. (1997). Natural killer cell cytolytic activity is inhibited by NKG2-A and activated by NKG2-C. *Journal of Immunology*, 158(8), 3603-3609.

Hsu, K.C.; Keever-Taylor, C.A.; Wilton, A.; Pinto, C.; Heller, G.; Arkun, K.; O'Reilly, R.J.; Horowitz, M.M. & Dupont, B. (2005). Improved outcome in HLA-identical sibling hematopoietic stem-cell transplantation for acute myelogenous leukemia predicted by KIR and HLA genotypes. *Blood*, 105(12), 4878-4884.

Igarashi, T.; Wynberg, J.; Srinivasan, R.; Becknell, B.; McCoy, J.P.; Takahashi, Y.; Suffredini, D.A.; Linehan, W.M.; Caligiuri, M.A. & Childs, R.W. (2004). Enhanced cytotoxicity of allogeneic NK cells with killer immunoglobulin -like receptor (KIR) ligand incompatibility against melanoma and renal cell carcinoma cells. *Blood*, 104(1), 170-177.

Iyengar, R.; Handgretinger, R.; Babarin-Dorner, A.; Leimig, T.; Otto, M.; Geiger, T.L.; Holladay, M.S.; Houston, J. & Leung, W. (2003). Purification of human natural killer cells using a clinical-scale immunomagnetic method. *Cytotherapy*, 5(6), 479-484.

Kao, I.T.; Yao, C.L.; Kong, Z.L.; Wu, M.L.; Chuang, T.L. & Hwang, S.M. (2007). Generation of natural killer cells from serum-free, expanded human umbilical cord blood CD34+ cells. *Stem Cells and Development,* 16(6), 1043-1051.

Kärre, K.; Ljunggren, H.G.; Piontek, G. & Kiessling, R. (1986a). Selective rejection of H-2-deficient lymphoma variants suggests alternative immune defence strategy. *Nature,* 319(6055), 675-678.

Kärre, K.; Ljunggren, H.G.; Piontek, G. & Kiessling, R. (1986b). Selective rejection of H-2-deficient lymphoma variants suggests alternative immune defence strategy. *Nature,* 319(6055), 675-678.

Kiessling, R.; Klein, E.; Pross, H. & Wigzell, H. (1975a). "Natural" killer cells in the mouse. II. Cytotoxic cells with specificity for mouse Moloney leukemia cells. Characteristics of the killer cell. *European Journal of Immunology,* 5(2), 117-121.

Kiessling, R.; Klein, E. & Wigzell, H. (1975b). "Natural" killer cells in the mouse. I. Cytotoxic cells with specificity for mouse Moloney leukemia cells. Specificity and distribution according to genotype. *European Journal of Immunology,* 5(2), 112-117.

Kim, D.H.; Sohn, S.K.; Lee, N.Y.; Baek, J.H.; Kim, J.G.; Won, D.I.; Suh, J.S.; Lee, K.B. & Shin, I.H. (2005a). Transplantation with higher dose of natural killer cells associated with better outcomes in terms of non-relapse mortality and infectious events after allogeneic peripheral blood stem cell transplantation from HLA-matched sibling donors. *European Journal of Hematology,* 75(4), 299-308.

Kim, S.; Poursine-Laurent, J.; Truscott, S.M.; Lybarger, L.; Song, Y.J.; Yang, L.; French, A.R.; Sunwoo, J.B.; Lemieux, S.; Hansen, T.H. & Yokoyama, W.M. (2005b). Licensing of natural killer cells by host major histocompatibility complex class I molecules. *Nature,* 436(7051), 709-713.

Kim, D.H.; Won, D.I.; Lee, N.Y.; Sohn, S.K.; Suh, J.S. & Lee, K.B. (2006). Non-CD34(+) Cells, Especially CD8(+) Cytotoxic T Cells and CD56(+) Natural Killer Cells, Rather Than CD34 Cells, Predict Early Engraftment and Better Transplantation Outcomes in Patients with Hematologic Malignancies after Allogeneic Peripheral Stem Cell Transplantation. *Biology of Blood and Marrow Transplantation,* 12(7), 719-728.

Klingemann, H.G. (2005). Natural killer cell-based immunotherapeutic strategies. *Cytotherapy,* 7(1), 16-22.

Klingemann, H.G. & Martinson, J. (2004). Ex vivo expansion of natural killer cells for clinical applications. *Cytotherapy,* 6(1), 15-22.

Koehl, U.; Esser, R.; Zimmermann, S.; Tonn, T.; Kotchetkov, R.; Bartling, T.; Sorensen, J.; Gruttner, H.P.; Bader, P.; Seifried, E.; Martin, H.; Lang, P.; Passweg, J.R.; Klingebiel, T. & Schwabe, D. (2005). Ex vivo expansion of highly purified NK cells for immunotherapy after haploidentical stem cell transplantation in children. *Klinische Pädiatrie,* 217(6), 345-350.

Kolb, H.J.; Simoes, B. & Schmid, C. (2004). Cellular immunotherapy after allogeneic stem cell transplantation in hematologic malignancies. *Current Opinion in Oncology,* 16(2), 167-173.

Lakshmikanth, T.; Burke, S.; Ali, T.H.; Kimpfler, S.; Ursini, F.; Ruggeri, L.; Capanni, M.; Umansky, V.; Paschen, A.; Sucker, A.; Pende, D.; Groh, V.; Biassoni, R.; Hoglund, P.; Kato, M.; Shibuya, K.; Schadendorf, D.; Anichini, A.; Ferrone, S.; Velardi, A.; Karre, K.; Shibuya, A.; Carbone, E. & Colucci, F. (2009). NCRs and DNAM-1 mediate NK cell recognition and lysis of human and mouse melanoma cell lines in vitro and in vivo. *Journal of Clinical Investigation,* 119(5), 1251-1263.

Lanier, L.L.; Corliss, B.C.; Wu, J.; Leong, C. & Phillips, J.H. (1998). Immunoreceptor DAP12 bearing a tyrosine-based activation motif is involved in activating NK cells. *Nature,* 391(6668), 703-707.

Lanier, L.L.; Ruitenberg, J.J. & Phillips, J.H. (1988). Functional and biochemical analysis of CD16 antigen on natural killer cells and granulocytes. *Journal of Immunology,* 141(10), 3478-3485.

Le, D.E.; Vely, F.; Olcese, L.; Cambiaggi, A.; Guia, S.; Krystal, G.; Gervois, N.; Moretta, A.; Jotereau, F. & Vivier, E. (1998). Inhibition of antigen-induced T cell response and antibody-induced NK cell cytotoxicity by NKG2A: association of NKG2A with SHP-1 and SHP-2 protein-tyrosine phosphatases. *European Journal of Immunology,* 28(1), 264-276.

Leung, W.; Iyengar, R.; Triplett, B.; Turner, V.; Behm, F.G.; Holladay, M.S.; Houston, J. & Handgretinger, R. (2005). Comparison of killer Ig-like receptor genotyping and phenotyping for selection of allogeneic blood stem cell donors. *Journal of Immunology,* 174(10), 6540-6545.

Leung, W.; Iyengar, R.; Turner, V.; Lang, P.; Bader, P.; Conn, P.; Niethammer, D. & Handgretinger, R. (2004). Determinants of antileukemia effects of allogeneic NK cells. *Journal of Immunology,* 172(1), 644-650.

Ljunggren, H.G. & Kärre, K. (1990). In search of the 'missing self': MHC molecules and NK cell recognition. *Immunology Today,* 11(7), 237-244.

Ljunggren, H.G.; Sturmhofel, K.; Wolpert, E.; Hammerling, G.J. & Kärre, K. (1990). Transfection of beta 2-microglobulin restores IFN-mediated protection from natural killer cell lysis in YAC-1 lymphoma variants. *Journal of Immunology,* 145(1), 380-386.

Lundqvist, A.; McCoy, J.P.; Samsel, L. & Childs, R. (2007). Reduction of GVHD and enhanced antitumor effects after adoptive infusion of alloreactive Ly49-mismatched NK cells from MHC-matched donors. *Blood,* 109(8), 3603-3606.

Mandelboim, O.; Lieberman, N.; Lev, M.; Paul, L.; Arnon, T.I.; Bushkin, Y.; Davis, D.M.; Strominger, J.L.; Yewdell, J.W. & Porgador, A. (2001). Recognition of haemagglutinins on virus-infected cells by NKp46 activates lysis by human NK cells. *Nature,* 409(6823), 1055-1060.

McKenna, D.H., Jr.; Sumstad, D.; Bostrom, N.; Kadidlo, D.M.; Fautsch, S.; McNearney, S.; Dewaard, R.; McGlave, P.B.; Weisdorf, D.J.; Wagner, J.E.; McCullough, J. & Miller, J.S. (2007). Good manufacturing practices production of natural killer cells for immunotherapy: a six-year single-institution experience. *Transfusion,* 47(3), 520-528.

Meyer-Monard, S.; Passweg, J.; Siegler, U.; Kalberer, C.; Koehl, U.; Rovo, A.; Halter, J.; Stern, M.; Heim, D.; ois Gratwohl, J.R. & Tichelli, A. (2009). Clinical-grade purification of natural killer cells in haploidentical hematopoietic stem cell transplantation. *Transfusion,* 49(2), 362-371.

Miller, J.S.; Soignier, Y.; Panoskaltsis-Mortari, A.; McNearney, S.A.; Yun, G.H.; Fautsch, S.K.; McKenna, D.; Le, C.; Defor, T.E.; Burns, L.J.; Orchard, P.J.; Blazar, B.R.; Wagner, J.E.; Slungaard, A.; Weisdorf, D.J.; Okazaki, I.J. & McGlave, P.B. (2005). Successful adoptive transfer and in vivo expansion of human haploidentical NK cells in patients with cancer. *Blood,* 105(8), 3051-3057.

Miller, J.S.; Verfaillie, C. & McGlave, P. (1992). The generation of human natural killer cells from CD34+/DR- primitive progenitors in long-term bone marrow culture. *Blood,* 80(9), 2182-2187.

Moretta, A.; Poggi, A.; Pende, D.; Tripodi, G.; Orengo, A.M.; Pella, N.; Augugliaro, R.; Bottino, C.; Ciccone, E. & Moretta, L. (1991). CD69-mediated pathway of lymphocyte activation: anti-CD69 monoclonal antibodies trigger the cytolytic activity of different lymphoid effector cells with the exception of cytolytic T lymphocytes expressing T cell receptor alpha/beta. *Journal of Experimental Medicine,* 174(6), 1393-1398.

Moretta, A.; Sivori, S.; Vitale, M.; Pende, D.; Morelli, L.; Augugliaro, R.; Bottino, C. & Moretta, L. (1995). Existence of both inhibitory (p58) and activatory (p50) receptors for HLA-C molecules in human natural killer cells. *Journal of Experimental Medicine,* 182(3), 875-884.

Neumann, F.; Graef, T.; Tapprich, C.; Vaupel, M.; Steidl, U.; Germing, U.; Fenk, R.; Hinke, A.; Haas, R. & Kobbe, G. (2005). Cyclosporine A and Mycophenolate Mofetil vs Cyclosporine A and Methotrexate for graft-versus-host disease prophylaxis after stem cell transplantation from HLA-identical siblings. *Bone Marrow Transplantation,* 35(11), 1089-1093.

Ohata, K.; Espinoza, J.L.; Lu, X.; Kondo, Y. & Nakao, S. (2011). Mycophenolic Acid inhibits natural killer cell proliferation and cytotoxic function: a possible disadvantage of including mycophenolate mofetil in the graft-versus-host disease prophylaxis regimen. *Biology of Blood and Marrow Transplantation,* 17(2), 205-213.

Olcese, L.; Lang, P.; Vely, F.; Cambiaggi, A.; Marguet, D.; Blery, M.; Hippen, K.L.; Biassoni, R.; Moretta, A.; Moretta, L.; Cambier, J.C. & Vivier, E. (1996). Human and mouse killer-cell inhibitory receptors recruit PTP1C and PTP1D protein tyrosine phosphatases. *Journal of Immunology,* 156(12), 4531-4534.

Olson, J.A.; Leveson-Gower, D.B.; Gill, S.; Baker, J.; Beilhack, A. & Negrin, R.S. (2010). NK cells mediate reduction of GVHD by inhibiting activated, alloreactive T cells while retaining GVT effects. *Blood,* 115(21), 4293-4301.

Orr, M.T.; Murphy, W.J. & Lanier, L.L. (2010). 'Unlicensed' natural killer cells dominate the response to cytomegalovirus infection. *Nature Immunoly,* 11(4), 321-327.

Papamichail, M.; Perez, S.A.; Gritzapis, A.D. & Baxevanis, C.N. (2004). Natural killer lymphocytes: biology, development, and function. *Cancer Immunology, Immunotherapy,* 53(3), 176-186.

Parham, P. (2005). MHC class I molecules and KIRs in human history, health and survival. *Nature Reviews Immunology,* 5(3), 201-214.

Parham, P. (2006). Taking license with natural killer cell maturation and repertoire development. *Immunological Reviews,* 214, 155-160.

Passweg, J.R.; Stern, M.; Koehl, U.; Uharek, L. & Tichelli, A. (2005). Use of natural killer cells in hematopoetic stem cell transplantation. *Bone Marrow Transplantation,* 35(7), 637-643.

Passweg, J.R.; Tichelli, A.; Meyer-Monard, S.; Heim, D.; Stern, M.; Kuhne, T.; Favre, G. & Gratwohl, A. (2004). Purified donor NK-lymphocyte infusion to consolidate engraftment after haploidentical stem cell transplantation. *Leukemia,* 18(11), 1835-1838.

Pawelec, G.; Da, S.P.; Max, H.; Kalbacher, H.; Schmidt, H.; Bruserud, O.; Zugel, U.; Baier, W.; Rehbein, A. & Pohla, H. (1995). Relative roles of natural killer- and T cell-mediated anti-leukemia effects in chronic myelogenous leukemia patients treated with interferon-alpha. *Leukemia and Lymphoma,* 18(5-6), 471-478.

Peggs, K.S.; Thomson, K.; Hart, D.P.; Geary, J.; Morris, E.C.; Yong, K.; Goldstone, A.H.; Linch, D.C. & Mackinnon, S. (2004). Dose-escalated donor lymphocyte infusions following reduced intensity transplantation: toxicity, chimerism, and disease responses. *Blood,* 103(4), 1548-1556.

Pende, D.; Cantoni, C.; Rivera, P.; Vitale, M.; Castriconi, R.; Marcenaro, S.; Nanni, M.; Biassoni, R.; Bottino, C.; Moretta, A. & Moretta, L. (2001). Role of NKG2D in tumor cell lysis mediated by human NK cells: cooperation with natural cytotoxicity receptors and capability of recognizing tumors of nonepithelial origin. *European Journal of Immunology.*

Pende, D.; Parolini, S.; Pessino, A.; Sivori, S.; Augugliaro, R.; Morelli, L.; Marcenaro, E.; Accame, L.; Malaspina, A.; Biassoni, R.; Bottino, C.; Moretta, L. & Moretta, A. (1999). Identification and molecular characterization of NKp30, a novel triggering receptor involved in natural cytotoxicity mediated by human natural killer cells. *Journal of Experimental Medicine,* 190(10), 1505-1516.

Pierson, B.A. & Miller, J.S. (1996). CD56+bright and CD56+dim natural killer cells in patients with chronic myelogenous leukemia progressively decrease in number, respond less to stimuli that recruit clonogenic natural killer cells, and exhibit decreased proliferation on a per cell basis. *Blood,* 88(6), 2279-2287.

Raulet, D.H. & Vance, R.E. (2006). Self-tolerance of natural killer cells. *Nature Reviews Immunology,* 6(7), 520-531.

Raulet, D.H.; Vance, R.E. & McMahon, C.W. (2001). Regulation of the natural killer cell receptor repertoire. *Annual Review of Immunology,* 19, 291-330.

Ruggeri, L.; Aversa, F.; Martelli, M.F. & Velardi, A. (2006). Allogeneic hematopoietic transplantation and natural killer cell recognition of missing self. *Immunological Reviews,* 214, 202-218.

Ruggeri, L.; Capanni, M.; Casucci, M.; Volpi, I.; Tosti, A.; Perruccio, K.; Urbani, E.; Negrin, R.S.; Martelli, M.F. & Velardi, A. (1999). Role of natural killer cell alloreactivity in HLA-mismatched hematopoietic stem cell transplantation. *Blood,* 94(1), 333-339.

Ruggeri, L.; Capanni, M.; Mancusi, A.; Urbani, E.; Perruccio, K.; Burchielli, E.; Tosti, A.; Topini, F.; Aversa, F.; Martelli, M.F. & Velardi, A. (2004). Alloreactive natural killer cells in mismatched hematopoietic stem cell transplantation. *Blood Cells, Molecules and Diseases,* 33(3), 216-221.

Ruggeri, L.; Capanni, M.; Urbani, E.; Perruccio, K.; Shlomchik, W.D.; Tosti, A.; Posati, S.; Rogaia, D.; Frassoni, F.; Aversa, F.; Martelli, M.F. & Velardi, A. (2002). Effectiveness of donor natural killer cell alloreactivity in mismatched hematopoietic transplants. *Science,* 295(5562), 2097-2100.

Ruggeri, L.; Mancusi, A.; Capanni, M.; Urbani, E.; Carotti, A.; Aloisi, T.; Stern, M.; Pende, D.; Perruccio, K.; Burchielli, E.; Topini, F.; Bianchi, E.; Aversa, F.; Martelli, M.F. & Velardi, A. (2007). Donor natural killer cell allorecognition of missing self in haploidentical hematopoietic transplantation for acute myeloid leukemia: challenging its predictive value. *Blood,* 110(1), 433-440.

Salcedo, M.; Diehl, A.D.; Olsson-Alheim, M.Y.; Sundback, J.; Van, K.L.; Karre, K. & Ljunggren, H.G. (1997). Altered expression of Ly49 inhibitory receptors on natural killer cells from MHC class I-deficient mice. *Journal of Immunology*, 158(7), 3174-3180.

Savani, B.N.; Mielke, S.; Adams, S.; Uribe, M.; Rezvani, K.; Yong, A.S.; Zeilah, J.; Kurlander, R.; Srinivasan, R.; Childs, R.; Hensel, N. & Barrett, A.J. (2007). Rapid natural killer cell recovery determines outcome after T-cell-depleted HLA-identical stem cell transplantation in patients with myeloid leukemias but not with acute lymphoblastic leukemia. *Leukemia*, 10, 2145-2152.

Schaap, N.; Schattenberg, A.; Bar, B.; Preijers, F.; Geurts van, K.A.; van der, M.R.; de, B.T. & de, W.T. (1997). Outcome of transplantation for standard-risk leukaemia with grafts depleted of lymphocytes after conditioning with an intensified regimen. *British Journal of Haematology*, 98(3), 750-759.

Schaap, N.; Schattenberg, A.; Bar, B.; Preijers, F.; van de Wiel van Kemenade & de Witte, T. (2001). Induction of graft-versus-leukemia to prevent relapse after partially lymphocyte-depleted allogeneic bone marrow transplantation by pre-emptive donor leukocyte infusions. *Leukemia*, 15(9), 1339-1346.

Schleuning, M.; Judith, D.; Jedlickova, Z.; Stubig, T.; Heshmat, M.; Baurmann, H. & Schwerdtfeger, R. (2008). Calcineurin inhibitor-free GVHD prophylaxis with sirolimus, mycophenolate mofetil and ATG in Allo-SCT for leukemia patients with high relapse risk: an observational cohort study. *Bone Marrow Transplantation*, 43(9), 717-723.

Seaman, W.E. (2000). Natural killer cells and natural killer T cells. *Arthritis & Rheumatism*, 43(6), 1204-1217.

Sentman, C.L.; Olsson, M.Y. & Karre, K. (1995). Missing self recognition by natural killer cells in MHC class I transgenic mice. A 'receptor calibration' model for how effector cells adapt to self. *Seminars in Immunology*, 7(2), 109-119.

Shibuya, A.; Campbell, D.; Hannum, C.; Yssel, H.; Franz-Bacon, K.; McClanahan, T.; Kitamura, T.; Nicholl, J.; Sutherland, G.R.; Lanier, L.L. & Phillips, J.H. (1996). DNAM-1, a novel adhesion molecule involved in the cytolytic function of T lymphocytes. *Immunity*, 4(6), 573-581.

Sivori, S.; Parolini, S.; Falco, M.; Marcenaro, E.; Biassoni, R.; Bottino, C.; Moretta, L. & Moretta, A. (2000). 2B4 functions as a co-receptor in human NK cell activation. *European Journal of Immunology*, 30(3), 787-793.

Sivori, S.; Vitale, M.; Morelli, L.; Sanseverino, L.; Augugliaro, R.; Bottino, C.; Moretta, L. & Moretta, A. (1997). p46, a novel natural killer cell-specific surface molecule that mediates cell activation. *Journal of Experimental Medicine*, 186(7), 1129-1136.

Snell, G.D. (1976). Recognition structures determined by the H-2 complex. *Transplantation Proceedings*, 8(2), 147-156.

Spanholtz, J.; Preijers, F.; Tordoir, M.; Trilsbeek, C.; Paardekooper, J.; de, W.T.; Schaap, N. & Dolstra, H. (2011). Clinical-grade generation of active NK cells from cord blood hematopoietic progenitor cells for immunotherapy using a closed-system culture process. *PLoS ONE*, 6(6), e20740.

Spanholtz, J.; Tordoir, M.; Eissens, D.; Preijers, F.; van der, M.A.; Joosten, I.; Schaap, N.; de Witte, T.M. & Dolstra, H. (2010). High Log-Scale Expansion of Functional Human

Natural Killer Cells from Umbilical Cord Blood CD34-Positive Cells for Adoptive Cancer Immunotherapy. *PLoS ONE,* 5(2), e9221.

Spits, H.; Lanier, L.L. & Phillips, J.H. (1995). Development of human T and natural killer cells. *Blood,* 85(10), 2654-2670.

Sutherland, C.L.; Rabinovich, B.; Chalupny, N.J.; Brawand, P.; Miller, R. & Cosman, D. (2006). ULBPs, human ligands of the NKG2D receptor, stimulate tumor immunity with enhancement by IL-15. *Blood,* 108(4), 1313-1319.

Tam, Y.K.; Martinson, J.A.; Doligosa, K. & Klingemann, H.G. (2003). Ex vivo expansion of the highly cytotoxic human natural killer-92 cell-line under current good manufacturing practice conditions for clinical adoptive cellular immunotherapy. *Cytotherapy,* 5(3), 259-272.

Thomas, E.D. & Blume, K.G. (1999). Historical markers in the development of allogeneic hematopoietic cell transplantation. *Biology of Blood and Marrow Transplantation,* 5(6), 341-346.

Ugolini, S. & Vivier, E. (2001). Multifaceted roles of MHC class I and MHC class I-like molecules in T cell activation. *Nature Immunology,* 2(3), 198-200.

Vales-Gomez, M.; Reyburn, H.T.; Erskine, R.A. & Strominger, J. (1998a). Differential binding to HLA-C of p50-activating and p58-inhibitory natural killer cell receptors. *Proceedings of the National Academy of Sciences,* 95(24), 14326-14331.

Vales-Gomez, M.; Reyburn, H.T.; Mandelboim, M. & Strominger, J.L. (1998b). Kinetics of interaction of HLA-C ligands with natural killer cell inhibitory receptors. *Immunity,* 9(3), 337-344.

Valiante, N.M.; Uhrberg, M.; Shilling, H.G.; Lienert, W.K.; Arnett, K.L.; D'Andrea, A.; Phillips, J.H.; Lanier, L.L. & Parham, P. (1997). Functionally and structurally distinct NK cell receptor repertoires in the peripheral blood of two human donors. *Immunity,* 7(6), 739-751.

van der Meer, A.; Schaap, N.P.M.; Schattenberg, A.V.M.B.; van Cranenbroek, B.; Tijssen, H.J. & Joosten, I. (2008). KIR2DS5 is associated with leukemia free survival after HLA identical stem cell transplantation in chronic myeloid leukemia patients. *Molecular Immunology,* 45(13), 3631-3638.

van Stijn, A.; Rowshani, A.T.; Yong, S.L.; Baas, F.; Roosnek, E.; ten Berge, I.J.M. & van Lier, R.A.W. (2008). Human Cytomegalovirus Infection Induces a Rapid and Sustained Change in the Expression of NK Cell Receptors on CD8+ T Cells. *The Journal of Immunology,* 180(7), 4550-4560.

Vilches, C. & Parham, P. (2002). KIR: diverse, rapidly evolving receptors of innate and adaptive immunity. *Annual Review of Immunology,* 20, 217-251.

Vitale, M.; Falco, M.; Castriconi, R.; Parolini, S.; Zambello, R.; Semenzato, G.; Biassoni, R.; Bottino, C.; Moretta, L. & Moretta, A. (2001). Identification of NKp80, a novel triggering molecule expressed by human NK cells. *European Journal of Immunology,* 31(1), 233-242.

Vivier, E. (2006). What is natural in natural killer cells? *Immunology Letters,* 107(1), 1-7.

Vivier, E. & Daeron, M. (1997). Immunoreceptor tyrosine-based inhibition motifs. *Immunology Today,* 18(6), 286-291.

Vivier, E.; Tomasello, E.; Baratin, M.; Walzer, T. & Ugolini, S. (2008). Functions of natural killer cells. *Nature Immunology,* 9(5), 503-510.

Vogelsang, G.B. & Arai, S. (2001). Mycophenolate mofetil for the prevention and treatment of graft-versus-host disease following stem cell transplantation: preliminary findings. *Bone Marrow Transplantation*, 27(12), 1255-1262.

Wang, H.; Grzywacz, B.; Sukovich, D.; McCullar, V.; Cao, Q.; Lee, A.B.; Blazar, B.R.; Cornfield, D.N.; Miller, J.S. & Verneris, M.R. (2007). The unexpected effect of cyclosporin A on CD56+CD16- and CD56+CD16+ natural killer cell subpopulations. *Blood*, 110(5), 1530-1539.

Wu, J.; Cherwinski, H.; Spies, T.; Phillips, J.H. & Lanier, L.L. (2000). DAP10 and DAP12 form distinct, but functionally cooperative, receptor complexes in natural killer cells. *Journal of Experimental Medicine*, 192(7), 1059-1068.

Wu, J.; Song, Y.; Bakker, A.B.; Bauer, S.; Spies, T.; Lanier, L.L. & Phillips, J.H. (1999). An activating immunoreceptor complex formed by NKG2D and DAP10. *Science*, 285(5428), 730-732.

7

Mesenchymal Stem Cells as Immunomodulators in Transplantation

Nadia Zghoul[1], Mahmoud Aljurf[2] and Said Dermime[1]
[1]Immunology & Innovative Cell Therapy Unit,
Department of Biomedical Research, Dasman Diabetes Institute
[2]Adult Haematology/Oncology, King Faisal Specialist
Hospital and Research Centre,
[1]Kuwait
[2]Kingdom of Saudi Arabia

1. Introduction

In recent years it has become evident that mesenchymal stem cells (MSCs), also termed mesenchymal stromal cells, have potent immunomodulatory effects in addition to their known ability of organ regeneration and recruitment to sites of injured or inflamed tissue (Caplan 1991; Garin, Chu et al. 2007; Nauta and Fibbe 2007; Bianco, Robey et al. 2008; Shi, Hu et al. 2010). While the ability of MSCs to mediate tissue and organ repair replacing damaged tissue has initially been attributed to their multilineage differentiation potential, it is now widely attributed to their ability to home to site of injury secreting cytokines and growth factors that mediate the repair process inducing proliferation and differentiation of progenitor cells (Karp and Leng Teo 2009; Hoogduijn, Popp et al. 2010; Sordi, Melzi et al. 2010). Whether MSCs migrate from the bone marrow in case of injury or if the stem cell niche available in the diseased organ replaces dying cells remains to be elucidated.

MSCs have been demonstrated to exhibit a profound immunomodulatory effect on T cells, B cells, and Natural Killer (NK) cells. This effect has been recently shown to be mediated via soluble factors, and this can be enhanced further if direct cell–cell contact between the MSCs and immune cells is allowed (Ren, Zhao et al. 2010). Via these factors, MSCs inhibit T cell proliferation (Di Nicola, Carlo-Stella et al. 2002; Aggarwal and Pittenger 2005), maturation and differentiation of B cells (Corcione, Benvenuto et al. 2006; Tabera, Perez-Simon et al. 2008; Asari, Itakura et al. 2009), maturation of dendritic cells (DCs) (Nauta, Kruisselbrink et al. 2006), generation of cytotoxic T cells (Angoulvant, Clerc et al. 2004) and proliferation and cytotoxic activity of NK cells (Rasmusson, Ringden et al. 2003; Sotiropoulou, Perez et al. 2006; Spaggiari, Capobianco et al. 2008), while inducing regulatory T cells (Tregs) (Prevosto, Zancolli et al. 2007; Di Ianni, Del Papa et al. 2008; Crop, Baan et al. 2010).

MSCs have been shown to induce immunologic peripheral tolerance, suggesting their potential application in a therapeutic approach for immune mediated disorders. In this context, MSCs can be used to support the function of standard pharmacological immunosuppressants to reduce their dosage or even replace such toxic immunosuppressants promoting long-term survival of the transplanted organ (Crop, Baan et al. 2009).

Limited information is available about the molecular mechanisms responsible for the immunomodulation By MSCs and there is no single mechanism responsible for their observed tolerogenic effect. However, MSCs have been considered to potentially work through multiple mechanisms and have the ability to affect immunological, inflammatory and regenerative pathways supporting or replacing current pharmacological agents.

Considering their immunosuppressive properties in addition to their low inherent immunogenicity (Rasmusson, Uhlin et al. 2007) makes MSCs an attractive treatment option in cell and organ transplantation potentially improving the graft outcome and eliminating a long immunosuppressive treatment regimen (Ryan, Barry et al. 2005; Eggenhofer, Steinmann et al. 2011). Both the immunosuppressive effects of MSCs and their regenerative potential participate to facilitate grafting of a transplanted organ as well as repair and regeneration of the organ after transplantation.

In both allogeneic hematopoietic stem cell transplantation (AHSCT) and organ transplantation setting, major problems exist due to the lack of suitable donors. High histo-incompatability between donor and recipient is often associated with an increased risk of graft rejection or graft versus host disease which MSCs might ameliorate if infusion of MSCs along with the organ transplant increases organ engraftment making this immunoprivilege useful for transplantation. Indeed, in one of the first in vivo studies showing the advantageous immunosuppressive effect of MSCs, allogeneic MSCs were demonstrated to prolong (MHC)-mismatched skin allograft survival in baboons (Bartholomew, Sturgeon et al. 2002).

Furthermore, the immunosuppressive properties of MSCs, in addition to their low immunogenicity features, have prompted researchers to investigate co-transplantation of these cells in AHSCT setting to promote hematopoietic stem cells (HSCs) engraftment and to prevent graft versus host reactions as well as host versus graft reactivity. Additionally, MSCs provide support for the growth and development of HSCs further promoting engraftment. In this, MSCs were shown to interact with HSCs through production of growth factors that influence HSCs-homing and –differentiation (Krampera, Cosmi et al. 2006). This effect was attributed via either cell-cell contact or production of soluble factors by MSCs such as the CXCL12 chemokine which may attract HSCs through its interaction with the CXCR4 ligand (Krampera, Cosmi et al. 2006) hence improving HSCs engraftment.

First clinical trials have been undertaken to assess the safety of MSCs administration as well as a potential treatment option for graft versus host disease (GvHD). Encouraging results have been obtained in patients with steroid resistant GvHD and in the management of chronic GvHD after AHSCT. Interestingly, MSCs treatment improved the overall outcome and successfully attenuated GvHD in these patients (Le Blanc, Rasmusson et al. 2004; Ringden and Le Blanc 2011).

MSCs were shown to attenuate graft rejection and in combination with immunosuppressive therapy were able to prolong cardiac allograft survival when co-administered with immunosuppressive therapy. Indeed, they promote donor-specific graft tolerance and ameliorate the alloimmune response where the use of low dose therapy alone was not sufficient to maintain the graft; only combination therapy with MSCs maintained the cardio graft (Ge, Jiang et al. 2009).

MSCs have also been suggested as a promising cell immunotherapy tool to promote tolerance for organ transplants and to control allograft rejection in post-transplant therapy settings facilitating both transplant acceptance and physiologic functions (Crop, Baan et al. 2009; Dahlke, Hoogduijn et al. 2009). MSCs have also been recently shown to have an ameliorating effect in a model of acute lung injury were transplantation of MSCs resulted in a significant increase in the level of protective/immunomodulatory Tregs (Sun, Han et al. 2011). Finally, clinical trials are ongoing to determine the efficacy of MSCs as an effective tool for the treatment of autoimmune diseases, such as multiple sclerosis, inflammatory bowel diseases, rheumatoid arthritis, and type 1 diabetes.

2. The biology and originality of mesenchymal stem cells and their generation and expansion in vitro for therapeutic use

MSCs are a self-renewing heterogeneous population of multipotent cells, originally isolated from bone marrow as shown in pioneer experiments by Friedenstein and colleagues and first referred to as colony-forming unit fibroblasts (Friedenstein, Chailakhyan et al. 1974). Since then, MSCs have been isolated from many other adult tissues such a umbilical cord blood, placenta, amniotic fluid, peripheral blood, adipose tissue and various other somatic tissues sharing the regenerative as well as the immunomodulatory properties of MSCs (In 't Anker, Scherjon et al. 2004; Zuk 2010; Bianco 2011) but have mainly been characterized after isolation from bone marrow.

MSCs can be expanded in vitro as plastic adherent cells with a fibroblast-like morphology and can be differentiated into cells of mesodermal lineage (osteocytes, chondrocytes and adipocytes) (Pittenger, Mackay et al. 1999) as well as cells from other embryonic lineages (Sanchez-Ramos 2006; Schwartz, Brick et al. 2008). At present, MSCs lack a definitive marker and no single marker has been identified distinguishing MSCs however the International Society for Stem Cell Research has outlined minimal criteria to characterize human MSCs, these cells have been reported to be positive for CD73, CD90, CD105 and major histocompatibility complex class I (HLA-ABC). They are devoid of the hematopoietic markers such as CD14, CD 19, CD34, CD45 and for major histocompatibility complex class II, (HLA-DR) (Dominici, Le Blanc et al. 2006).

An attractive characteristic of MSCs is that they can be easily expanded maintaining a relatively stable phenotype and karyotype along with their potential to differentiate into multiple mesodermal tissues. The possibility that MSCs might undergo malignant transformation does exist, however this might be directly linked to the origin of the tissue. Interestingly, it has been shown that human bone marrow derived MSCs could be expanded in vitro and despite decreased proliferative capacity upon prolonged expansion and eventual cell senescence, no chromosomal abnormalities were detected rendering these cells suitable for cell therapeutic approaches (Bernardo, Zaffaroni et al. 2007).

However, there is a general consensus that MSCs should be used at low passages when applied in cell therapy as chromosomal modifications and loss of function can occur after prolonged in vitro expansion.

3. The Immunomodulatory properties of mesenchymal stem cells and their role in transplantation

Understanding the mechanisms by which MSCs exert their immunomodulatory effects will have profound therapeutic implications in designing new therapies that can lead to more efficient use of these cells in novel treatment regimens. Currently, there is no single clear mechanism which clearly clarifies the immunomodulatory effect of MSCs and several mechanisms which sometimes seem paradoxical, have been suggested. Several in vitro experimental studies have shown that the immunosuppressive effect of MSCs is sustained in transwell experiments suggesting that soluble factors are responsible for such inhibition (Di Nicola, Carlo-Stella et al. 2002; Meisel, Zibert et al. 2004; Aggarwal and Pittenger 2005; Gao, Wu et al. 2008; Ren, Zhang et al. 2008; Selmani, Naji et al. 2008), while other studies have claimed a required cell-cell contact which may be due to the use of different systems and cells by the individual research groups (Quaedackers, Baan et al. 2009; Ren, Zhao et al. 2010).

MSCs have been shown to modulate the immune response mainly by inhibiting the proliferation of effector immune cells preventing further damage to injured tissue allowing repair after injury (Uccelli, Moretta et al. 2008). Moreover, MSCs can stimulate the activation and proliferation of Tregs which in turn have a beneficial immunosuppressive effect (Crop, Baan et al. 2010).

When MSCs home to site of tissue inflammation or injury, they release various growth factors which enhance repair at site of defect including : fibroblast growth factor, epidermal growth factor, platelet-derived growth factor, transforming growth factor-β, vascular endothelial growth factor and insulin-like growth factor (Ng, Boucher et al. 2008). MSCs mediated inhibition of effector T cell proliferation seems to be dependent on the microenvironment. In this respect, the presence of pro-inflammatory cytokines such as IFN-γ activates MSCs and this was more effective for the treatment of GvHD (Polchert, Sobinsky et al. 2008). Indeed, it has been shown, that the immunosuppressive capacity of MSCs was enhanced strongly under inflammatory conditions while their differentiation capacity was preserved and suggested that in vitro preconditioning provides MSCs with improved properties for immediate clinical immune therapy (Crop, Baan et al. 2010).

MSCs have been shown to affect almost all cell types of the immune system. It has been demonstrated that MSCs can alter the cytokine secretion profile of immune cells such as decreasing TNF-α and IFN-γ secretion and increasing the secretion of suppressive cytokines (IL-4 and IL-10) and this shift from a pro-inflammatory to a beneficial anti-inflammatory response is of therapeutic advantage for the management of GvHD (Dahlke, Hoogduijn et al. 2009; Hoogduijn, Popp et al. 2010). Moreover, several studies have demonstrated that the MSCs immunoregulatory properties are partially mediated by transforming growth factor (TGF-β), prostaglandin E2 (PGE2), hepatocyte growth factor (HGF) and Indoleamine 2, 3-dioxgenase (IDO) secreted by MSCs in addition to their induction and activation of Tregs all of which can lead to amplification of an effective immunosuppressive response (English, Ryan et al. 2009; Kim, Wee et al. 2011).

3.1 MSC–soluble factors and immunosuppression induction

Different studies have attributed the immunosuppressive effect of MSCs to several immunosuppressive factors leading to different mechanisms of immune cell inhibition. These include, IDO (Meisel, Zibert et al. 2004; DelaRosa, Lombardo et al. 2009), PGE2 (Aggarwal and Pittenger 2005), TGF-β and HGF (Di Nicola, Carlo-Stella et al. 2002), HLA-G (Selmani, Naji et al. 2008), nitric oxide (Ren, Zhang et al. 2008), interleukin (IL)-10 (Gao, Wu et al. 2008) and haeme oxygenase-1 (Chabannes, Hill et al. 2007). One important mechanism is that MSCs suppression is mediated by IDO, a tryptophan catabolising enzyme (Meisel, Zibert et al. 2004). In this, activated T cells or NK cells produce elevated levels of IFN-γ which in turn stimulates MSCs to produce IDO. IDO metabolizes tryptophan to kynurenine leading to essential tryptophan depletion and accumulation of metabolites in the medium which in turn inhibits proliferation of activated T cells and NK cells (Meisel, Zibert et al. 2004). Competitive inhibition of IDO activity did not completely abrogate MSC mediated immunosuppression and inhibition of IFN-γ was required for complete abrogation (Krampera, Cosmi et al. 2006; DelaRosa, Lombardo et al. 2009). This suggests that co-administration of MSCs with graft T cells-derived IFN-γ activates the immunomodulatory properties of MSCs. Furthermore, there is a species variation in the immunosuppressive mechanisms mediated by MSCs. It has been shown that while human IDO is a major effector molecule for MSCs immunosuppression, mouse MSCs mediate their inhibitory effect of immune responses via nitric oxide playing a central role in such immunosuppression (Sato, Ozaki et al. 2007; Ren, Zhang et al. 2008).

3.2 MSC-immune cell interaction and immunosuppression induction
MSCs have been demonstrated to exhibit a profound immunomodulatory effect on Tregs, cytotoxic and T helper cells, NK cells, B cells and dendritic cells.

3.2.1 Regulatory T cells
Tregs are a subset of T cells that regulate the immune response by suppressing the proliferation and cytokine production of effector T cells. Tregs are thus important for protecting our body by suppressing auto-reactive T cells (Thornton and Shevach 1998; Ng, Duggan et al. 2001). Tregs were shown to be upregulated in the presence of MSCs suggesting that MSCs constitute a suitable niche for Tregs (Crop, Baan et al. 2010). MSCs have been suggested to play a role in Tregs recruitment, regulating and maintaining the T regulatory phenotype and function over time (Prevosto, Zancolli et al. 2007; Di Ianni, Del Papa et al. 2008). Tregs induction has been suggested to be mediated by PGE2, synthesized by cyclooxygenase enzymes (COX) which are expressed by MSCs (Le Blanc and Ringden 2007). Furthermore, Treg induction has been shown to be mediated by direct cell-cell contact between MSCs and CD4+ T cells and the presence of soluble MSC derived factors such as TGF-β1 and PGE2 (English, Ryan et al. 2009). In a recent interesting study by (Sundin, D'Arcy et al. 2011) it was demonstrated for the first time that MSCs share features with regulatory T cells , such as the expression of the Tregs specific transcription factor FOXP3 (Yagi, Nomura et al. 2004) at variable levels. However, the MSC immunosuppressive function is not as tightly linked to FOXP3 expression as is the case for Tregs (Sundin, D'Arcy et al. 2011).

3.2.2 Cytotoxic T cells and T helper cells
MSCs were shown to inhibit the proliferation of CD4+ T helper cells (Di Nicola, Carlo-Stella et al. 2002; Aggarwal and Pittenger 2005). In addition to indirect inhibitory factors produced by MCSs such as TGF-β1, HGF, IL-10, IFN-γ and TNF-α, there is evidence that cell-membrane interaction between MCSs and T helper cells (Quaedackers, Baan et al. 2009) via the intracellular adhesion molecule (ICAM-1) or vascular cell adhesion molecule (VCAM-1) play a crucial role in such immunosuppression (Ren, Zhao et al. 2010). MSCs have also been shown to suppress the induction of cytotoxic T cell response to allo-antigens (Angoulvant, Clerc et al. 2004). However, once cytotoxic T cells are activated, MSCs show no inhibitory effect (Rasmusson, Ringden et al. 2003; Le Blanc and Ringden 2007). On the other hand, it is

not clear how helper and cytotoxic T cells affect MSCs development and function. It has been shown that MSCs have a low immunophenotype as they express low levels of HLA class I, no HLA class II, no co-stimulatory molecules such as CD80 and CD86, and therefore do not induce immune responses (Beggs, Lyubimov et al. 2006; Rasmusson, Uhlin et al. 2007). This should make MSCs transplantable across HLA barriers (Le Blanc, Tammik et al. 2003). However, in contrast to these data, there is evidence that MSCs are immunogenic and can induce memory T-cell responses both in animals (Badillo, Beggs et al. 2007) and human studies (Nauta, Westerhuis et al. 2006). Furthermore, it has recently been reported that MSCs are susceptible for lysis by CD8+ cytotoxic T cells (Crop, Korevaar et al. 2011). Designing tools to escape allogeneic MSCs destruction by cytotoxic T cells should render MSCs a promising therapeutic option for transplantation across MHC barriers.

3.2.3 Natural Killer cells
MSCs have been shown to inhibit NK cell proliferation, and cytotoxicity (Sotiropoulou, Perez et al. 2006). It has been demonstrated that MSCs can mediate this inhibitory effect trough inhibition of cytokine production in addition to the central role played by IDO and PGE2 (Spaggiari, Capobianco et al. 2008). Inversely, it has been shown that MSCs are susceptible for lysis by NK cells (Spaggiari, Capobianco et al. 2006; Crop, Korevaar et al. 2011) as MSCs express the activating NK cell-receptor ligands NKG2D and UL16 (Poggi, Prevosto et al. 2007). Moreover, intravenously administered MSCs have been demonstrated to disappear within days after infusion in immunocompetent mice (Popp, Eggenhofer et al. 2008). It is possible that lysis by cytotoxic T cells (and not NK cells) is responsible for the disappearance of the infused MSCs (Eliopoulos, Stagg et al. 2005). The demonstration of tumour engraftment after administration of autologous MSCs in immunodeficient mice (NK cells intact) further strengthens this possibility.

3.2.4 B cells
MSCs have been shown to suppress B cell terminal differentiation (Asari, Itakura et al. 2009) and modulate their function (Corcione, Benvenuto et al. 2006; Tabera, Perez-Simon et al. 2008). Human MSCs were shown to inhibit antibody production induced in vitro by allo-stimulation (Comoli, Ginevri et al. 2008; English, French et al. 2010). They have the ability to regulate Immunoglobulin production by B cells through soluble factors affecting B cells directly or through an indirect MSCs effect by altering the amount of free alloantigen due to the overall suppression of graft damage (Ge, Jiang et al. 2009).

3.2.5 Dendritic cells
MSCs inhibit monocyte maturation into dendritic cells (Jiang, Zhang et al. 2005), the most potent antigen presenting cells, inhibiting their migration to lymph nodes and thereby reducing their ability to activate allo-reactive T cells (Aggarwal and Pittenger 2005). In this, MSCs were shown to reduce secretion of pro-inflammatory cytokines such as IFN-γ, IL-12 and TNF-α by DCs while IL-10, a suppressive cytokine, was increased leading to the inhibition of DCs maturation and the inability to activate allo-reactive T cells resulting in a state of an immunologic tolerance. The inhibitory effect of MSCs on DC differentiation is mainly mediated through cell-cell contact involving activation of the Notch signalling pathway (Li, Paczesny et al. 2008) as well via soluble factors (Nauta, Kruisselbrink et al. 2006). Moreover, PGE2 produced by MSCs following TNF-α or IFN-γ

stimulation blocks differentiation of monocytes into DCs and stimulates macrophages to produce Il-10.

3.3 MSCs-Galectins and immunosuppression induction

Recently, Sioud et al (Sioud, Mobergslien et al. 2010; Sioud 2011)and Gieseke et al (Gieseke, Bohringer et al. 2010) have described another mechanism of MSCs immunosuppression that involves a family of beta galactosidase-binding proteins named Galectins which are involved in immune tolerance (Garin, Chu et al. 2007). It has been demonstrated that Galectin-1, Galectin-3, Galectin-8 and Galectin-9 are constitutively expressed by human bone marrow MSCs with Galectin-1 and Galectin -3 being further secreted and expressed on the outer plasma membrane (Wada and Makino 2001). New evidence has shown the involvement of Galectin-3 as a regulator of MSCs immunosuppression function inhibiting allogeneic T cell proliferation by MSCs (Sioud 2011). This group demonstrated that gene knockdown of Galectin-3 resulted in less immunosuppressive effect on T cell proliferation (Sioud, Mobergslien et al. 2010). Galectins were also shown to regulate the secretion of pro-inflammatory cytokines and promote expansion of IL-10 producing peripheral Tregs (Sioud 2011). Gieseke et al have also reported that galectin-1 is expressed by MSCs and has immunosuppressive activity on both CD4+ and CD8+ T cells (Gieseke, Bohringer et al. 2010).

4. Clinical prospects of mesenchymal stem cells

Currently suggested clinical uses of MSCs include; differentiation and repairing of damaged tissue e.g. in osteogenesis imperfecta, promoting hematopoietic cell engraftment in AHSCT e.g. in leukaemia and their immunosuppressive abilities in autoimmune-induced inflammatory bowel disease, GvHD induced upon allogeneic cell or organ transplantation as well as autoimmune diseases. Treating autoimmunity with MSCs was first investigated for experimental autoimmune encephalomyelitis as a model for multiple sclerosis in preclinical studies followed by collagen-induced arthritis, autoimmune type 1 diabetes, experimental colitis and lupus nephritis (Uccelli and Prockop 2010).

Still, very little is known about the mechanisms underlying the MSCs immunomodulatory effect in vivo and survival of MSCs upon injection and whether they remain present after systemic injection or local transplantation remains unresolved. However, the clinical studies performed so far look encouraging but still the mechanisms as to how the MSCs regulate immune cells in vivo are still missing. Furthermore, direct methods to assess MSCs mobilization and homing in response to injury or inflammation is essential to eventually understand the underlying mechanism (Karp and Leng Teo 2009).

MSCs are immune-privileged and were shown in most studies to 'escape' the immune system and be tolerated when transplanted across MHC barriers engrafting and failing to induce an immune response. It is important to mention that most of these clinical studies have used MSCs from HLA-identical or near identical donors (Le Blanc and Ringden 2007).

It has been reported that AHSCT recipients have specific tolerance, immune-unresponsiveness, directed towards MSCs but not to other cells from the MSC donor (Sundin, Barrett et al. 2009). This suggests that totally HLA mismatched MSCs from one donor can be expanded ex vivo, cryopreserved and used for the treatment of multiple patients. Furthermore, the inability of MSCs to induce donor specific tolerance suggests that

MSCs co-transplantation with a solid organ most probably facilitates engraftment through the immunosuppressive action of MSCs and not by inducing specific tolerance to the transplant (Sundin, D'Arcy et al. 2011).

4.1 Graft versus Host Disease
GvHD occurs in donated organ recipients and patho-physiologically presents itself as damage in skin, mucosa, gastrointestinal tract, the liver, connective tissue and exocrine glands. It is considered chronic when it persists more than 100 days after transplantation and it is distinguished from acute GvHD which often cannot be ameliorated because of a coexistent immunosuppression. It results from the attack of donor own T cells in the graft on recipient tissues after activation by recipient MHC molecules as well as activation of cytotoxic T cells, antigen presenting cells and NK cells. In GvHD the observation of an increased secretion of pro-inflammatory cytokines such as TNF-α, IFN-γ, IL-1, IL-2 and IL-12 suggests that therapeutic approaches to inhibit these cytokines should lead to a decreased severity of GvHD (Aggarwal and Pittenger 2005).

The immunosuppressive effects of MSCs have been evidenced in a successful clinical trial reported by Ringden et al (Ringden and Le Blanc 2011) in patients presented with acute GvHD after AHSCT and resistant to conventional immunosuppressive therapy. This study showed a dramatic improvement after MSCs infusion with acute GvHD disappearing completely in patients with steroid resistant GvHD suggesting that MSCs could be considered as a promising alternative immunosuppressive therapy with improved long term outcome for the treatment of GvHD (Le Blanc, Rasmusson et al. 2004; English, French et al. 2010; Ringden and Le Blanc 2011; Tolar, Villeneuve et al. 2011).

4.2 Type 1 diabetes
MSCs have been suggested as a prospective cell therapy of autoimmune type 1 diabetes known to be associated with an inflammation in the pancreas and degeneration of β cells. In a preclinical study, it has been shown that co-transplantation of bone marrow cells and syngeneic or allogeneic MSCs initiated endogenous pancreatic regeneration and improved blood glucose levels in streptozotocin induced diabetic mice (Ulicna, Danisovic et al. 2009). The success in the treatment was suggested to be due to MSCs aiding in the regeneration of recipient derived pancreatic beta cells, as well as maintaining the β cell reserve through MSC inhibition of T cell-mediated immune responses against the newly formed β cells preventing further cell degeneration (Voltarelli, Couri et al. 2007; Couri and Voltarelli 2009; Ulicna, Danisovic et al. 2009; Sordi, Melzi et al. 2010). Hence, despite of the persisting hostile autoimmune response in the pancreas, when MSCs are applied at an early stage of the disease they potentially protect and allow the endogenous regeneration of the remaining intact β cell reserve.

4.3 Solid organ transplantation
In solid organ transplantation (e.g. liver transplant), rejection of a transplanted organ is typically caused by induction of T cell proliferation and presentation of allo-antigens to naive and memory T cells by antigen presenting cells (both host and donor) leading to activation and differentiation into effector T cells (Popp, Renner et al. 2009). Both the regenerative and immunomodulatory properties of MSCs are of medical importance in organ transplantation studies. MSCs have been shown to home to site of allograft and help

the body accommodate the new organ through immunosuppression or preventing rejection and acquisition of a state of tolerance (English, French et al. 2010). Furthermore, the regenerative properties of MSCs possibly maintain the organ to be transplanted stretching its lifespan in case of delayed transplantation (Hematti 2008; Hoogduijn, Popp et al. 2010).

For MSCs to be used as a sole therapy or as a combination therapy replacing immunosuppressive drugs, reducing the burden on the patient and the risk for long term side effects, further investigation will be needed to fully explain the immunomodulatory properties of MSCs. However, MSCs were shown to increase immunosuppression when co-administered complementing the therapy (Sundin, D'Arcy et al. 2011). In this regard, an interesting animal study of allogeneic heart graft transplantation that MSCs combined with the immunosuppressive drug mycophenolate mofetil (MMF) promoted the elimination of activated T cells in secondary lymphatic organs, delayed antigen presenting cells activation, and protected the graft from cellular infiltration by modulating the endothelium (Eggenhofer, Steinmann et al. 2011).

5. Quality considerations and regulations in MSC based therapy

Clinical use of MSCs for cellular therapeutic approaches will require that the bio-safety of these cells has to be adequately optimised. This requires the absence of chromosomal, functional, and phenotypical alterations in ex vitro expanded MSCs before considering their injection in patients. The safety of these cells has to be guaranteed upon their administration as immunocompromised patients might have an increased risk of tumour induction or the potential risk of stimulating the growth of a previously undetected cancer. The risk of tumorigenicity and genomic instability remains an obstacle for any given stem-cell based therapy product and will have to be adequately assessed prior to approval for human use (Dittmar, Simann et al. 2010). In this respect, the first clinical trials have been undertaken to assess the safety of MSC administration and potential treatment options for GvHD and it has been reported that autologous and allogeneic MSCs are safe to be injected in patients with life threatening acute GvHD not responding to conventional immunosuppressive therapy without acute toxicity and no signs of ectopic tissue formation (Lazarus, Koc et al. 2005).

MSCs administered for therapy might carry viruses (e.g. herpes simplex virus, cytomegalo virus (CMV), Epstein-Barr Virus (EBV)) transmitted from the donor to the host tissue especially when the patient is immunocompromised. Interestingly, MSCs were shown to exert differential effects on alloantigen and virus-specific T cell responses (Karlsson, Samarasinghe et al. 2008). In this regard, it has been reported that despite MSC infusion as a cellular immunotherapy for GvHD, effector functions of virus specific T cells were retained with very little effect on T cell responses to pathogenic CMV and EBV contrasting the strong immunosuppressive effect on allo-reactive T cells suggesting that MSCs to be a promising cellular immunotherapy (Karlsson, Samarasinghe et al. 2008). This is an important advantageous aspect of MSCs therapy especially since after allogeneic organ transplantation; infections are a major cause of morbidity and mortality in immunocompromised patients. Therefore, MSCs can be safely administered without exacerbating their susceptibility to infectious pathogens.

Currently large clinical trials are being carried out in using MSCs for the treatment of autoimmune diseases including diabetes as well as to treat or ameliorate symptoms of GvHD. Further, clinical trials are also testing the MSCs ability to facilitate the prevention of the rejection upon organ transplantation thereby reducing or completely eliminating the need for immunosuppressive therapies. Reviewing the clinical trials registered by the U.S. National Institutes of Health (NIH) in the United States and around the world (U.S. National Institutes of Health, http://clinicaltrials.gov/), 168 registered studies (with a start date between September 2004 and March 2011) were found upon entering the search criteria mesenchymal + stem + cells including clinical trials in regenerating organs (e.g. bone fractures, diabetic foot and foot ulcer), liver failure, the administration of MSCs for the treatment of type 1 Diabetes Mellitus as well as Type 2, acute GvHD including studies with patients who have failed to respond to steroid therapy (or with steroid resistance) and poor graft function. In addition to these trials, ongoing clinical studies investigating the safety and efficacy of MSCs promoting engraftment of allogeneic hematopoietic stem cells are in hand (Le Blanc, Rasmusson et al. 2004).

The translation into cellular therapies satisfying safety and efficacy criteria by the regulatory authorities will have to ensure the identity, purity, potency, and lack of tumorigenicity. Questions regarding the expansion of MSCs in vitro and the passage at which they are used as well as the culture conditions containing foetal calf serum, optimal dosing, timing and HLA matching still remain to be answered (Le Blanc, Samuelsson et al. 2007; Sundin, Ringden et al. 2007).

Scientists and clinicians should adhere to local, national and international guidelines and regulations that govern transfer of cells into patients. The clinical trial and the eventual cell therapeutic product is assessed and approved by a national regulatory agency, such as the European Medicines Agency (EMA) or the U.S. Food and Drug Administration (FDA).The International Society for Stem Cell Research (ISSCR) has published guidelines for the clinical translation of stem cells emphasising on the scientific, clinical and ethical issues that should be addressed for a responsible translation of basic stem cell research into suitable clinical applications. The guidelines give attention to the main areas of clinical translational stem cell research namely, cell processing and manufacture, the necessity of preclinical studies and clinical research promoting maximum safety and quality of the cells to be used (Hyun, Lindvall et al. 2008).

6. Conclusion

Understanding the immunomodulatory properties of MSCs and possibly identifying genes that regulate MSC inhibitory function, and genes regulating inflammation which play a major role in transplant rejection and inflammatory processes should help in developing applicable MSC based cellular therapies for solid organ transplantation, GvHD and autoimmune diseases.

The currently available data, in vitro and in vivo, suggest that MSCs can be applied in a wide range of clinical approaches, ranging from tissue repair and regeneration, drug or gene delivery to injured tissue, treatment and prevention of GvHD and AHSCT engraftment offering a promising option for treating autoimmune mediated disorders as well as organ transplantation. Administration of MSCs provides novel modalities for the treatment of patients with allograft rejection with fewer side effects than existing immunosuppressive therapies following organ transplantation.

There is an enormous amount of excitement and the scope of possible stem cell based therapies has expanded in the recent years due to rapid advances in stem cell research. But today the range of diseases where stem cell treatments have been shown to be beneficial in responsibly conducted clinical trials is still extremely restricted.

The best defined and most extensively used is hematopoietic stem cell transplantation in blood malignancies and aplastic anaemia. To design safe and effective cellular therapies, the long term effects of MSCs injection will still need to be shown in relevant clinical trials and further studies are needed to optimize cell-dosing, time of injection and the combination with immunosuppressive drugs to confirm both efficacy and safety of this cell therapy, are still needed within the careful regulations of the EMA and FDA.

7. References

Aggarwal, S. and M. F. Pittenger (2005). "Human mesenchymal stem cells modulate allogeneic immune cell responses." Blood 105(4): 1815-1822.

Angoulvant, D., A. Clerc, et al. (2004). "Human mesenchymal stem cells suppress induction of cytotoxic response to alloantigens." Biorheology 41(3-4): 469-476.

Asari, S., S. Itakura, et al. (2009). "Mesenchymal stem cells suppress B-cell terminal differentiation." Exp Hematol 37(5): 604-615.

Badillo, A. T., K. J. Beggs, et al. (2007). "Murine bone marrow stromal progenitor cells elicit an in vivo cellular and humoral alloimmune response." Biol Blood Marrow Transplant 13(4): 412-422.

Bartholomew, A., C. Sturgeon, et al. (2002). "Mesenchymal stem cells suppress lymphocyte proliferation in vitro and prolong skin graft survival in vivo." Exp Hematol 30(1): 42-48.

Beggs, K. J., A. Lyubimov, et al. (2006). "Immunologic consequences of multiple, high-dose administration of allogeneic mesenchymal stem cells to baboons." Cell Transplant 15(8-9): 711-721.

Bernardo, M. E., N. Zaffaroni, et al. (2007). "Human bone marrow derived mesenchymal stem cells do not undergo transformation after long-term in vitro culture and do not exhibit telomere maintenance mechanisms." Cancer Res 67(19): 9142-9149.

Bianco, P. (2011). "Back to the future: Moving beyond "mesenchymal stem cells"." J Cell Biochem 112(7): 1713-1721.

Bianco, P., P. G. Robey, et al. (2008). "Mesenchymal stem cells: revisiting history, concepts, and assays." Cell Stem Cell 2(4): 313-319.

Caplan, A. I. (1991). "Mesenchymal stem cells." J Orthop Res 9(5): 641-650.

Chabannes, D., M. Hill, et al. (2007). "A role for heme oxygenase-1 in the immunosuppressive effect of adult rat and human mesenchymal stem cells." Blood 110(10): 3691-3694.

Comoli, P., F. Ginevri, et al. (2008). "Human mesenchymal stem cells inhibit antibody production induced in vitro by allostimulation." Nephrol Dial Transplant 23(4): 1196-1202.

Corcione, A., F. Benvenuto, et al. (2006). "Human mesenchymal stem cells modulate B-cell functions." Blood 107(1): 367-372.

Couri, C. E. and J. C. Voltarelli (2009). "Stem cell therapy for type 1 diabetes mellitus: a review of recent clinical trials." Diabetol Metab Syndr 1(1): 19.

Crop, M. J., C. C. Baan, et al. (2009). "Donor-derived mesenchymal stem cells suppress alloreactivity of kidney transplant patients." Transplantation 87(6): 896-906.

Crop, M. J., C. C. Baan, et al. (2010). "Inflammatory conditions affect gene expression and function of human adipose tissue-derived mesenchymal stem cells." Clin Exp Immunol 162(3): 474-486.

Crop, M. J., C. C. Baan, et al. (2010). "Human adipose tissue-derived mesenchymal stem cells induce explosive T-cell proliferation." Stem Cells Dev 19(12): 1843-1853.

Crop, M. J., S. S. Korevaar, et al. (2011). "Human mesenchymal stem cells are susceptible to lysis by CD8+ T-cells and NK cells." Cell Transplant.

Dahlke, M. H., M. Hoogduijn, et al. (2009). "Toward MSC in solid organ transplantation: 2008 position paper of the MISOT study group." Transplantation 88(5): 614-619.

DelaRosa, O., E. Lombardo, et al. (2009). "Requirement of IFN-gamma-mediated indoleamine 2,3-dioxygenase expression in the modulation of lymphocyte proliferation by human adipose-derived stem cells." Tissue Eng Part A 15(10): 2795-2806.

Di Ianni, M., B. Del Papa, et al. (2008). "Mesenchymal cells recruit and regulate T regulatory cells." Exp Hematol 36(3): 309-318.

Di Nicola, M., C. Carlo-Stella, et al. (2002). "Human bone marrow stromal cells suppress T-lymphocyte proliferation induced by cellular or nonspecific mitogenic stimuli." Blood 99(10): 3838-3843.

Dittmar, K. E., M. Simann, et al. (2010). "Quality of Cell Products: Authenticity, Identity, Genomic Stability and Status of Differentiation." Transfus Med Hemother 37(2): 57-64.

Dominici, M., K. Le Blanc, et al. (2006). "Minimal criteria for defining multipotent mesenchymal stromal cells. The International Society for Cellular Therapy position statement." Cytotherapy 8(4): 315-317.

Eggenhofer, E., J. F. Steinmann, et al. (2011). "Mesenchymal stem cells together with mycophenolate mofetil inhibit antigen presenting cell and T cell infiltration into allogeneic heart grafts." Transpl Immunol 24(3): 157-163.

Eliopoulos, N., J. Stagg, et al. (2005). "Allogeneic marrow stromal cells are immune rejected by MHC class I- and class II-mismatched recipient mice." Blood 106(13): 4057-4065.

English, K., A. French, et al. (2010). "Mesenchymal stromal cells: facilitators of successful transplantation?" Cell Stem Cell 7(4): 431-442.

English, K., J. M. Ryan, et al. (2009). "Cell contact, prostaglandin E(2) and transforming growth factor beta 1 play non-redundant roles in human mesenchymal stem cell induction of CD4+CD25(High) forkhead box P3+ regulatory T cells." Clin Exp Immunol 156(1): 149-160.

Friedenstein, A. J., R. K. Chailakhyan, et al. (1974). "Stromal cells responsible for transferring the microenvironment of the hemopoietic tissues. Cloning in vitro and retransplantation in vivo." Transplantation 17(4): 331-340.

Gao, F., D. Q. Wu, et al. (2008). "In vitro cultivation of islet-like cell clusters from human umbilical cord blood-derived mesenchymal stem cells." Transl Res 151(6): 293-302.

Garin, M. I., C. C. Chu, et al. (2007). "Galectin-1: a key effector of regulation mediated by CD4+CD25+ T cells." Blood 109(5): 2058-2065.

Ge, W., J. Jiang, et al. (2009). "Infusion of mesenchymal stem cells and rapamycin synergize to attenuate alloimmune responses and promote cardiac allograft tolerance." Am J Transplant 9(8): 1760-1772.

Gieseke, F., J. Bohringer, et al. (2010). "Human multipotent mesenchymal stromal cells use galectin-1 to inhibit immune effector cells." Blood 116(19): 3770-3779.

Hematti, P. (2008). "Role of mesenchymal stromal cells in solid organ transplantation." Transplant Rev (Orlando) 22(4): 262-273.

Hoogduijn, M. J., F. Popp, et al. (2010). "The immunomodulatory properties of mesenchymal stem cells and their use for immunotherapy." Int Immunopharmacol 10(12): 1496-1500.

Hoogduijn, M. J., F. C. Popp, et al. (2010). "Advancement of mesenchymal stem cell therapy in solid organ transplantation (MISOT)." Transplantation 90(2): 124-126.

Hyun, I., O. Lindvall, et al. (2008). "New ISSCR guidelines underscore major principles for responsible translational stem cell research." Cell Stem Cell 3(6): 607-609.

In 't Anker, P. S., S. A. Scherjon, et al. (2004). "Isolation of mesenchymal stem cells of fetal or maternal origin from human placenta." Stem Cells 22(7): 1338-1345.

Jiang, X. X., Y. Zhang, et al. (2005). "Human mesenchymal stem cells inhibit differentiation and function of monocyte-derived dendritic cells." Blood 105(10): 4120-4126.

Karlsson, H., S. Samarasinghe, et al. (2008). "Mesenchymal stem cells exert differential effects on alloantigen and virus-specific T-cell responses." Blood 112(3): 532-541.

Karp, J. M. and G. S. Leng Teo (2009). "Mesenchymal stem cell homing: the devil is in the details." Cell Stem Cell 4(3): 206-216.

Kim, Y. H., Y. M. Wee, et al. (2011). "IL-10 induced by CD11b+cells and IL-10 activated regulatory T cells play a role in immune modulation of mesenchymal stem cells in rat islet allograft." Mol Med.

Krampera, M., L. Cosmi, et al. (2006). "Role for interferon-gamma in the immunomodulatory activity of human bone marrow mesenchymal stem cells." Stem Cells 24(2): 386-398.

Lazarus, H. M., O. N. Koc, et al. (2005). "Cotransplantation of HLA-identical sibling culture-expanded mesenchymal stem cells and hematopoietic stem cells in hematologic malignancy patients." Biol Blood Marrow Transplant 11(5): 389-398.

Le Blanc, K., I. Rasmusson, et al. (2004). "Treatment of severe acute graft-versus-host disease with third party haploidentical mesenchymal stem cells." Lancet 363(9419): 1439-1441.

Le Blanc, K. and O. Ringden (2007). "Immunomodulation by mesenchymal stem cells and clinical experience." J Intern Med 262(5): 509-525.

Le Blanc, K., H. Samuelsson, et al. (2007). "Generation of immunosuppressive mesenchymal stem cells in allogeneic human serum." Transplantation 84(8): 1055-1059.

Le Blanc, K., C. Tammik, et al. (2003). "HLA expression and immunologic properties of differentiated and undifferentiated mesenchymal stem cells." Exp Hematol 31(10): 890-896.

Li, Y. P., S. Paczesny, et al. (2008). "Human mesenchymal stem cells license adult CD34+ hemopoietic progenitor cells to differentiate into regulatory dendritic cells through activation of the Notch pathway." J Immunol 180(3): 1598-1608.

Meisel, R., A. Zibert, et al. (2004). "Human bone marrow stromal cells inhibit allogeneic T-cell responses by indoleamine 2,3-dioxygenase-mediated tryptophan degradation." Blood 103(12): 4619-4621.

Nauta, A. J. and W. E. Fibbe (2007). "Immunomodulatory properties of mesenchymal stromal cells." Blood 110(10): 3499-3506.

Nauta, A. J., A. B. Kruisselbrink, et al. (2006). "Mesenchymal stem cells inhibit generation and function of both CD34+-derived and monocyte-derived dendritic cells." J Immunol 177(4): 2080-2087.

Nauta, A. J., G. Westerhuis, et al. (2006). "Donor-derived mesenchymal stem cells are immunogenic in an allogeneic host and stimulate donor graft rejection in a nonmyeloablative setting." Blood 108(6): 2114-2120.

Ng, F., S. Boucher, et al. (2008). "PDGF, TGF-beta, and FGF signaling is important for differentiation and growth of mesenchymal stem cells (MSCs): transcriptional profiling can identify markers and signaling pathways important in differentiation of MSCs into adipogenic, chondrogenic, and osteogenic lineages." Blood 112(2): 295-307.

Ng, W. F., P. J. Duggan, et al. (2001). "Human CD4(+)CD25(+) cells: a naturally occurring population of regulatory T cells." Blood 98(9): 2736-2744.

Pittenger, M. F., A. M. Mackay, et al. (1999). "Multilineage potential of adult human mesenchymal stem cells." Science 284(5411): 143-147.

Poggi, A., C. Prevosto, et al. (2007). "NKG2D and natural cytotoxicity receptors are involved in natural killer cell interaction with self-antigen presenting cells and stromal cells." Ann N Y Acad Sci 1109: 47-57.

Polchert, D., J. Sobinsky, et al. (2008). "IFN-gamma activation of mesenchymal stem cells for treatment and prevention of graft versus host disease." Eur J Immunol 38(6): 1745-1755.

Popp, F. C., E. Eggenhofer, et al. (2008). "Mesenchymal stem cells can induce long-term acceptance of solid organ allografts in synergy with low-dose mycophenolate." Transpl Immunol 20(1-2): 55-60.

Popp, F. C., P. Renner, et al. (2009). "Mesenchymal stem cells as immunomodulators after liver transplantation." Liver Transpl 15(10): 1192-1198.

Prevosto, C., M. Zancolli, et al. (2007). "Generation of CD4+ or CD8+ regulatory T cells upon mesenchymal stem cell-lymphocyte interaction." Haematologica 92(7): 881-888.

Quaedackers, M. E., C. C. Baan, et al. (2009). "Cell contact interaction between adipose-derived stromal cells and allo-activated T lymphocytes." Eur J Immunol 39(12): 3436-3446.

Rasmusson, I., O. Ringden, et al. (2003). "Mesenchymal stem cells inhibit the formation of cytotoxic T lymphocytes, but not activated cytotoxic T lymphocytes or natural killer cells." Transplantation 76(8): 1208-1213.

Rasmusson, I., M. Uhlin, et al. (2007). "Mesenchymal stem cells fail to trigger effector functions of cytotoxic T lymphocytes." J Leukoc Biol 82(4): 887-893.

Ren, G., L. Zhang, et al. (2008). "Mesenchymal stem cell-mediated immunosuppression occurs via concerted action of chemokines and nitric oxide." Cell Stem Cell 2(2): 141-150.

Ren, G., X. Zhao, et al. (2010). "Inflammatory cytokine-induced intercellular adhesion molecule-1 and vascular cell adhesion molecule-1 in mesenchymal stem cells are critical for immunosuppression." J Immunol 184(5): 2321-2328.

Ringden, O. and K. Le Blanc (2011). "Mesenchymal stem cells for treatment of acute and chronic graft-versus-host disease, tissue toxicity and hemorrhages." Best Pract Res Clin Haematol 24(1): 65-72.

Ryan, J. M., F. P. Barry, et al. (2005). "Mesenchymal stem cells avoid allogeneic rejection." J Inflamm (Lond) 2: 8.

Sanchez-Ramos, J. (2006). "Stem cells from umbilical cord blood." Semin Reprod Med 24(5): 358-369.

Sato, K., K. Ozaki, et al. (2007). "Nitric oxide plays a critical role in suppression of T-cell proliferation by mesenchymal stem cells." Blood 109(1): 228-234.

Schwartz, P. H., D. J. Brick, et al. (2008). "Differentiation of neural lineage cells from human pluripotent stem cells." Methods 45(2): 142-158.

Selmani, Z., A. Naji, et al. (2008). "Human leukocyte antigen-G5 secretion by human mesenchymal stem cells is required to suppress T lymphocyte and natural killer function and to induce CD4+CD25highFOXP3+ regulatory T cells." Stem Cells 26(1): 212-222.

Shi, Y., G. Hu, et al. (2010). "Mesenchymal stem cells: a new strategy for immunosuppression and tissue repair." Cell Res 20(5): 510-518.

Sioud, M. (2011). "New insights into mesenchymal stromal cell-mediated T-cell suppression through galectins." Scand J Immunol 73(2): 79-84.

Sioud, M., A. Mobergslien, et al. (2010). "Evidence for the involvement of galectin-3 in mesenchymal stem cell suppression of allogeneic T-cell proliferation." Scand J Immunol 71(4): 267-274.

Sordi, V., R. Melzi, et al. (2010). "Mesenchymal cells appearing in pancreatic tissue culture are bone marrow-derived stem cells with the capacity to improve transplanted islet function." Stem Cells 28(1): 140-151.

Sotiropoulou, P. A., S. A. Perez, et al. (2006). "Interactions between human mesenchymal stem cells and natural killer cells." Stem Cells 24(1): 74-85.

Spaggiari, G. M., A. Capobianco, et al. (2008). "Mesenchymal stem cells inhibit natural killer-cell proliferation, cytotoxicity, and cytokine production: role of indoleamine 2,3-dioxygenase and prostaglandin E2." Blood 111(3): 1327-1333.

Spaggiari, G. M., A. Capobianco, et al. (2006). "Mesenchymal stem cell-natural killer cell interactions: evidence that activated NK cells are capable of killing MSCs, whereas MSCs can inhibit IL-2-induced NK-cell proliferation." Blood 107(4): 1484-1490.

Sun, J., Z. B. Han, et al. (2011). "Intrapulmonary Delivery of Human Umbilical Cord Mesenchymal Stem Cells Attenuates Acute Lung Injury by Expanding CD4CD25(+) Forkhead Boxp3 (FOXP3) (+) Regulatory T Cells and Balancing Anti- and Pro-inflammatory Factors." Cell Physiol Biochem 27(5): 587-596.

Sundin, M., A. J. Barrett, et al. (2009). "HSCT recipients have specific tolerance to MSC but not to the MSC donor." J Immunother 32(7): 755-764.

Sundin, M., P. D'Arcy, et al. (2011). "Multipotent mesenchymal stromal cells express FoxP3: a marker for the immunosuppressive capacity?" J Immunother 34(4): 336-342.

Sundin, M., O. Ringden, et al. (2007). "No alloantibodies against mesenchymal stromal cells, but presence of anti-fetal calf serum antibodies, after transplantation in allogeneic hematopoietic stem cell recipients." Haematologica 92(9): 1208-1215.

Tabera, S., J. A. Perez-Simon, et al. (2008). "The effect of mesenchymal stem cells on the viability, proliferation and differentiation of B-lymphocytes." Haematologica 93(9): 1301-1309.

Thornton, A. M. and E. M. Shevach (1998). "CD4+CD25+ immunoregulatory T cells suppress polyclonal T cell activation in vitro by inhibiting interleukin 2 production." J Exp Med 188(2): 287-296.

Tolar, J., P. Villeneuve, et al. (2011). "Mesenchymal stromal cells for graft-versus-host disease." Hum Gene Ther 22(3): 257-262.

Uccelli, A., L. Moretta, et al. (2008). "Mesenchymal stem cells in health and disease." Nat Rev Immunol 8(9): 726-736.

Uccelli, A. and D. J. Prockop (2010). "Why should mesenchymal stem cells (MSCs) cure autoimmune diseases?" Curr Opin Immunol 22(6): 768-774.

Ulicna, M., L. Danisovic, et al. (2009). "Diabetes--adult stem cells as an future alternative therapy?" Bratisl Lek Listy 110(12): 773-776.

Voltarelli, J. C., C. E. Couri, et al. (2007). "Autologous nonmyeloablative hematopoietic stem cell transplantation in newly diagnosed type 1 diabetes mellitus." JAMA 297(14): 1568-1576.

Wada, J. and H. Makino (2001). "Galectins, galactoside-binding mammalian lectins: clinical application of multi-functional proteins." Acta Med Okayama 55(1): 11-17.

Yagi, H., T. Nomura, et al. (2004). "Crucial role of FOXP3 in the development and function of human CD25+CD4+ regulatory T cells." Int Immunol 16(11): 1643-1656.

Zuk, P. A. (2010). "The adipose-derived stem cell: looking back and looking ahead." Mol Biol Cell 21(11): 1783-1787.

8

Dendritic Cells in Hematopoietic Stem Cell Transplantation

Yannick Willemen[1,*], Khadija Guerti[1,2,3,*], Herman Goossens[2],
Zwi Berneman[1], Viggo Van Tendeloo[1] and Evelien Smits[1]

*[1]Laboratory of Experimental Hematology, Vaccine
and Infectious Disease Institute*
*[2]Laboratory of Medical Microbiology, Vaccine
and Infectious Disease Institute*
[3]Laboratory of Immunology, Antwerp University Hospital
University of Antwerp
Belgium

1. Introduction

Dendritic cells (DC) are highly specialized antigen-presenting cells (APC) that are pivotal in regulating the balance between immune tolerance and protective immunity. This functional versatility is highlighted in the context of allogeneic hematopoietic stem cell transplantation (allo-HSCT), where DC are crucial for the induction and modulation of graft-versus-host reactions. Furthermore, in the process of immune restoration after allo-HSCT, DC play a central role in generating protective immunity against pathogens. The importance of DC in directing the immune system during the complex immunological situation after allo-HSCT warrants further research, aimed at uncovering the therapeutic potential they hold in this setting.

2. Role of dendritic cells in the development of acute graft-versus-host disease following allogeneic hematopoietic stem cell transplantation

Allo-HSCT is a well-established and valuable therapeutic option for a variety of life-threatening malignant and non-malignant diseases (Gratwohl et al., 2010). In cancer, allo-HSCT has been mainly applied to treat leukemia and lymphoma patients (Gratwohl et al., 2010). Immunologic graft-versus-leukemia (GVL) effects mediated by allogeneic lymphocytes present in the graft are major contributors to its success. A number of distinct donor cell subsets have been identified that may play a role in the GVL responses after allo-HSCT. These include natural killer cells (Gill et al., 2009; Ruggeri et al., 2007), T cells reactive to tumor-specific or tumor-associated antigens (TAA; Molldrem et al., 2002; K. Rezvani & Barrett, 2008), and T cells reactive to host minor histocompatibility (miHC) antigens (Falkenburg et al., 2002, 2003; Riddell et al., 2002, 2003).

---

* Both authors contributed equally

2.1 Development of acute graft-versus-host disease following allogeneic hematopoietic stem cell transplantation

A major obstacle that substantially limits the therapeutic potential of allo-HSCT is the occurrence of graft-versus-host reactions against healthy host tissues, resulting in graft-versus-host disease (GVHD). GVHD is a major cause of morbidity and mortality following allo-HSCT. The overall incidence lies between 30% and 60% with a mortality rate of approximately 50% (Barton-Burke et al., 2008). It is a complex multi-step process, involving innate and adaptive immunity and affecting many organs, including skin, liver and the gastrointestinal tract (Ball & Egeler, 2008; Ferrara et al., 2009).

Billingham was the first to describe GVHD (Billingham, 1966). According to the Billingham criteria, three conditions must exist in order for GVHD to occur after allogeneic transplantation: (1) the donor graft must contain viable and immunologically functional effector cells, (2) the donor and recipient must be histoincompatible, and (3) the recipient must be immunocompromised.

The series of events that contribute to the development of acute GVHD (as described by Ferrara & Reddy, 2006; Goker et al., 2001) can be divided in three phases (Goker et al., 2001). The first phase – conditioning phase – starts before the engraftment. This phase involves tissue damage caused by pre-transplantation myeloablative radiation/chemotherapy regimens, followed by release of lipopolysaccharide and secretion of proinflammatory cytokines, upregulation of adhesion molecules and enhanced expression of major histocompatibility complex (MHC) molecules on recipient tissues. The proinflammatory environment will also activate APC. The second phase – induction and expansion phase – starts with the recognition of the histoincompatible host tissue antigens by donor T cells. This phase involves T cell activation, stimulation, proliferation and differentiation. Activated host APC play a key role in the second phase of the graft-versus-host reaction by presenting mismatched recipient antigens to donor T cells. The first two phases constitute the afferent phase of GVHD. Finally, the third phase – effector phase – represents the actual clinical phase of acute GVHD and involves direct and indirect damage to host cells contributing to aggravation of GVHD.

From these models, it is clear that donor T cells play a crucial role in evoking GVHD after allo-HSCT. Simultaneously, donor T cells represent major mediators of GVL effects. Therefore, research efforts are aimed at separating GVL reactions from GVHD (Li et al., 2009a; Mackinnon et al., 1995; A.R. Rezvani & Storb, 2008). A key question is whether GVL activity and GVHD are fundamentally different mechanisms, or whether they are both clinical manifestations of similar graft-versus-host reactions.

Preclinical model systems and clinical trials designed to investigate the possibility of selectively activating graft-versus-host reactions that result in GVL effects without GVHD, have led to new insights in the pathophysiology of GVL responses and GVHD after allo-HSCT (Li et al., 2009a; A.R. Rezvani & Storb, 2008). In a more complex model of human GVHD and GVL pathophysiology (Li et al., 2009a), differentiation of activated T cells into the distinct subsets T helper (Th)1/cytotoxic T cell (Tc)1, Th2/Tc2, Th17 or regulatory T (Treg) cells is taken into account. These T cell subsets differ both in cytokine profiles and in their graft-versus-host activities. Activated Th1/Tc1 cells can directly attack host tissue and initiate specific inflammatory immune responses that lead to both GVL responses and acute GVHD. Th2 cells on the other hand, evoke antigen-specific cellular and humoral immune responses resulting in GVL responses, but also in chronic GVHD. Notably, Th2 cytokines may inhibit the development of acute GVHD. Activated Th17 cells potentiate inflammation and lead to acute GVHD, whereas the Th1 cytokine interferon (IFN)-γ can suppress Th17 responses to decrease GVHD. Donor Treg cells suppress GVHD, but the effect of Treg cells on GVL responses remains to be further elucidated. The T cell subsets that are most likely associated with shifting the balance away from GVHD towards GVL responses are Th1/Tc1, γδ T and Treg cells (Li et al., 2009a).

2.2 Dendritic cells in the development of acute graft-versus-host disease

Early models have mainly focused on the central role of T cell activation and cytokine release in the pathophysiologic process of GVHD. The 1966 Billingham criteria clearly accounted for the presence of viable and immunologically functional effector cells as a prerequisite for the development of GVHD (Billingham, 1966). More recent models of GVHD (Choi et al., 2010; Ferrara & Reddy, 2006; Goker et al., 2001; Li et al., 2009a) also take into account the key role of antigen presentation in its development by stating that activation of APC precedes activation and clonal expansion of T cells in the immune cascade. Host APC play a crucial role in the graft-versus-host reaction by presenting mismatched recipient antigens to donor T cells (Goker et al., 2001). In allo-HSCT with a histocompatible donor, the relevant antigens are miHC antigens (Falkenburg et al., 2002, 2003; Ridell et al., 2002, 2003). APC digest miHC antigens into short peptides that are linked to MHC molecules and presented on the surface of APC as allopeptide-MHC complexes. Physical interaction between the allopeptide-MHC complexes and antigen-specific T cell receptors (TCR) then leads to recognition and activation of antigen-specific T cells (Clark & Chakraverty, 2002; Goker et al., 2001).

Following allo-HSCT, a unique situation is created in which both host- and donor-derived APC co-exist within the host. Thus, foreign miHC antigens can be presented by either host-derived or donor-derived APC. The latter case implies effective cross-presentation of recipient miHC antigens by donor-derived APC (Shlomchik, 2003). The roles of host- and donor-derived APC in the development of GVHD have been examined in experimental mouse studies. In a murine allogeneic bone marrow transplantation (BMT) model, Shlomchik and colleagues showed that host-derived APC were necessary and sufficient to initiate GVHD (Shlomchik et al., 1999). Donor APC on the other hand, while redundant for the onset of GVHD, were required to maximize the GVHD (Matte et al., 2004). A model focusing on the role of host-derived APC in the effector phase of GVHD demonstrated that tissue-resident APC control migration of alloreactive donor T cells into the tissues and subsequent local development of GVHD (Zhang et al., 2002).

APC represent a heterogeneous population of cells with varying antigen-presenting capacities. As the most specialized and professional APC of the immune system, DC are highly efficient in processing and presenting antigens (Mellman & Steinman, 2001). The role of DC in GVHD has been investigated and confirmed in various experimental settings (Mohty, 2007; Mohty & Gaugler, 2008; Xu et al., 2008).

Allo-HSCT can change the origin (host- versus donor-derived), number, lineage and activation level of DC in the host (Clark & Chakraverty, 2002). Several studies have examined the role of DC counts and subsets in the development and severity of GVHD. Based on their immunophenotype and functional properties, DC can be classified into myeloid conventional DC (cDC) and plasmacytoid DC (pDC) (Liu, 2001). A murine BMT model demonstrated that host-derived DC are necessary and sufficient for priming donor T cells to cause acute GVHD (Duffner et al., 2004). In humans, peripheral blood DC chimerism experiments have been performed following allo-HSCT to analyze the contribution of different DC subsets to GVHD (Boeck et al., 2006; Chan et al., 2003; Pihusch et al., 2005). Findings of Chan et al (Chan et al., 2003) confirmed the importance of host DC, because persistence of the DC at day 100 after allo-HSCT was correlated with GVHD. On the other hand, graft-versus-host reactions were also detected in patients that had DC exclusively of donor origin (Boeck et al., 2006). Lower counts of cDC and pDC in patients were associated with an increased risk for acute GVHD (Horváth et al., 2009; Lau et al., 2007; Rajasekar et al., 2008; Reddy et al., 2004; Vakkila et al., 2005). In addition, higher numbers of donor pDC following allo-HSCT decreased the risk of developing chronic GVHD, but also increased the risk of relapse, possibly due to interference with GVL reactions (Waller et al., 2001). In contrast to these data, higher pDC numbers in the graft or in the recipient after allo-HSCT have also been found to correlate with the development of chronic GVHD (Clark et al., 2003; Rossi et al., 2002). Next to absolute numbers, also activation status can be predictive of GVHD, with activated cDC being highly correlated with acute GVHD (Lau et al., 2007). Taken together, experimental data suggest that different DC subsets have different effects on GVHD and GVL reactions, but further research is required to unravel the exact role of each subset.

3. Dendritic cell-based therapy and allogeneic hematopoietic stem cell transplantation

Over the past decade several approaches of DC-based therapy in allo-HSCT settings have been scrutinized, yielding some promising results with regard to decreasing GVHD, optimizing GVL reactions and restoring protective immunity against pathogens.

3.1 Dendritic cell-based therapy to reduce graft-versus-host-disease and enhance graft-versus-leukemia effects

Allogeneic T cells have the capacity to kill residual malignant cells in the host, but also to destruct normal host tissue contributing to GVHD, which can be life-threatening and limits the use of allo-HSCT. While T cell depletion of the graft is a very effective way of reducing the risk of GVHD, it also diminishes the GVL effect, thereby increasing the risk of relapse. Hence, a more refined approach is needed to balance graft-versus-host reactions after allo-HSCT. Given the inherent key regulatory function of DC, DC-based therapy is considered an attractive approach to shift the balance in favor of GVL reactions.

3.1.1 Dendritic cell-based therapy to reduce graft-versus-host-disease

The finding in murine BMT models that host APC are necessary for GVHD to develop (Matte et al., 2004; Shlomchik et al., 1999), led the authors to suggest that depletion of host APC before the conditioning regimen should prevent GVHD without the need for prolonged immunosuppressive treatment.

Antibody-mediated depletion of DC was investigated in a chimeric human/mouse model of GVHD, in which severe combined immunodeficient (SCID) mice received a xenogeneic transplantation with human peripheral blood mononuclear cells (PBMC) (Wilson et al., 2009). Antibodies against the DC activation marker CD83 were injected in host mice 3 hours before injection of human PBMC. This therapeutic intervention almost completely prevented lethal GVHD, whereas negative control mice all developed severe GVHD.

Moreover, mice treated with anti-CD83 antibodies required no further immunosuppressive therapy and possessed functional T cell immunity *in vitro* (Wilson et al., 2009).

These data support further investigation of *in vivo* depletion of host and/or donor APC as a way of preventing GVHD in allo-HSCT recipients. This strategy makes redundant both T cell depletion, thereby preserving the memory T cell pool, and T cell-targeted immunosuppression, which greatly hampers GVL responses and protective immunity. However, the effect of DC depletion on GVL responses still needs to be investigated in animal allo-HSCT models including *in vivo* leukemic challenge. Some concern can be raised about potential interference of DC depletion with the GVL effect, because in mice studies antigen-presentation by host APC has been shown to be important in mediating GVL responses following donor lymphocyte infusions (DLI) (Chakraverty et al., 2006; Mapara et al., 2002). Furthermore, DC depletion might result in a delayed restorage of immunity against pathogens (Clark & Chakraverty, 2002).

More thorough elucidation of the role of distinct DC subsets in allo-antigen responses after allo-HSCT will pave the way to depletion of undesirable or expansion of desirable DC subsets. In this context, a study of Li et al. (Li et al., 2009b) has shown that manipulating the content of donor APC subsets in allo-HSCT grafts can enhance the GVL effect without increasing GVHD. In their study, leukemia-bearing mice that received hematopoietic stem cells (HSC) and CD11b-negative donor APC had substantially enhanced survival compared to recipients of HSC alone, HSC and T cells, or HSC and CD11b-positive APC.

Another promising strategy to modulate allo-antigen responses following allo-HSCT involves DC engineered to boost their tolerogenic or regulatory capacities.

In a study of Reichardt et al (Reichardt et al., 2008), DC were isolated directly from mice bone marrow and spleen cells using positive magnetic cell selection and exposed to rapamycin for 24 hours. Adoptive transfer of rapamycin-treated DC of host origin, but not donor origin, administered together with the bone marrow transplant, reduced GVHD severity and led to improved survival of recipient mice in a dose-dependent way. The reduced expansion of alloreactive T cells could account for the beneficial effects on GVHD and survival, but carries the risk of reducing the GVL effect.

In two other studies with similar methodology (Chorny et al., 2006; Sato et al., 2003), DC were generated from murine bone marrow cells using granulocyte macrophage colony-stimulating factor (GM-CSF) and either interleukin (IL)-10 and transforming growth factor (TGF)-β1 or vasoactive intestinal peptide (VIP) for 6 days. Then, lipopolysaccharide (LPS) was added for 2 days to induce activation, followed by injection of the DC 2 days after BMT. Results of both studies demonstrated that host-matched DC, but not host-mismatched DC, prevented the onset of severe GVHD in recipient mice in a dose-dependent way. In order to study the effect of DC therapy on GVL responses, mice were challenged with P815 or A20 malignant cells. BMT recipient mice that received host-matched DC were not only protected from lethal GVHD, but also maintained a strong GVL effect and survived significantly longer than control animals (Chorny et al., 2006; Sato et al., 2003).

In conclusion, the administration of specifically engineered DC appears to be a favorable means of modulating alloreactivity after allo-HSCT, because they are able to reduce the risk of severe GVHD, while maintaining the benefits of the GVL effect. Clinical trials will have to show if these beneficial effects can also be seen in humans. Considering that only host-matched DC were able to protect the recipient from severe GVHD and conserve a strong GVL effect in these murine models, it seems likely that the DC will have to be tailored to every individual patient. Although this will be costly and labor-intensive, it can be cost-effective if proven beneficial in allo-HSCT.

3.1.2 Dendritic cell-based therapy to enhance the graft-versus-leukemia effect without aggravating graft-versus-host-disease

Donor alloreactive T cells responsible for the GVL effect target a broad range of allogeneic antigens and may thereby lead to GVHD. Hence, there is much interest in developing strategies that can direct the immune reaction towards specific antigens only or primarily expressed on malignant cells, so-called TAA.

As key regulators of the immune system, DC are inherently capable of inducing tumor-specific immune responses (Steinman & Banchereau, 2007). Various clinical studies have already explored the use of DC loaded with TAA as cellular cancer vaccines for hematological malignancies (Smits et al., 2011; Van de Velde et al., 2008). Thus far, results are often modest, but there is proof of principle that a DC vaccine can lead to eradication of malignant cells in an antigen-specific manner. Promisingly, in a phase I/II study by our group, vaccination with autologous monocyte-derived DC loaded with Wilms' tumor 1 (WT1) protein-encoding mRNA was able to convert partial remission into complete molecular remission in two patients in the absence of any other therapy (Van Tendeloo et al., 2010). These clinical responses were correlated with vaccine-associated increases in WT1-specific CD8+ T cell frequencies.

While DC vaccines are thoroughly being investigated in clinical trials for their capacity to induce tumor-specific immune responses, only few trials addressed their use in the setting of HSCT. In the context of autologous hematopoietic stem cell transplantation (auto-HSCT) for multiple myeloma (MM), a clinical trial in 27 patients suggested a benefit in overall survival of vaccination with autologous idiotype-pulsed APC, given at 4 time points after auto-HSCT, compared to historical controls (Lacy et al., 2009).

In allo-HSCT, the dynamic immunological situation that follows transplantation due to the scollision of donor and host immune system adds complexity to the development of DC-based therapy. Hitherto, it is unclear whether donor- or host-derived DC would be best suited for use in immunotherapy aimed at increasing GVL responses. In this regard, murine models demonstrated that host APC are crucial for GVL reactions and that donor APC, although not strictly necessary, can contribute to the GVL effect (Matte et al., 2004; Reddy et al., 2005). This is similar to what is observed in GVHD, which is not surprising given that both are manifestations of graft-versus-host immunity. Therefore, avoiding aggravation of GVHD is an important concern when developing DC-based strategies aiming to augment GVL immunity after allo-HSCT.

Next to GVHD, another concern regarding DC vaccination to boost GVL responses is its effectiveness when given shortly after allo-HSCT, considering the immunosuppressive state of patients at that time. Murine vaccination studies have shown, however, that tumor lysate-pulsed bone marrow-derived DC administered early after auto- or allo-HSCT can elicit effective anti-tumor immunity (Asavaroengchai et al., 2002; Moyer et al., 2006). Furthermore, DC vaccination around the time of HSCT could have some benefits, such as lower tumor burden, donor T cells that are not tolerant to host antigens and low numbers of host Treg cells (Hashimoto et al., 2011).

A total of 6 patients have been involved in three clinical reports of DC vaccines after allo-HSCT. Donor monocyte-derived DC were used for vaccination, pulsed with recipient tumor cells (Fujii et al., 2001; Tatsugami et al., 2004) or with WT1 peptide (Kitawaki et al., 2008). Only one trial reported clinical, but transient responses in 4 relapsed patients with hematological malignancies in the absence of GVHD (Fujii et al., 2001). There were no detectable responses nor GVHD in the other two cases (renal cell carcinoma and acute myeloid leukemia). In the trial reporting clinical responses, patients were infused both with donor monocyte-derived DC pulsed with irradiated patient tumor cells and with donor T cells primed by these DC, which might both have contributed to the observed responses.

A fourth study involving 20 MM patients investigated DLI and/or host-derived DC vaccination (Levenga et al., 2010). The authors concluded that partial T cell-depleted allo-HSCT can be combined with pre-emptive DLI and recipient monocyte-derived DC vaccination to increase graft-versus-myeloma effects with limited GVHD.

In conclusion, early results of clinical DC vaccination in the context of HSCT are promising with no or limited GVHD, but because of the small study populations and lack of controls, further research is required.

Instead of engineering DC *ex vivo* and then transferring them to patients, another approach is to directly target them *in vivo*. To our knowledge, this approach has not been tested yet in the allo-HSCT setting.

However, in 8 patients with Hodgkin disease, non-Hodgkin lymphoma or advanced-stage breast cancer, auto-HSCT was followed by immunotherapy with fms-like tyrosine kinase receptor-3-ligand (Flt3-L) for 6 weeks (Chen et al., 2005). Flt3-L is a hematopoietic growth factor, essential for the development of DC from progenitor cells. This phase I study demonstrated that vaccination with Flt3-L was safe and well-tolerated, resulting in increased frequencies and absolute numbers of circulating immature DC and their precursors in patients' blood without affecting other mature cell lineages. The expanded DC were mostly pDC and were shown here to enhance T cell activation and NK cell cytotoxicity against tumor cells *in vitro* after Toll-like receptor 9-ligand administration, but are also known to play a role in antiviral immunity and in preventing GVHD (Arpinati et al., 2003). In correspondence with these data, others have also suggested that mobilization of specific DC subsets through Flt3-L administration might be a feasible way to target DC *in vivo* (Eto et al., 2002; Teshima et al., 2002), but more research is needed to unravel the functional diversity of these mobilized DC.

3.2 Dendritic cell-based therapy to restore protective immunity against pathogens

Viral and fungal infections are an important cause of morbidity and mortality in patients following HSCT (Gratwohl et al., 2005). These patients have increased susceptibility for primary infection, reinfection and also reactivation of latent viruses due to hampering of their immune system by two main factors (Smits & Berneman, 2010). Firstly, there is the immunosuppressed state accompanying HSCT, often further increased by medication given to prevent GVHD. Secondly, the intense pre-transplantation chemotherapy conditioning regimen, intended to destroy a large part of blood cells, is believed to eliminate memory T cells. Furthermore, early after HSCT dysfunctional DC lead to severely impaired development of antigen-specific T cells (Safdar, 2006). Considering their central role in innate and adaptive immunity, DC seem the ideal candidate for immunotherapy aimed at bringing about the swift restoration of immunity against pathogens in this particular setting. With regard to DC-based therapy for antifungal immunity after allo-HSCT, much knowledge was obtained from research by the group of Romani. They showed in murine models of allo-HSCT that DC discriminate between different fungal morphotypes or their corresponding RNA with regard to maturation, cytokine production and Th1 cell priming both *in vitro* and *in vivo* (Bacci et al., 2002; Bozza et al., 2003; d'Ostiani et al., 2000). Similarly, also human monocyte-derived DC were found to react differently in terms of cytokine production and activation of IFN-γ-producing T cells.

Subcutaneous vaccination of mice with DC pulsed with Candida yeasts or Aspergillus conidia (or transfected with the corresponding RNA) on days 1 and 7 after T cell-depleted allo-BMT dramatically increased the recovery of antifungal resistance to subsequent fungal challenge (Bacci et al., 2002; Bozza et al., 2003).

They also demonstrated that Flt3-L-expanded and thymosin α1-treated IL-4-expanded monocyte-derived DC were capable of inducing antifungal immunity as well as allogeneic transplant tolerance (Romani et al., 2006). Overall, the findings of the group of Romani suggest a role for active DC vaccination very shortly after allo-HSCT to restore antifungal immunity and show that expansion of distinct DC might allow more specific regulation of post-transplantation immunity (Montagnoli et al., 2008; Perruccio et al., 2004).

Over the last 10 years, DC have established a firm foothold in immune-based strategies aimed at restoring antiviral (and especially anti-CMV) immunity following allo-HSCT. Monocyte-derived DC from CMV-seropositive HSCT donors pulsed with CMV peptide/lysate or transfected with an adenoviral vector encoding CMV-peptide, have been used with great success to expand CMV-specific cytotoxic T lymphocytes (CTL) *ex vivo* (Micklethwaite et al., 2008; Peggs et al., 2001; Szmania et al., 2001). Clinical trials examining adoptive transfer of these DC-expanded CMV-specific CTL to allo-HSCT recipients demonstrated that this is a safe method capable of restoring functional anti-CMV immunity early after transplantation (Micklethwaite et al., 2007, 2008; Peggs et al., 2009). Although a minority of the patients developed GVHD after adoptive transfer of CMV-specific CTL, this was most likely not related to the infusion itself.

Another study showed that DC transfected with CMV pp65-encoding RNA can successfully expand autologous CMV-specific CTL *in vitro* from both seropositive and -negative patients after allo-HSCT, suggesting that CMV-loaded DC vaccination could provide a valid clinical alternative to adoptive CTL transfer (Heine et al., 2006).

Also for measles virus (MV), DC vaccination could be a favorable approach as results of an *in vitro* study with MV-loaded DC from HSCT patients showed that these DC significantly induced autologous MV-specific T cells from the naïve repertoire (Nashida et al., 2006). Clinical trials are needed, however, to validate whether viral antigen-loaded DC vaccination can indeed live up to the promising results obtained with adoptive virus-specific CTL transfer.

4. Conclusion

DC have been the subject of intensive investigation in mouse models to reduce the occurrence of GVHD and enhance GVL reactions following allo-HSCT. Also in humans, it is clear that DC play an important role in initiating and balancing graft-versus-host reactions. Further clarification of differences between DC subsets in their capacity to shift the balance away from GVHD towards GVL and anti-microbial reactions will help to translate the promising mouse data into clinical success. Questions to be solved are which would be the best time frame and strategy of immunotherapy to use in allotransplant patients. DC-based approaches to be further investigated include DC vaccines, adoptive transfer of *in vitro* primed T cells and *in vivo* targeting of DC.

5. Acknowledgment

E.S. is postdoctoral researcher of the Research Foundation Flanders (FWO-Vlaanderen). This work was supported in part by research grants of the FWO-Vlaanderen (G.0082.08), the Belgian Foundation against Cancer, the Vlaamse Liga tegen Kanker, the National Cancer Plan Action 29, the Agency for Innovation by Science and Technology (IWT-TBM) and the Methusalem program of the Flemish Government.

6. References

Arpinati, M.; Chirumbolo, G.; Urbini, B.; Perrone, G.; Rondelli, D. & Anasetti, C. (2003). Role of plasmacytoid dendritic cells in immunity and tolerance after allogeneic hematopoietic stem cell transplantation. *Transplant Immunology*, Vol.11, No.3-4, (July-September 2003), pp. 345-356, ISSN 0966-3274

Asavaroengchai, W.; Kotera, Y. & Mulé, J.J. (2002). Tumor lysate-pulsed dendritic cells can elicit an effective antitumor immune response during early lymphoid recovery. *Proceedings of the National Academy of Sciences of the United States of America*, Vol.99, No.2, (January 2002), pp. 931-936, ISSN 0027-8424

Bacci, A.; Montagnoli, C.; Perruccio, K.; Bozza, S.; Gaziano, R.; Pitzurra, L.; Velardi, A.; d'Ostiani, CF.; Cutler, J.E. & Romani, L. (2002). Dendritic cells pulsed with fungal RNA induce protective immunity to Candida albicans in hematopoietic transplantation. *Journal of Immunology*, Vol.168, No.6, (March 2002), pp. 2904-2913, ISSN 0022-1767

Ball, L.M. & Egeler, R.M. (2008). Acute GvHD: pathogenesis and classification. *Bone Marrow Transplantation*, Vol.41, Suppl.2, (June 2008), pp. 58-64, ISSN 0268-3369

Barton-Burke, M.; Dwinell, D.M.; Kafkas, L.; Lavalley, C.; Sands, H.; Proctor, C. & Johnson E. (2008). Graft-versus-host disease: a complex long-term side effect of hematopoietic stem cell transplant. *Oncology Williston Park NY*, Vol.22, No.11, (October 2008), pp. 31-45, ISSN 0890-9091

Billingham, R.E. (1966). The biology of graft-versus-host reactions. *Harvey Lectures 1966-67*, Vol.62, pp. 21-78, ISSN 0073-0874

Boeck, S.; Hamann, M.; Pihusch, V.; Heller, T.; Diem, H.; Rolf, B.; Pihusch, R.; Kolb, H.J. & Pihusch, M. (2006). Kinetics of dendritic cell chimerism and T cell chimerism in allogeneic stem cell recipients. *Bone Marrow Transplantation*, Vol.37, No.1, (January 2006), pp. 57-64, ISSN 0268-3369

Bozza, S.; Perruccio, K.; Montagnoli, C.; Gaziano, R.; Bellocchio, S.; Burchielli, E.; Nkwanyuo, G.; Pitzurra, L.; Velardi, A. & Romani, L. (2003). A dendritic cell vaccine against invasive aspergillosis in allogeneic hematopoietic transplantation. *Blood*, Vol.102, No.10, (November 2003), pp. 3807-3814, ISSN 0006-4971

Chakraverty, R.; Eom, H.S.; Sachs, J.; Buchli, J.; Cotter, P.; Hsu, R.; Zhao, G. & Sykes, M. (2006). Host MHC class II+ antigen-presenting cells and CD4 cells are required for CD8-mediated graft-versus-leukemia responses following delayed donor leukocyte infusions. *Blood*, Vol.108, No.6, (September 2006), pp. 2106-2113, ISSN 0006-4971

Chan, G.W.; Gorgun, G.; Miller, K.B. & Foss, F.M. (2003). Persistence of host dendritic cells after transplantation is associated with graft-versus-host disease. *Biology of Blood and Marrow Transplantation*, Vol.9, No.3, (March 2003), pp. 170-176, ISSN 1083-8791

Chen, W.; Chan, A.S.; Dawson, A.J.; Liang, X.; Blazar, B.R. & Miller, J.S. (2005). FLT3 ligand administration after hematopoietic cell transplantation increases circulating dendritic cell precursors that can be activated by CpG oligodeoxynucleotides to enhance T-cell and natural killer cell function. *Biology of Blood and Marrow Transplantation*, Vol.11, No.1, (January 2005), pp. 23-34, ISSN 1083-8791

Choi, S.W.; Levine, J.E. & Ferrara, J.L. (2010). Pathogenesis and management of graft-versus-host disease. *Immunology and Allergy Clinics of North America*, Vol.30, No.1, (February 2010), pp. 75-101, ISSN 0889-8561

Chorny, A.; Gonzalez-Rey, E.; Fernandez-Martin, A.; Ganea, D. & Delgado, M. (2006). Vasoactive intestinal peptide induces regulatory dendritic cells that prevent acute graft-versus-host disease while maintaining the graft-versus-tumor response. *Blood*, Vol.107, No.9, (May 2006), pp. 3787-3794, ISSN 0006-4971

Clark, F.J. & Chakraverty R. (2002). Role of dendritic cells in graft-versus-host disease. *Journal of Hematotherapy & Stem Cell Research*, Vol.11, No.4, (August 2002), pp. 601-616, ISSN 1061-6128

Clark, F.J.; Freeman, L.; Dzionek, A.; Schmitz, J.; McMullan, D.; Simpson, P.; Mason, J.; Mahedra, P.; Craddock, C.; Griffiths, M.; Moss, P.A. & Chakraverty, R. (2003). Origin and subset distribution of peripheral blood dendritic cells in patients with chronisch graft-versus-host disease. *Transplantation*, Vol.75, No.2, (January 2003), pp. 221-225, ISSN 0041-1337

d'Ostiani, C.F.; Del Sero, G.; Bacci, A.; Montagnoli, C.; Spreca, A.; Mencacci, A.; Ricciardi-Castagnoli, P. & Romani, L. (2000). Dendritic cells discriminate between yeasts and hyphae of the fungus Candida albicans. Implications for initiation of T helper cell immunity in vitro and in vivo. *The Journal of Experimental Medicine*, Vol.191, No.10, (May 2000), pp. 1661-1674, ISSN 0022-1007

Duffner, U.A.; Maeda, Y.; Cooke, K.R.; Reddy, P.; Ordemann, R.; Liu, C.; Ferrara, J.L. & Teshima, T. (2004). Host dendritic cells alone are sufficient to initiate acute graft-versus-host disease. *The Journal of Immunology*, Vol.172, No.12, (June 2004), pp. 7393-7398, ISSN 0022-1767

Eto, M.; Hackstein, H.; Kaneko, K.; Nomoto, K. & Thomson, A.W. (2002). Promotion of skin graft tolerance across MHC barriers by mobilization of dendritic cells in donor hemopoietic cell infusions. *The Journal of Immunology*, Vol.169, No.5, (September 2002), pp. 2390-2396, ISSN 0022-1767

Falkenburg, J.H.; Marijt, W.A.; Heemskerk, M.H. & Willemze, R. (2002). Minor histocompatibility antigens as targets of graft-versus-leukemia reactions. *Current Opinion in Hematology*, Vol.9, No.6, (November 2002), pp. 497-502, ISSN 1065-6251

Falkenburg, J.H.; van de Corput, L.; Marijt, E.W. & Willemze, R. (2003). Minor histocompatibility antigens in human stem cell transplantation. *Experimental Hematology*, Vol.31, No.9, (September 2003), pp. 743-751, ISSN 0301-472X

Ferrara, J.L. & Reddy, P. (2006). Pathophysiology of graft-versus-host disease. *Seminars in Hematology*, Vol.43, No.1, (January 2006), pp. 3-10, ISSN 0037-1963

Ferrara, J.L.; Levine, J.E.; Reddy, P. & Holler E. (2009). Graft-versus-host disease. *The Lancet*, Vol.373, No.9674, (May 2009), pp. 1550-1561, ISSN 0140-6736

Fujii, S.; Shimizu, K.; Fujimoto, K.; Kiyokawa, T.; Tsukamoto, A.; Sanada, I. & Kawano, F. (2001). Treatment of post-transplanted, relapsed patients with hematological malignancies by infusion of HLA-matched, allogeneic-dendritic cells (DCs) pulsed with irradiated tumor cells and primed T cells. *Leukemia & Lymphoma*, Vol.42, No.3, (July 2001), pp. 357-369, ISSN 1026-8022

Gill, S.; Olson, J.A. & Negrin, R.S. (2009). Natural killer cells in allogeneic transplantation: effect on engrafment, graft-versus-tumor, and graft-versus-host responses. *Biology of Blood and Marrow Transplantation*, Vol.15, No.7, (July 2009), pp. 765-776, ISSN 1083-8791

Goker, H.; Haznedaroglu, I.C. & Chao, N.J. (2001). Acute graft-vs-host disease: pathobiology and management. *Experimental Hematology*, Vol.29, No.3, (March 2001), pp. 259-277, ISSN 0301-472X

Gratwohl, A.; Brand, R.; Frassoni, F.; Rocha, V.; Niederwieser, D.; Reusser, P.; Einsele, H. & Cordonnier, C. (2005). Cause of death after allogeneic haematopoietic stem cell transplantation (HSCT) in early leukaemias: an EBMT analysis of lethal infectious complications and changes over calendar time. *Bone Marrow Transplantation*, Vol.36, No.9, (November 2005), pp. 757-769, ISSN 0268-3369

Gratwohl, A.; Baldomero, H.; Aljurf, M.; Pasquini, M.C.; Bouzas, L.F.; Yoshimi, A.; Szer, J.; Lipton, J.; Schwendener, A.; Gratwohl, M.; Frauendorfer, K.; Niederwieser, D.; Horowitz, M. & Kodera, Y. (2010). Hematopoietic stem cell transplantation: a global perspective. *Journal of the American Medical Association*, Vol.303, No.16, (April 2010), pp. 1617-1624, ISSN 0098-7484

Hashimoto, D. & Merad, M. (2011). Harnessing dendritic cells to improve allogeneic hematopoietic cell transplantation outcome. *Seminars in Immunology*, Vol.23, No.1, (February 2011), pp. 50-57, ISSN 1044-5323

Heine, A.; Grünebach, F.; Holderried, T.; Appel, S.; Weck, M.M.; Dörfel, D.; Sinzger, C. & Brossart, P. (2006). Transfection of dendritic cells with in vitro-transcribed CMV RNA induces polyclonal CD8+- and CD4+-mediated CMV-specific T cell responses. *Molecular Therapy*, Vol.13, No.2, (February 2006), pp. 280-288, ISSN 1525-0016

Horváth, R.; Budinský, V.; Kayserová, J.; Kalina, T.; Formánková, R.; Starý, J.; Bartůňková, J.; Sedláček, P. & Špíšek, R. (2009). Kinetics of dendritic cells reconstitution and costimulatory molecules expression after myeloablative allogeneic haematopoetic stem cell transplantation: implications for the development of acute graft-versus-host disease. *Clinical Immunology*, Vol.131, No.1, (April 2009), pp. 60-69, ISSN 1521-6616

Kitawaki, T.; Kadowaki, N.; Kondo, T.; Ishikawa, T.; Ichinohe, T.; Teramukai, S.; Fukushima, M.; Kasai, Y.; Maekawa, T. & Uchiyama, T. (2008). Potential of dendritic-cell immunotherapy for relapse after allogeneic hematopoietic stem cell transplantation, shown by WT1 peptide- and keyhole-limpet-hemocyanin-pulsed, donor-derived dendritic-cell vaccine for acute myeloid leukemia. *American Journal of Hematology*, Vol.83, No.4, (April 2008), pp. 315-317, ISSN 0361-8609

Lacy, M.Q.; Mandrekar, S.; Dispenzieri, A.; Hayman, S.; Kumar, S.; Buadi, F.; Dingli, D.; Litzow, M.; Wettstein, P.; Padley, D.; Kabat, B.; Gastineau, D.; Rajkumar, S.V. & Gertz, M.A. (2009). Idiotype-pulsed antigen-presenting cells following autologous transplantation for multiple myeloma may be associated with prolonged survival.

American Journal of Hematology, Vol.84, No.12, (December 2009), pp. 799-802, ISSN 0361-8609

Lau, J.; Sartor, M.; Bradstock, K.F.; Vuckovic S.; Munster, D.J. & Hart, D.N. (2007). Activated circulating dendritic cells after hematopoietic stem cell transplantation predict acute graft-verus-host disease. *Transplantation*, Vol.83, No.7, (April 2007), pp. 839-846, ISSN 0041-1337

Levenga, H.; Schaap, N.; Maas, F.; Esendam, B.; Fredrix, H.; Greupink-Draaisma, A.; de Witte, T.; Dolstra, H. & Raymakers, R. (2010). Partial T cell-depleted allogeneic stem cell transplantation following reduced-intensity conditioning creates a platform for immunotherapy with donor lymphocyte infusion and recipient dendritic cell vaccination in multiple myeloma. *Biology of Blood and Marrow Transplantation*, Vol.16, No.3, (March 2010), pp. 320-332, ISSN 1083-8791

[a]Li, J.M.; Giver, C.R.; Lu, Y.; Hossain, M.S.; Akhtari, M. & Waller, E.K. (2009). Separating graft-versus-leukemia from graft-versus-host disease in allogeneic hematopoietic stem cell transplantation. *Immunotherapy*, Vol.1, No.4, (July 2009), pp. 599-621, ISSN 1750-743X

[b]Li, J.M.; Southerland, L.T.; Lu, Y.; Darlak, K.A.; Giver, C.R.; McMillin, D.W.; Harris, W.A.; Jaye, D.L. & Waller, E.K. (2009). Activation, immune polarization, and graft-versus-leukemia activity of donor T cells are regulated by specific subsets of donor bone marrow antigen-presenting cells in allogeneic hemopoietic stem cell transplantation. *Journal of Immunology*, Vol.183, No.12, (December 2009), pp. 7799-7809, ISSN 0022-1767

Liu, Y.J. (2001). Dendritic cell subsets and lineages, and their functions in innate and adaptive immunity. *Cell*, Vol.106, No.3, (August 2001), pp. 259-262, ISSN 0092-8674

Mackinnon, S.; Papadopoulos, E.B.; Carabasi, M.H.; Reich, L.; Collins, N.H.; Boulad, F.; Castro-Malaspina, H.; Childs, B.H.; Gillio, A.P.; Kernan, N.A.; Small, T.N.; Young, J.W. & O'Reilly, R.J. (1995). Adoptive immunotherapy evaluating escalating doses of donor leukocytes for relapse of chronic myeloid leukemia after bone marrow transplantation: separation of graft-versus-leukemia responses from graft-versus-host disease. *Blood*, Vol.86, No.4, (August 1995), pp. 1261-8, ISSN 0006-4971

Mapara, M.Y.; Kim, Y.M.; Wang, S.P.; Bronson, R.; Sachs, D.H. & Sykes, M. (2002). Donor lymphocyte infusions mediate superior graft-versus-leukemia effects in mixed compared to fully allogeneic chimeras: a critical role for host antigen-presenting cells. *Blood*, Vol.100, No.5, (September 2002), pp. 1903-1909, ISSN 0006-4971

Matte, C.C.; Liu, J.; Cormier, J.; Anderson, B.E.; Athanasiadis, I.; Jain, D.; McNiff, J. & Shlomchik, W.D. (2004). Donor APCs are required for maximal GVHD but not for GVL. *Nature Medicine*, Vol.10, No.9, (September 2004), pp. 987-992, ISSN 1078-8956

Mellman, I. & Steinman, R.M. (2001). Dendritic cells: specialized and regulated antigen processing mahines. *Cell*, Vol.106, No.3, (August 2001), pp. 255-258, ISSN 0092-8674

Micklethwaite, K.; Hansen, A.; Foster, A.; Snape, E.; Antonenas, V.; Sartor, M.; Shaw, P.; Bradstock, K. & Gottlieb, D. (2007). Ex vivo expansion and prophylactic infusion of CMV-pp65 peptide-specific cytotoxic T-lymphocytes following allogeneic hematopoietic stem cell transplantation. *Biology of Blood and Marrow Transplantation*, Vol.13, No.6, (June 2007), pp. 707-714, ISSN 1083-8791

Micklethwaite, K.P.; Clancy, L.; Sandher, U.; Hansen, A.M.; Blyth, E.; Antonenas, V.; Sartor, M.M.; Bradstock, K.F. & Gottlieb, D.J. (2008). Prophylactic infusion of cytomegalovirus-specific cytotoxic T lymphocytes stimulated with Ad5f35pp65 gene-modified dendritic cells after allogeneic hemopoietic stem cell transplantation. *Blood,* Vol.112, No.10, (November 2008), pp. 3974-3981, ISSN 0006-4971

Mohty, M. (2007). Dendritic cells and acute graft-versus-host disease after allogeneic stem cell transplantation. *Leukemia & Lymphoma,* Vol.48, No.9, (September 2007), pp. 1696-1701, ISSN 1042-8194

Mohty, M. & Gaugler, B. (2008). Inflammatory cytokines and dendritic cells in acute graft-versus-host disease after allogeneic stem cell transplantation. *Cytokine & Growth Factor Reviews,* Vol.19, No.1, (February 2008), pp. 53-63, ISSN 1359-6101

Molldrem, J.J.; Komanduri, K. & Wieder, E. (2002). Overexpressed differentiation antigens as targets of graft-versus-leukemia reactions. *Current Opinion in Haematology,* Vol.9, No.6, (November 2002), pp. 503-508, ISSN 1065-6251

Montagnoli, C.; Perruccio, K.; Bozza, S.; Bonifazi, P.; Zelante, T.; De Luca, A.; Moretti, S.; D'Angelo, C.; Bistoni, F.; Martelli, M.; Aversa, F.; Velardi, A. & Romani, L. (2008). Provision of antifungal immunity and concomitant alloantigen tolerization by conditioned dendritic cells in experimental hematopoietic transplantation. *Blood cells, Molecules & Diseases,* Vol.40, No.1, (January-February 2008), pp. 55-62, ISSN 1079-9796

Moyer, J.S.; Maine, G. & Mulé, J.J. (2006). Early vaccination with tumor-lysate-pulsed dendritic cells after allogeneic bone marrow transplantation has antitumor effects. *Biology of Blood and Marrow Transplantation,* Vol.12, No.10, (October 2006), pp. 1010-1019, ISSN 1083-8791

Nashida, Y.; Kumamoto, T.; Azuma, E.; Hirayama, M.; Araki, M.; Yamada, H.; Dida, F.; Iwamoto, S.; Tamaki, S.; Ido, M.; Ihara, T. & Komada, Y. (2006). Development of a dendritic cell vaccine against measles for patients following hematopoietic cell transplantation. *Transplantation,* Vol.82, No.8, (October 2006), pp. 1104-1107, ISSN 0041-1337

Peggs, K.; Verfuerth, S. & Mackinnon, S. (2001). Induction of cytomegalovirus (CMV)-specific T-cell responses using dendritic cells pulsed with CMV antigen: a novel culture system free of live CMV virions. *Blood,* Vol.97, No.4, (February 2001), pp. 994-1000, ISSN 0006-4971

Peggs, K.S.; Verfuerth, S.; Pizzey, A.; Chow, S.L.; Thomson, K. & Mackinnon, S. (2009). Cytomegalovirus-specific T cell immunotherapy promotes restoration of durable functional antiviral immunity following allogeneic stem cell transplantation. *Clinical Infectious Diseases,* Vol.49, No.12, (December 2009), pp. 1851-1860, ISSN 1058-4838

Perruccio, K.; Bozza, S.; Montagnoli, C.; Bellocchio, S.; Aversa, F.; Martelli, M.; Bistoni, F.; Velardi, A. & Romani, L. (2004). Prospects for dendritic cell vaccination against fungal infections in hematopoietic transplantation. *Blood cells, Molecules & Diseases,* Vol.33, No.3, (November-December 2004), pp. 248-255, ISSN 1079-9796

Pihusch, M.; Boeck, S.; Hamann, M.; Pihusch, V.; Heller, T.; Diem, H.; Rolf, B.; Pihusch, R.; Andreesen, R.; Holler, E. & Kolb, H.J. (2005). Peripheral dendritic cell chimerism in allogeneic stem cell recipients. *Transplantation,* Vol.80, No.6, (September 2005), pp. 843-849, ISSN 0041-1337

Rajasekar, R.; Mathews, V.; Lakshmi, K.M.; Sellathamby, S.; George, B.; Viswabandya, A.; Daniel, D.; Chandy, M. & Srivastava, A. (2008). Plasmacytoid dendritic cell count on day 28 in HLA-matched related allogeneic peripheral blood stem cell transplant predicts the incidence of acute and chronic GVHD. *Biology of Blood and Marrow Transplantation*, Vol.14, No.3, (March 2008), pp. 344-350, ISSN 1083-8791

Reddy, V.; Iturraspe, J.A.; Tzolas, A.C.; Meier-Kriesche, H.U.; Schold, J. & Wingard, J.R. (2004). Low dendritic cell count after allogeneic hematopoietic stem cell transplantation predicts relapse, death, and acute graft-versus-host disease. *Blood*, Vol.103, No.11, (June 2004), pp. 4330-4335, ISSN 0006-4971

Reddy, P.; Maeda, Y.; Liu, C.; Krijanovski, O.I.; Korngold, R. & Ferrara, J.L. (2005). A crucial role for antigen-presenting cells and alloantigen expression in graft-versus-leukemia responses. *Nature Medicine*, Vol.11, No.11, (November 2005), pp. 1244-1249, ISSN 1078-8956

Reichardt, W.; Dürr, C.; von Elverfeldt, D.; Jüttner, E.; Gerlach, U.V.; Yamada, M.; Smith, B.; Negrin, R.S. & Zeiser, R. (2008). Impact of mammalian target of rapamycin inhibition on lymphoid homing and tolerogenic function of nanoparticle-labeled dendritic cells following allogeneic hematopoietic cell transplantation. *Journal of Immunology*, Vol.181, No.7, (October 2008), pp. 4770-4779, ISSN 0022-1767

Rezvani, A.R. & Storb, R.F. (2008). Separation of graft-vs.-tumor effects from graft-vs.-host disease in allogeneic hematopoietic cell transplantation. *Journal of Autoimmunity*, Vol.30, No.3, (May 2008), pp. 172-179, ISSN 0896-8411

Rezvani, K. & Barrett, A.J. (2008). Characterizing and optimizing immune responses to leukaemia antigens after allogeneic stem cell transplantation. *Best Practice and Research Clinical Haematology*, Vol.21, No.3, (September 2008), pp. 437-453, ISSN 1521-6926

Riddell, S.R.; Murata, M.; Bryant, S. & Warren, E.H. (2002). Minor histocompatibility antigens - targets of graft versus leukemia responses. *International Journal of Hematology*, Vol.76, Suppl.2, (August 2002), pp. 155-161, ISSN 0925-5710

Riddell, S.R.; Berger, C.; Murata, M.; Randolph, S. & Warren, E.H. (2003). The graft versus leukemia response after allogeneic hematopoietic stem cell transplantation. *Blood Reviews*, Vol.17, No.3, (September 2003), pp. 153-162, ISSN 0268-960X

Romani, L.; Bistoni, F.; Perruccio, K.; Montagnoli, C.; Gaziano, R.; Bozza, S.; Bonifazi, P.; Bistoni, G.; Rasi, G.; Velardi, A.; Fallarino, F.; Garaci, E. & Puccetti, P. (2006). Thymosin alpha1 activates dendritic cell tryptophan catabolism and establishes a regulatory environment for balance of inflammation and tolerance. *Blood*, Vol.108, No.7, (October 2006), pp. 2265-2274, ISSN 0006-4971

Rossi, M.; Arpinati, M.; Rondelli, D. & Anasetti, C. (2002). Plasmacytoid dendritic cells: do they have a role in immune responses after hematopoietic cell transplantation? *Human immunology*, Vol.63, No.12, (December 2002), pp. 1194-1200, ISSN 0198-8859

Ruggeri, L.; Mancusi, A.; Burchielli, E.; Aversa, F.; Martelli, M.F. & Velardi, A. (2007). Natural killer cell alloreactivity in allogeneic hematopoietic transplantation. *Current Opinion in Oncology*, Vol.19, No.2, (March 2007), pp. 142-147, ISSN 1040-8746

Safdar, A. (2006). Strategies to enhance immune function in hematopoietic transplantation recipients who have fungal infections. *Bone Marrow Transplantation*, Vol.38, No.5, (September 2006), pp. 327-337, ISSN 0268-3369

Sato, K.; Yamashita, N.; Yamashita, N.; Baba, M. & Matsuyama, T. (2003). Regulatory dendritic cells protect mice from murine acute graft-versus-host disease and leukemia relapse. *Immunity,* Vol.18, No.3, (March 2003), pp. 367-379, ISSN 1074-7613

Shlomchik, W.D.; Couzens, M.S.; Tang, C.B.; McNiff, J.; Robert, M.E.; Liu, J.; Shlomchik M.J. & Emerson, S.G. (1999). Prevention of graft versus host disease by inactivation of host antigen-presenting cells. *Science,* Vol.285, No.5426, (July 1999), pp. 412-415, ISSN 0036-8075

Shlomchik, W.D. (2003). Antigen presentation in graft-vs-host disease. *Experimental Hematology,* Vol.31, No.12, (December 2003), pp. 1187-1197, ISSN 0301-472X

Smits, E.L. & Berneman, Z.N. (2010). Viral infections following allogeneic stem cell transplantation: how to cure the cure? *Leukemia & Lymphoma,* Vol.51, No.6, (June 2010), pp. 965-966, ISSN 1026-8022

Smits, E.L.; Lee, C.; Hardwick, N.; Brooks, S.; Van Tendeloo, V.F.; Orchard, K.; Guinn, B.A. (2011) Clinical evaluation of cellular immunotherapy in acute myeloid leukaemia. *Cancer Immunology Immunotherapy,* Vol.60, No.6, (June 2011), pp. 757-769, ISSN 1432-0851

Steinman, R.M. & Banchereau, J. (2007). Taking dendritic cells into medicine. *Nature,* Vol.449, No.7161, (September 2007), pp. 419-426, ISSN 0028-0836

Szmania, S.; Galloway, A.; Bruorton, M.; Musk, P.; Aubert, G.; Arthur, A.; Pyle, H.; Hensel, N.; Ta, N.; Lamb, L.Jr.; Dodi, T.; Madrigal, A.; Barrett, J.; Henslee-Downey, J. & van Rhee, F. (2001). Isolation and expansion of cytomegalovirus-specific cytotoxic T lymphocytes to clinical scale from a single blood draw using dendritic cells and HLA-tetramers. *Blood,* Vol.98, No.3, (August 2001), pp. 505-512, ISSN 0006-4971

Tatsugami, K.; Eto, M.; Harano, M.; Nagafuji, K.; Omoto, K.; Katano, M.; Harada, M. & Naito, S. (2004). Dendritic-cell therapy after non-myeloablative stem-cell transplantation for renal-cell carcinoma. *The Lancet Oncology,* Vol.5, No.12, (December 2004), pp. 750-752, ISSN 1470-2045

Teshima, T.; Reddy, P.; Lowler, K.P.; KuKuruga, M.A.; Liu, C.; Cooke, K.R. & Ferrara, J.L. (2002). Flt3 ligand therapy for recipients of allogeneic bone marrow transplants expands host CD8 alpha(+) dendritic cells and reduces experimental acute graft-versus-host disease. *Blood,* Vol.99, No.5, (March 2002), pp. 1825-1832, ISSN 0006-4971

Vakkila, J.; Thomson, A.W.; Hovi, L.; Vettenranta, K. & Saarinen-Pihkala, U.M. (2005). Circulating dendritic cell subset levels after allogeneic stem cell transplantation in children correlate with time post transplant and severity of acute graft-versus-host disease. *Bone Marrow Transplantation,* Vol.35, No.5, (March 2005), pp. 501-507, ISSN 0268-3369

Van de Velde, A.; Berneman, Z.N.; Van Tendeloo, V.F. (2008) Immunotherapy of hematological malignancies using dendritic cells. *Bulletin du Cancer,* Vol.95, No.3, (March 2008), pp. 320-326, ISSN 0007-4551

Van Tendeloo, V.F.; Van de Velde, A.; Van Driessche, A.; Cools, N.; Anguille, S.; Ladell, K.; Gostick, E.; Vermeulen, K.; Pieters, K.; Nijs, G.; Stein, B.; Smits, E.L.; Schroyens, W.A.; Gadisseur, A.P.; Vrelust, I.; Jorens, P.G.; Goossens, H.; de Vries, I.J.; Price, D.A.; Oji, Y.; Oka, Y.; Sugiyama, H. & Berneman, Z.N. (2010). Induction of complete and molecular remissions in acute myeloid leukemia by Wilms' tumor 1 antigen-targeted dendritic cell vaccination. *Proceedings of the National Academy of Sciences of the United States of America,* Vol.107, No.31, (August 2010), pp. 13824-13829, ISSN 0027-8424

Waller, E.K.; Rosenthal, H.; Jones, T.W.; Peel, J.; Lonial, S.; Langston, A.; Redei, I.; Jurickova, I.; Boyer, M.W. (2001). Larger numbers of CD4(bright) dendritic cells in donor bone marrow are associated with increased relapse after allogeneic bone marrow transplantation. *Blood,* Vol.97, No.10, (May 2001), pp. 2948-2956, ISSN 0006-4971

Wilson, J.; Cullup, H.; Lourie, R.; Sheng, Y.; Palkova, A.; Radford, K.J.; Dickinson, A.M.; Rice, A.M.; Hart, D.N. & Munster, D.J. (2009). Antibody to the dendritic cell surface activation antigen CD83 prevents acute graft-versus-host disease. *The Journal of Experimental Medicine,* Vol.206, No.2, (February 2009), pp. 387-398, ISSN 0022-1007

Xu, J.; Zhou, T. & Zhang, Y. (2008). Role of dendritic cells and chemokines in acute graft-versus-host disease. *Frontiers in Bioscience,* Vol.13, (January 2008), pp. 2065-2074, ISSN 1093-9946

Zhang, Y.; Shlomchik, W.D.; Joe, G.; Louboutin, J.P.; Zhu, J.; Rivera, A.; Giannola, D. & Emerson, S.G. (2002). APCs in the liver and spleen recruit activated allogeneic CD8+ T cells to elicit hepatic graft-versus-host disease. *The Journal of Immunology,* Vol.169, No.12, (December 2002), pp. 7111-7118, ISSN 0022-1767

9

Endovascular Methods for Stem Cell Transplantation

Johan Lundberg and Staffan Holmin

Department of Clinical Neuroscience, Karolinska Institutet and Department of Neuroradiology, Karolinska University Hospital, Stockholm, Sweden

1. Introduction

Results from cell transplantation research have received interest and attention both from a clinical, a scientific and a public point of view. This chapter discusses new endovascular transplantation methods for different cell systems. First different cell based therapies are presented, followed by an overview of pathological conditions wherein several cell based strategies are implemented. Thereafter the delivery of cells in broad terms, and then specifically by endovascular technique compared to surgical technique, is presented. A general description of the active process of diapedesis is provided, as it is understood for immunological cells, since this is most probably a fundamental process for endovascular transplantation of cells as well.

1.1 Cell based therapies

Cell based strategies are sought after as a way of repairing or facilitating self renewal in pathological organ systems that have little or no intrinsic regenerative capacity. The plethora of different diseases in organ systems that might have a regenerative capacity, but is limited through physiological processes, is almost boundless (Bajada et al. 2008). Cell based therapies have been successfully used in the clinical practice for distinct pathological conditions during a relatively long period of modern medicine. One of the broadest success stories are the transplantation of cells to patients suffering from hematological diseases (Buckner et al. 1974; Thomas et al. 1975; Thomas et al. 1975; Slavin et al. 1998). Hematological stem cell transplantation has also been expanded to comprise autologous transplantations following chemotherapy of solid tumor forms (Childs et al. 2000). Following the isolation of stem cell lines from human blastocysts (Thomson et al. 1998) and other adult sources such as the central nervous system (CNS) (Johansson et al. 1999), bone marrow (Bruder et al. 1997), multi-lineage mesenchymal (Pittenger et al. 1999), adipose tissue (Zuk et al. 2001) among others, new cell based approaches to disease treatment can be envisioned. The potential for *in vivo* expansion of these cells followed by transplantation, re-implantation and/or tissue engineering becomes possible (Vacanti et al. 1999). These findings open up possibilities for strategies aimed at ameliorating disease burden, or in the long run, obtaining curative goals through cell therapies in a clinical setting. Proposed treatments can broadly be divided into stimulation of an endogenous population or transplantation of cells (Lindvall et al. 2006), be them homologous, from a donor or across the xeno-barrier. The wider implications of the prospect of cell based treatments are summarized in a review article where the coining of the effort and/or subject of Regenerative Medicine is presented (Daar et al. 2007).

The CNS has attracted attention since the potential of restored function could be very valuable for patients. Particularly since pathological conditions in the CNS can be severely disabling. Cell based therapies are in clinical trials in *e.g.* Parkinsons Disease (Freed et al. 2001; Gordon et al. 2004), ischemic stroke (Kondziolka et al. 2000; Bang et al. 2005) and spinal cord lesions (Sykova et al. 2006). Outside the CNS, other clinical trials with cell based therapies aimed at *e.g.* muscle dystrophy (Gussoni et al. 1997; Miller et al. 1997), ischemic heart disease (Stamm et al. 2003), graft versus host disease (Le Blanc et al. 2004; Ringden et al. 2006) and type I diabetes mellitus (Scharp et al. 1991; Shapiro et al. 2000; Korsgren et al. 2008) have yielded promising results. So far, many of the cell therapies are still in trials since both safety and effects must be thoroughly evaluated.

In many areas of pre-clinical, and to some extent clinical research, cell based therapies deliver positive results. However, as with the definition of stem cells/progenitor cells (Potten et al. 1990) the field of cell based therapies are a very heterogeneous one (Bajada et al. 2008). One feasible way of applying taxonomy to this field is by discussing different basic components in the treated diseases. The first example would be in pathological conditions with a definable population of cells being defect. Examples of diseases with certain cell types being depleted are Morbus Parkinson - dopamine producing cells, (Lindvall et al.), muscle dystrophy -satellite cells of the muscles (Gussoni et al. 1997) and type I diabetes - insulin producing cells (White et al. 2001). Such specialized cells might be easier to replace than the second general idea of cell transplantation wherein attempts of transplantation is aimed at more intricately functioning physiological systems. The complexity increases steeply when transplanted cells must differentiate into subpopulations of cell and/or interact within networks (*e.g.* the CNS). An example of that would be the transplantation of neural progenitor cells with the aim of full neural integration (Nikolic et al. 2009). A third strategy is to exert effects on existing cells/organs through transplantation but without functional integration. This strategy might explain some of the results from studies aimed at integration of cells, but without engraftment in the target organ, albeit with positive functional results observed (Borlongan et al. 2004). One explanation for that phenomenon is that in more complex situations, such as following CNS insults, some of the reported beneficial effects might be associated with immune modulation or local secretion of growth factors, thereby rescuing cells from apoptosis. Examples of immune modulation could be Fas-ligand expressing cells (Ghio et al. 1999; Nagata 1999; Lee et al. 2008) whereas secretion of growth factors could be exemplified by an over-expression of IGF-1 from transplanted mesenchymal cells (Haider et al. 2008). Modulation of the immunological response by cell transplantation has also been shown to favorably treat graft versus host reactions in clinical practice (Le Blanc et al. 2004; Ringden et al. 2006). The concept of transplantation of cells serving as self renewing, local, biologically active, pharmacological factories are attractive for many parts of regenerative medicine (Amar et al. 2003). Local, self-sustaining, treatments that are only affecting niche parts of organs have many benefits that might include, but are not limited to, higher local concentration, less risk of adverse events and customization to different pathological conditions.

1.2 Delivery of cells

For cell transplantation, different percutaneous techniques assisted by modern imaging are viable through minimal invasive methods (Bale et al. 2007) and most parts and locales of the human body can be reached with that approach. On the other hand, for organs with less accessible anatomical location, parenchymal access can be associated with significant surgical risks (Villiger et al. 2005; Ben-Haim et al. 2009). In situations where engraftment rate after intravenous or intra-arterial cell administration is low and when a high anatomical specificity is required, such as the scenario when replacing a distinct cell type, direct puncture of the parenchyma might be preferable. For CNS applications this can be done with stereotactic needle puncture or in a combination with open surgery (Hagell et al. 2002; Wennersten et al. 2004).

Direct parenchymal access can also be achieved by endovascular technique. An example of this is a system that adds a possibility to, via large veins, administrate cells to the heart parenchyma (Thompson et al. 2003). The design of that system, requiring a large diameter catheter and without a closure device for the penetration site makes it usable only in large vessels on the venous side, more specifically, in the coronary sinus of the heart (Thompson et al. 2003; Siminiak et al. 2005). Other organs that might be difficult to reach, such as the CNS and the pancreas, are not reachable by the transvenous technique due to the design of that system requiring a large catheter diameter. Furthermore, venous navigation to most parts of the CNS and the pancreas, and to certain parts of the heart, is very difficult due to the more unpredictable venous anatomy and the venous valves.

Insulin producing cells are today transplanted by a hybrid method with percutaneous access to the portal vein and then intra-luminal cell release in the bloodstream. The concept of the intra portal transplantation is considered superior to open surgical techniques, due to the un-acceptable risk of adverse events (Kandaswamy et al. 1999; Humar et al. 2000). The risk-analysis naturally differs substantially for different surgical procedures and transplantations, both with respect to organs and cells. Risks with portal vein transplantation include portal vein thrombosis, hemorrhages, and transient increase of transaminase values (Shapiro et al. 1995; Ryan et al. 2001). A continuous work of reaching a balance between the risk of bleeding after the procedure and portal vein thrombosis is of utmost importance for portal vein transplantations and results are improving steadily in clinical trials. Further adding to the risk side of the comparison is the need for immunosuppressant treatment after transplantation. The potential benefit of the procedure must also, as in the case with diabetes and insulin producing cells, be compared to the standard treatment of insulin injection and or pumps. Patients eligible for portal vein transplantation of insulin producing cells are thus: patients already subject to immunosuppressive therapy due to previous transplantations, patients with unstable glycemia, unawareness hypoglycemia, or patients with progressive chronic complications despite intensive insulin treatment (Bertuzzi et al. 2006). It has been suggested that it would be of great benefit if insulin producing cells could be transplanted directly to the parenchyma of the pancreas. Advantages with pancreas as the target locale are e.g. the possibility of mimicking the physiological release of insulin and the more hospital micro-environment for the insulin producing cells; the pancreas has a higher oxygen tension compared to the liver (Merani et al. 2008).

Different strategies of cell based therapies are currently being evaluated in both pre-clinical and clinical trials but the cell delivery methods per se have received limited interest. One of the larger obstacles that have been observed, is that the lung acts as a kind of clearance filter for the intravenous cell infusion, resulting in pulmonary trapping (Barbash et al. 2003; Fischer et al. 2009). An intra-arterial selective approach would possibly result in higher transplantation efficiency in certain conditions. The versatility of cell suspensions must not be underestimated and limit the way of thinking when considering treatments with cell based approaches (Nikolic et al. 2009). The cell suspensions can easily be handled and administrated through tubing and catheters, thus providing the possibility to by-pass the lung and selectively reach designated target vessels/parenchyma with a first passage effect. Those possibilities of cell handling forms the basis for catheter based strategies for cell transplantation.

Endovascular treatments are continuously providing a third option to open surgical or percutaneous approaches. From the establishment of the Seldinger technique (Seldinger 1953) and the first use of digital subtraction angiography (DSA) (Meaney et al. 1980) to the modern interventional lab with 3D road maps (Soderman et al. 2005) and CT like capacities of the C-arm (Soderman et al. 2008) the path has been long but rapidly progressing. The driving force up until today, that has made the leap ward style of improvements possible, is both rapid developments in computational power and material sciences. The arteries and veins can today be regarded as "internal routes" for navigation, diagnosis and intervention. The shift from open surgical options is for example illustrated by the patients that used to undergo thoracotomy and that now are being referred for percutaneous coronary intervention or the established coiling of intracranial aneurysms instead of open neurosurgical operation.

1.3 Scaling from bench to bedside

As this chapter hopes to illustrate; the rapid development of endovascular technique has implications on cell transplantation methods as well. To illustrate these implications as opposed to organ transplantation, one can visualize a liver transplantation. The wound in the abdominal wall must at least be big enough for the liver to go into the patient. This severely limits the possibility of minimal invasive transplantation of organs. On the other hand, the versatility of cell suspensions could make intra-luminal techniques the natural way of access. In experimental trials, open surgical options are used in e.g. rodent models for transplantation with positive results. This presents a limitation of scalability for clinical translation. For instance, when evaluating pre clinical CNS transplantation schemes in rodents one or two burr holes are established and cells are transplanted. One or two injections in the rat brain covers a relatively large volume but when scaling that to the human brain following e.g. a middle cerebral artery ischemic event, a large number of percutaneous trajectories would be required to cover a human brain volume corresponding to the experimental situation. The migratory capacity for transplanted mesenchymal cells after stereo-tactical transplantation has been shown to be around two millimeter over 14 days (Chen et al. 2001). Furthermore, the mechanical neuronal injury and the risk for intracerebral hemorrhage would increase with each injection trajectory. In brain stimulation procedures, the literature is somewhat divergent; the risk for hemorrhage could be as high as 5% per injection (Ben-Haim et al. 2009). The easier clinical scalability of endovascular access comes in the terms of cells delivered to a larger volume of tissue by taking advantage of the already existing vascular system. If an ischemic stroke occurs due to a vessel occlusion at some point, it would be very tempting to intraluminally disperse cells from the same point via the vascular system in order to reach the affected parenchyma. A normal cell dose for a human adult would probably at least be hundredfold higher than in the rodent and needs to spread out over a vastly larger volume thus requiring many injection trajectories. The average human brain weight is quoted at around 1400 grams as opposed to the adult rat at 2 grams to give some sense to the scale proportions.

Endovascular intervention is not without risks either, exemplified by the risk of adverse events reported at 0 to 4.0%, commonly reported at 0.5%, in different cerebral interventions (Raymond et al. 1997; Cognard et al. 1998; Ng et al. 2002; Murayama et al. 2003; Gonzalez et al. 2004; Cronqvist et al. 2005). Added to the risk of the procedure *per se* is the risk of cell transplantations. The risk of intra-arterial transplantation has already been documented in humans for up to 24 months without severe complications, albeit in a small material (Sykova et al. 2006). Other pre-clinical studies with intra-arterial coronary injections performed in healthy dogs revealed micro-infarction of the heart parenchyma (Vulliet et al. 2004) whereas that has not been observed in clinical studies (Stamm et al. 2003). Factors that might be limiting are the size of the cells injected versus the size of the capillary system, the proportion of shunts in the microcirculation, the stickyness of the cells and the amount of cells administrated. Many of the cells have a much larger diameter (10 up to 70 μm) as opposed to the capillaries 5 to 8 μm (Chien et al. 1975). The shunting zones in the microcirculation could potentially lead also large cells to the post-capillary venules where diapedesis usually occurs (Tuma 2008). The main reason for leukocyte adhesion/diapedesis through venules is the usually restricted expression of adhesion molecules on venular but not arteriolar or capillary endothelium (Tuma 2008). In intravital microscopy studies, adipose mesenchymal cells have been shown to act as embolic material (Furlani et al. 2009). This risk could be speculated on to be lower than the comparable trauma of the surgical methods although a final risk assessment requires a randomized clinical trial.

1.4 Leaving the bloodstream - diapedesis

One limiting factor to specific intra-arterial and intravenous transplantations is that an intra-parenchymal approach yields a higher efficacy. It has been shown that when performing transplantations to a rodent stroke model and comparing intravenous, intra-ventricular and intra-striatal injections, the highest efficacy in sheer number of cells were obtained with the intra-striatal route (Jin et al. 2005). Further limiting the selective intra-luminal approach is the speculation that some cell systems, such as insulin producing cells, appear incapable of leaving the bloodstream (Hirshberg et al. 2002).

In all implementations aimed at intra-luminal administration (intra-luminal encompassing both intravenous and selective intra-arterial administration) the ability of the cells to leave the bloodstream, or perform diapedesis (Fulton et al. 1957) is fundamental. The diapedesis function has previously been studied predominantly in immunological cells (Fulton 1957), it is in fact the active process whereby cells leave the bloodstream. The diapedesis of immunologically active cells has been thoroughly studied since the discovery of the significant multistep, ordered, cross-talk procedure of leukocyte-endothelial cell interaction both *in vitro* and *in vivo* (Butcher 1991; Springer 1994).

The barricades limiting the cells from haphazardly leaving the bloodstream are many. All blood vessels contain an endothelium and several organized barriers. In the CNS for instance, tight junctions are located between endothelial cells, predominantly to permit the conservation of the water fraction of the blood stream. The liquid pressure gradient composed of the blood pressure can be broken down to one force directed with the axis of the laminar flow of blood and one force aimed perpendicular to the flow on to the wall (Glagov et al. 1992; Fay 1994), thereby providing an evolutionary rationale for sealing the blood stream tightly. Situated underneath the endothelial cells and forming their structural base is the basal layer; a specific protein structure composed of extra cellular matrix (ECM) proteins abundant with expression of elastin, laminin and collagen type I, III and IV (Mayne 1986). Collagen and elastin are the major structural components of blood vessels of all sizes throughout the mammalian body. The cross-banded fibrils in the tunica media and tunica adventitia, formed by type I and type III collagen, provide the tensile strength and comprise probably 80 to 90% of the total collagen present. The other major structural protein component in elastic arteries is elastin; the protein that provides the elastic component of the blood vessels (Mayne 1986). Around most capillaries, pericytes are situated which further seal the blood stream. The pericytes are less abundant in the post capillary venules where most of the diapedesis occurs. As a general note, the post capillary venules are the most "leaky" part of the vascular tree. It should be noted that blood vessels are not merely the plumbing in the mammal body, they are in all respects a vividly living part of the organism, reorganized as a response to stress and demand (Gibbons et al. 1994) and among other things have a self-generating electro potential towards the bloodstream that is important for the clotting cascade (Danon et al. 1976).

As previously mentioned, in a diverging literature, it has been speculated that some cells totally lack the function of exiting the blood stream, thereby limiting intra-luminal based techniques. Even though insulin producing cells appears incapable of leaving the bloodstream, they are still transplanted through the portal vein (Hirshberg et al. 2002). The mechanism of action is believed to be microembolization of the cells to the liver parenchyma in the low pressure system that the portal vein constitutes (Lehmann et al. 2007). It has been speculated that arterial blood from the hepatic artery pushes back into the portal vein during the mixing of the two flows which would stop the cells and create advantageous conditions for engraftment. The cells found functioning in the livers of transplanted patients are, however, situated as plaques in the hepatic artery tree thus adding yet another hurdle to the understanding of portal vein transplantation. The hypothesis is that the cells cannot perform diapedesis but are instead primarily forming a mural thrombus after, with low probability, being displaced against the blood flow into the arterial tree and then encapsulated by endothelial cells. The plaque formation can thereby provide capillary ingrowth, an absolute requirement for endocrine function (Korsgren et al. 2008). Such a hypothesis would also shed further light on the low efficacy of portal transplantations methods. Nevertheless, the portal vein approach to transplantation is today the golden standard since the existing open surgical options of total pancreatic transplantation carries a mortality risk of 10% during the first year of follow-up (Kandaswamy et al. 1999; Humar et al. 2000).

The process of diapedesis is basically divided into tethering, rolling and stopping of leukocytes prior to diapedesis into inflamed tissue. It is thought of as a multistep procedure involving complex crosstalk between cells in the bloodstream and the endothelial cells. On the endothelial side intra-cellular adhesion molecule -1 (ICAM-1) (Dustin et al. 1986; Rothlein et al. 1986), vascular cell adhesion molecule -1 (VCAM-1) (Elices et al. 1990; Pulido et al. 1991) and junctional adhesion molecule –A (JAM-A) have all been implicated to play crucial roles. Interestingly, all of these receptors are part of the Ig-super family. Leukocytes capacity for homing and diapedesis is pivotal for the development of the inflammatory response to injury and starts as a tightly controlled up-regulation of endothelial E- and P-selectins that stimulate the leukocytes (Vestweber et al. 1999). These leukocytes then respond by activation of G protein-coupled receptors that increase the affinity for endothelial VCAM-1 and ICAM-1 (Muller 2003). Interaction with VCAM-1 is maintained through the heterodimer CD29 and CD49d forming the cell surface antigen Very Late Antigen – 4 (VLA-4) (Elices et al. 1990) and the CD11aCD18 heterodimer interacting with ICAM-1 (Meerschaert et al. 1995). VCAM-1 and ICAM-1 have previously been shown to be up-regulated on the endothelium as a response to inflammation (Dustin et al. 1986; Pulido et al. 1991). This interaction starts the diapedesis itself wherein the leukocytes "crawl" through, either a para-cellular or a trans-cellular pathway interacting with both PECAM-1 and/or CD99 or members of the JAM family of proteins (Petri et al. 2006). Thus significant crosstalk is needed to initiate and execute the active process of diapedesis.

VCAM-1 is also implicated both as a model of treatment for immunological modulation of the inflammatory responses following CNS insults and as surface antigen for cell treatment of CNS insults. In one study, fluorescence activated cell sorting (FACS) was performed for the expression of CD49d and identifying it as one of the important factors for directing diapedesis (Guzman et al. 2008). This finding has received a lot of interest from different fields, among other it has been shown that VCAM-1 expression has a critical role in transplantation of cells in dystrophic muscle (Gavina et al. 2006). Another utilization of VCAM-1 is the selective blocking by the monoclonal antibody drug Natalizumab used in multiple sclerosis, thereby inhibiting diapedesis for immunologically active cells (Stuve et al. 2008). VCAM-1 blockade has also been tested for neuroprotective effects following ischemic events in pre-clinical trials with disappointing results (Justicia et al. 2006).

2. Results and discussion with emphasis on the central nervous system

In this chapter three different types of endovascular methods of cell transplantation are discussed. The first two are the selective intra-arterial and the intravenous methods, these are compared for efficacy. The third method is the trans-vessel wall technique by using the Extroducer; an endovascular catheter system developed within our group for penetrating the vessel wall from the inside to out, thereby creating a working channel to extravascular tissue.

For certain cell types, the selective intra-arterial method is superior to the intravenous one after TBI in the rat. This was measured by the level of engraftment of hMSC at one and five days following TBI, without thrombo-embolic complications (Lundberg et al. 2009). Selective intra-arterial transplantation method for rNPC after TBI in the rat is also superior compared to intravenous method. We were, however, not able to engraft hNPC, *ceteris paribus*, thus indicating that diapedesis and engraftment is an active process and that different cell systems have different capabilities to engraft following intraluminal delivery (Lundberg et al. 2011). We show, by indirect methods, that CD29CD49dVCAM-1 interactions might be one of the factors with impact on engraftment in an intra-luminal transplantation setting (Lundberg et al. 2011). Further, we show that it is possible to perform minimally invasive parenchymal injections by trans-vessel wall technique by the development of the Extroducer (Lundberg et al. 2010). The Extroducer have no adverse long term effects on the blood vessels up to 3 months following interventions (Lundberg et al. 2011) and it is feasible to use the system as a novel approach for transplantation of e.g. insulin producing cells to the CNS, to the pancreas or other cell types to organs that are difficult or risky to reach by traditional methods. The trans-vessel wall technique thereby adds a new possibility when transplanting cell populations without the necessary properties for performing diapedesis. The establishment of a working channel to the extravascular tissue, by endovascular method, also opens up several other possible applications, such as different methods for sampling.

2.1 Selective intra-arterial method versus intravenous method

We established a model for selective intra-arterial transplantation (Lundberg et al. 2009) that we applied to a model of TBI in the rat (Feeney et al. 1981). We compared the selective intra-arterial method to intra-venous methods for different cell systems in the same TBI setting. Several different variables were tested such as cell concentration, days post injury for transplantation, time for infusion, level of immunosuppressant drugs etc. The majority of transplantation experiments were not successful from the start and many different variables were tested before robust engraftments could be reached. Too few cells had a dire impact on the success of transplantation; 200.000 (unpublished results) and 500.000 hMSCs did only result in very low engraftment. The failure of low cell numbers can obviously be interpreted as an indication that the efficacy of the intra arterial method in this setting is quite low although it is still superior to intravenous alternatives.

Results of engraftment levels were obtained through IHC methods by counting engrafted cells in sectioned brains (Fig 1). We found that engraftment levels of rNPCs were more than five-fold higher than in the control group (p=0.034) and hMSC were more than fifteen-fold higher than the in control group in absolute values (p=0.007), with a large spread within the intra-arterial groups (Fig 2). Few studies compare selective intra-arterial and intravenous methods but recent clinical data suggest an advantage for the selective intra-arterial route (Sykova et al. 2006). A known problem with all intravenous methods is the fact that the lung acts as a kind of clearance filter during the first passage (Barbash et al. 2003; Fischer et al. 2009). Following intravenous cell infusion, the blood transports the cells after venous passage to the right ventricle and then through the lung where up to 80% of cells are trapped during the first passage (Fischer et al. 2009). Thus as low as 20% of the cells transplanted might be ejected for the first total body distribution through the aorta. Of all the blood leaving the left ventricle of the heart, only somewhere between 1.8 to 8.5 percent of the blood actually reaches the brain of the rat (Pannier et al. 1973) leaving only 0.01 to 1.7 percent of the initially transplanted cells to reach the brain in the first passage. All cells not distributed to the brain are then again re-transported for another passage through the lung, acting as a filter. This phenomenon has been studied *e.g.* by PET for mesenchymal stem cells

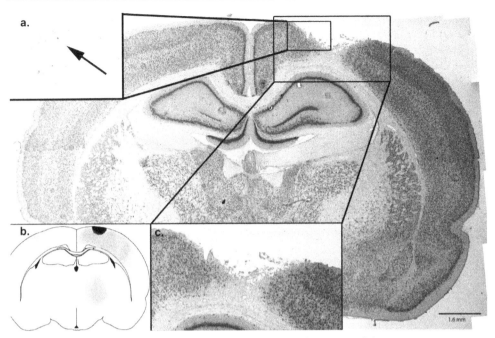

Fig. 1. Representation of intra-arterial transplantation in the TBI model

In the background is a reconstructed image showing a coronal section of the rat brain 2.5 mm posterior to bregma stained with GFAP (red) and NeuN (Brown) five days after traumatic brain injury. In blow-up a. a low magnification single staining with HuN (human nuclear antigen, MAB 1281) without any counterstaining, along the peri-lesional zone is shown. Brown dots represent HuN positive, transplanted cells (arrow indicates an example of a positive cell). In blow-up b. the black area represents the contusion zone and the grey areas represent primary localization of engrafted mesenchymal stem cells. In blow-up c. a magnification of the injury area itself is presented.

(Ma et al. 2005). This situation can readily be changed by placing a micro-catheter in the arteries supplying the organ of interest. An interesting finding in the present study is that our hMSCs predominantly were found in the spleen with few transplanted cells in the lung at 24 hours post injection, a bio-distribution phenomenon, from the lung to the spleen, previously described in rat following intravenous hMSC transplantation (Detante et al. 2009). To increase the understanding of the role of cell line properties for engraftment, we conducted a study with transplantation of different cell lines through either intra-arterial or intravenous routes. This analysis showed that there were dramatic differences between the different cell lines; hNPCs did not engraft at all after intra-luminal delivery whereas there was a significant difference between the hMSCs and the rNPCs using the same transplantation method. Noteworthy is the large variability in the engraftment levels of the latter two cell lines. One important factor that might contribute to this is that neither hMSC nor rNPCs are defined homologous cell lines, succinctly there can be important variations within the cell systems transplanted. The remarkable finding that no engraftment was obtained following hNPC transplantations is even more noteworthy since the hNPCs have previously been robustly transplanted by open surgical technique (Wennersten et al. 2004; Akesson et al. 2007).

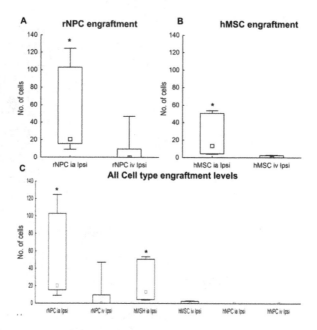

Fig. 2. Graph illustrating engraftment levels
Engrafted cells were counted per section and is reported with median (marker), quartiles (box) and max – min (whiskers). In A a significant difference between engraftment levels per section following selective intra-arterial and intravenous transplantation in the ipsilateral hemisphere of the rNPC group. In B a significant difference between engraftment levels per section following selective intra-arterial and intravenous transplantation in the ipsilateral hemisphere of the hMSC group and finally in C a panel of all engraftment levels per section in the ipsilateral hemispheres of all groups. * marks $p < 0.05$

2.2 Gene expression profiling of cell systems

After discovering that there were differences in engraftment capability between the different cell lines, the opportunity to investigate the bio-molecular basis of said differences presented itself. We started with characterizing and confirming earlier results (Clausen et al. 2007) that our TBI model leads to up-regulation of VCAM-1 expression in the endothelium. That result may suggest that the injured CNS parenchyma could provide cues for diapedesis and migration of engrafted cells in similar ways as immunological cells respond to inflammatory cues (Butcher 1991; Springer 1994). As a screening method, we started by performing microarray on the human cells. rNPCs were not included in the microarray analysis due to problems with cross-species comparisons in the microarray chips used. hMSCs showed a broad expression of integrins, commonly expressed by immune cells, that are important for diapedesis through the vessel endothelium and subsequent migration into the parenchyma. Specifically, analysis of the heterodimers forming receptors for ICAM-1 and VCAM-1 were analyzed, based on previous work indicating CD49d expression as important for successful intra-vasal transplantations (Guzman et al. 2008). Thus, probably the most interesting finding was the CD49d signal of 68 in hMSC as opposed to 0.4 in hNPC (p=0.0047). This was then confirmed with RT-qPCR data from all cell lines with average CD49d mRNA levels that were highest in the hMSC (0.98) followed by the rNPC (0.0057) and finally a dwindling finding in hNPC (0.0012). CD29 and CD49d forms a heterodimer named very late antigen -4 (VLA-4) which was expressed in falling order in hMSC, rNPC and hNPC (Fig 3). The difference in mRNA levels between rNPC and hNPC is not large but might reflect larger differences in protein translation. Further studies at the protein and functional level are required to elucidate the importance of CD49d for diapedesis of these cell systems. CD11a mRNA was detected in hNPC (0.0029) albeit with low CD18 mRNA (0.00025), suggesting that CD11a-CD18-ICAM-1 interaction may be dispensable for engraftment. In contrast, hMSC displayed high CD18 mRNA levels (0.43) but no detectable CD11a expression, suggesting neglectable ICAM-1 dependent engraftment in the hMSCs.

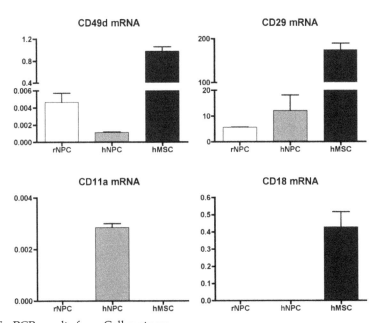

Fig. 3. RT-qPCR results from Cell systems
Bars represent relative levels of integrin CD49d, CD29, CD11a and CD18 mRNA expression in rNPC, hNPC and hMSC compared to respective endogenous TBP mRNA levels. Error bars represent the distribution between the biological replicates.

Finally, both our own findings regarding hNPCs and other previously known cells incapable of diapedesis, such as insulin producing cells (Hirshberg et al. 2002), shows the apparent need for surgical techniques. In some organs that are hard to reach and/or when surgical technique comes with a high risk of adverse events for the patients, the need for an alternative strategy becomes apparent. Thus, we also initiated the development of the trans-vessel wall approach.

2.3 Trans-vessel wall transplantation

An endovascularly based system that could penetrate the vessel wall would, in instances where the target parenchyma is either hard to reach or carries a significant surgical risk, be a method with both the merits of accurate placement and reduction of patient risk. Further, it would solve the problem for certain cells to leave the bloodstream. A proposed solution to this problem is a endovascular catheter system that we have named the Extroducer (Lundberg et al. 2010).

2.3.1 Extroducer in vivo testing - small animals

After extensive computer simulations and *ex vivo* testing, *in vivo* short term testing were performed in rat by creating arterial access from the medial tail artery and performing the Extroducer trans-vessel wall technique passage in either the subclavian or carotid artery. Two different stages of the procedure was tested; first the trans-vessel wall technique passage per se with surgical microscope monitoring of hemorrhage or other adverse events, and thereafter the deployment of the distal penetrating tip through the vascular wall and retracting the proximal part of the system. No cases of intra-operative hemorrhage or intra-luminal thrombosis occurred. Thus, the vascular penetration procedure was uneventful and the vessel wall completely sealed around the Extroducer, thereby preventing leakage of blood.

The second group with deposited Extroducer tips also showed absolute hemostasis during the primary intervention. Fourteen days post intervention, this group showed no signs of pain or discomfort. No signs of dissection of the vessels or impairment of blood-flow distal to intervention sites were observed and macroscopical analysis of the organ supplied by the vessel, showed no infarcts.

With computer-based flow simulations, we found that there should be no blood-flow through the detached Extroducer interior lumen at physiological blood pressure. This was also tested *in vivo* by cannulating the deployed distal tip of the prototypes with a nitinol mandrel. This was done to reassure that even when removing possible clotting inside the prototype, it still prevented bleeding from inside the vessel to the extravascular space. Furthermore, no signs of delayed hemorrhage were detected.

2.3.2 Extroducer in vivo testing - large animals

After successful trials in small animals, the Extroducer system was tested in large animals. An adaptation towards clinical use was that these prototypes were manufactured from a longer nitinol tube, 1700 mm *vis-à-vis* 300 mm that was used in the rat. We evaluated the prototypes in the rabbit together with standard clinical catheters and angiographical equipment.

The Extroducer prototypes within the microcatheters were visible at high magnification fluoroscopy and thereby maneuvered into the subclavian artery (SCA) (Fig 4). The rabbit SCA was chosen since it is close to the intended target vessel size of 0.5 to 3 millimeters, the SCA is fairly easy to access in order to perform simultaneous open surgical monitoring and it had been used in the rat. A slight amount of pressure was required on the protecting plastic catheter to advance the system through the microcatheter to the desired vessel wall, thereafter the Extroducer was gently advanced out through the vessel wall to the extra-vascular space. Hemorrhages were neither observed by simultaneous direct observation through a surgical microscope, nor by high resolution angiographical series (DSA), during and after the intervention (Fig 4). Further, no thromboembolic complications or vascular dissections were observed using high resolution DSA. No navigational problems were encountered with respect to Extroducer prototype integration with clinical catheters.

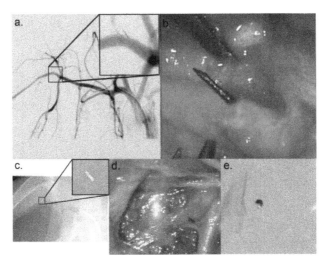

Fig. 4. Trans-vessel wall interventions
For full control over the procedure in the large animal trials, both a surgical microscope and high resolution angiographical series was used. In a. digital subtraction angiogram showing a detached Extroducer tip without hemorrhage, dissection or thromboembolic complications. In b. photograph showing the microsurgical view of the detached Extroducer tip. In c. x-ray image showing the detached Extroducer tip with guide catheter. In d. photograph from post-operative dissection showing the detached Extroducer tip with methylene blue injected in the surrounding tissue. In e. digital subtraction angiogram showing an extra vascular injection of 25 µl contrast agent through the Extroducer system.

Finally, electrolysis detachment of the distal Extroducer distal tip was tested in rabbit. We chose electrolysis since it was the easiest way of performing detachment in our hands. Our design was based on the work of the first detachable coils (Guglielmi et al. 1991). An important difference compared to the detachment zone in coils was, however, that we needed a hollow detachment zone which required additional development. After navigation to the designated intervention site and after methylene blue or contrast agent had been deposited in the extravascular space, a tension of 8V was applied and the distal tip was then detached after, on average, five minutes (range three to nine minutes). This was also un-eventful without observation of hemorrhage from around the body of the distal tip or through the inner lumen. The procedure was successfully performed both with simultaneous microscopical monitoring via surgical access, and with fluoroscopical/angiographical guidance solely. In a previous work describing a method for penetrating large veins (Thompson et al. 2003), that system design required a much larger catheter and also lacked a method for sealing the vessel wall, thus making penetration through the arteries impossible. This severely limits the use of that system to their testing vessel, i.e. the sinus coronarius of the heart, whereas the Extroducer is applicable in both arteries and veins of any sizes down to approximately 0.5 mm in diameter. Another system, in which vessel perforations are performed, is the trans-jugular intrahepatic portacaval stent shunt (TIPS) technique (Richter et al. 1990). That system also does not have the requirement of sealing the vessel wall when finishing the procedure, since a patent blood flow through the stent is the preferred result. On the contrary, thrombosis of the stent might be considered the main problem (Merli et al. 1998) which requires rigorous follow-up.

Thus, the Extroducer system is unique in the ways that it permits safe exit of both arteries and veins and that it is usable in vessels with large dimensions as well as in the microvasculature with inner lumen diameters down to approximately 0.5 mm.

2.2.3 Extroducer testing with long time follow up

In a long term follow up, the end points five days, one month and three months after the deployment of the device was selected. No stenosis or late hemorrhagic complications were noted in any animals. No alterations in behavior or other measures of discomfort were noted either (Lundberg et al. 2011).

The distribution of followed up animals were as follows; two at the five days end point , five at the 30 days end point and six at the 80 days end point with histological analysis of one resulting in a total number of 19 detached Extroducer tips.

In the follow up DSA we also found that four of 19 (21 %) of the detached tips were no longer placed through the vessel wall but had instead been "pushed" or "migrated" through the endothelium to the extravascular space immediately adjacent to the penetration site. No vascular stenosis or other adverse reactions were observed around those tips. Also for the rest of the tips, that were located through the vessel wall, no adverse reactions were detected. An important endpoint was biocompatibility of the detached tips. The nitinol alloy used was selected for its many advantageous properties. Nitinol is a nickel/titanium alloy with both memory and super elastic properties (Adler et al. 1990). These special properties are the foundation for the use of nitinol in stent fabrication in clinical practice. Thus, the excellent biocompatibility of nitinol (Castleman et al. 1976) has been extensively studied, especially with respect to vessel wall interactions in the use of stents (Stoeckel et al. 2004). However, the compatibility of nitinol when placed through arterial walls has, to our knowledge, not been studied. The parylene, used as coating in our device, is also FDA approved and CE marked when used in pacemaker electrodes. To evaluate interaction between the deposited tips and the endothelium, we performed histological analysis with the prototypes *in situ* by a specialized grind-cutting technique and then consulted an external, independent, evaluator with expertise in the field of titanium implants. This evaluation showed full biocompatibility with a very small fibrotic capsule (< 1 µm) formed around the detached distal tips (fig 5). No ongoing inflammation was observable around any of the distal tips. Around one (of the total number 14 left in place) of the day five animal implants, three macrophages were indentified in the area of the detached distal tip. Apart from those three macrophages, no other signs of inflammation were observed. The endothelia showed no signs of alterations adjacent to the deposited tips.

In conclusion, the biocompatibility of the distal tips was comparable to titanium implants. The interactions of nitinol with the interior of the vascular wall and the extra vascular space has not been as extensively studied since stents most often are positioned inside the vascular lumen with direct contact only with the bloodstream and the endothelium. Therefore, the present histological analysis in this new application and new position of nitinol, adds important knowledge about biocompatibility for possible future applications.

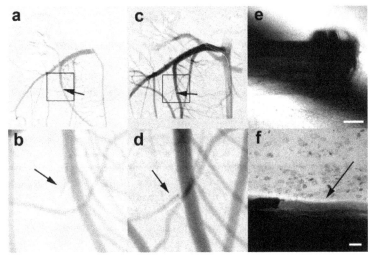

Fig. 5. Long term follow-up of the trans-vessel wall intervention
In a. the initial follow up angiogram directly following detachment in the Superior Mesenteric Artery (SMA) is shown with a square marking the blow-up in b. Arrows indicate the detached distal tip. In c. an SMA angiogram, performed 80 days after the intervention in the same animal, is shown with a square indicating the blow-up in d. Arrows indicate the detached distal tip. In e. a microphotograph of a histological van Geeson and toulene blue staining prepared by grind-cutting with the detached tip in situ, is shown. Scale bar = 100 μm. The blow-up in f shows the parylene coating surrounding the detached tip which is marked by an arrow. Note that no fibrous response or inflammation is observable. Scale bar = 4 μm.

The prototypes excluded due to failed detachment were analyzed by sweep electron microscopy (SEM), since monitoring of electric current gave limited prognostic information about the failure to detach. We found that, in failed detachments, large amounts of chloride were observed by surface spectroscopy (6-10 wt %) indicating titanium chloride ion formations in a passive layer, thus providing current transmission without electrolysis. Titanium chloride molecules can provide a surface area that lets electron pass through but without formation of soluble titanium or nickel ions. This problem is probably due to the simple technique used for creating the insulation defect in our hands. However, numerous available solutions for detachment are available on the market that can easily be integrated with the trans-vessel wall technique in an industrialized manufacturing process.

3. General discussion

The rationale for our previous studies within the field of endovascular cell transplantation is the path to translating cell based regenerative medicine to patients. In a translational perspective the actual route of transplantation will be important. For operative techniques there is a problem with scalability and for intravenous techniques there is a problem with efficacy. We show that by selective intra-arterial methods it is possible to increase the level of cerebral engraftment with certain cell types with six to fifteen fold yields. Further, not all cells are optimal for intra-luminal transplantation. It is, for example, known that insulin producing cells lack the capability to perform diapedesis (Hirshberg et al. 2002) and we show that hNPC, a cell system previously transplanted by open surgical means (Wennersten et al. 2004) also lacks the capability to perform diapedesis. For these cell systems, and other applications, we have developed the Extroducer as a tool to establish a direct, minimal invasive working channel with parenchymal access in organs that are difficult or risky to reach with traditional techniques.

The first passage of cells delivered through selective intra-arterial approaches, compared to systemic intravenous delivery, results in a higher local concentration, shorter blood stream exposure and less mechanical stress factors before cells reach the target site. These factors could be of importance for successful engraftment. Supporting that hypothesis are the present results showing significantly higher total cerebral uptake of cells after intra-arterial compared to intra-venous administration. The next supporting fact is the higher uptake of cells in the ipsilateral hemisphere after intra-arterial administration and by the absence of difference between the hemispheres after intravenous transplantation. Future studies are needed for elucidating molecules responsible for diapedesis, e.g by direct methods such as knock-ins, of for example CD49d, in non-functioning cell systems and knock down or blocking in other cell systems.

The absence of adverse effects in transplanted animals suggests that in the short term, the selective intra-arterial transplantation method is safe for delivering even high concentrations of cells. It has been reported ischemic events following intra-arterial approaches to the heart in dogs (Vulliet et al. 2004) thus indicating the need for thorough studies prior to translation into clinical practice. However, in clinical studies on intracoronary infusions (Stamm et al. 2003) and in spinal cord artery infusions (Sykova et al. 2006) no embolic events have been recorded. Connected to the need for safety studies, it could be argued that the higher engraftment rates in our intra-arterial groups would be a consequence of microembolization of cells. In that scenario we would, however, have detected ischemic histological changes and localization of the transplanted cells within arterioles and capillaries, which we did not.

For all intra-luminal approaches, this thesis shows that a thorough investigation must be performed to clarify if the cells actually can perform diapedesis prior to choosing transplantation strategy. hNPCs has previously been shown to have an impact on neurological outcome when transplanted with open surgical techniques, but in their present form they seem unsuitable for intra-luminal transplantation. Therefore, based on the findings in this thesis, considerations should be made that CD29CD49dVCAM-1 interaction is one of the best studied crosstalk mechanisms on how immunological cells leave the bloodstream to perform homing to disease ridden tissue where inflammation occurs (Elices et al. 1990). This line of reasoning is supported by other studies implicating VCAM-1 interaction in both ischemic stroke and muscle dystrophy pre-clinical studies (Gavina et al. 2006; Guzman et al. 2008). An interesting comparison can be made regarding diapedesis in cell systems aimed for transplantation compared to immunological cells. In such an exercise it could be considered blatantly ignorant to immediately dismiss the fylogenetically conserved mechanism of the immunological system and suggest a hitherto unknown method of diapedesis for these cells. Applying Occam's razor to the hypothesis of diapedesis for cell transplantation, two conclusions can potentially be made; i) the process of diapedesis is most probably an active process for cell systems transplanted, since there are no known inactive ways of diapedesis and ii) the most likely system for diapedesis crosstalk should be found within the same systems that are used by the immunological system, meaning that proteins are highly likely to come from the Ig-super family such as VCAM-1. The other, more complex, explanation would be that a hitherto unknown system for diapedesis exists. That it also unlikely since mutations in such a system would lead to genetical diseases that should be known, but without reasonable explanations. A research program dedicated on endovascular transplantation of different cell systems in different diseases should include a variety of diseases and cell systems to increase the understanding of both cell-endothelium interactions and the effects on target niches.

When designing both pre-clinical and clinical cell transplantation studies, consideration should be taken to how the cells are hypothesized to reach their designated targets. The first option might be open surgical techniques for small niche locations in a target parenchyma. Downsides to open surgical/percutaneous techniques are *e.g.* impracticalities of accruing the desired extent of target tissue volume, especially if the volume is relatively large, such as following a major CNS insult. Further, the patient risk for adverse events might be unacceptable in relation to a potential benefit, in particular for "difficult to reach" organs such as the CNS, the pancreas and/or the heart. If the disadvantages of open surgical/percutaneous techniques are unacceptable, intra-luminal options could be explored. For intra-luminal approaches, the concept of how transplanted cells are presumed to leave the blood stream becomes an issue with several potential solutions. For a cell system without the necessary features for diapedesis, one could use knock-in methods to provide the necessary adhesion molecule set up, otherwise intra-parenchymal injections must be considered. For knock-in methods, an intra-arterial approach would probably still have benefits in efficacy over intravenous methods through the first passage effect and by avoiding pulmonary trapping. As previously discussed, an interesting purely academical calculation when performing intravenous cell transplantations could result in such a low cell dose to the brain as 0.01 to 1.7% after intravenous injection, assuming that 80% of cells are trapped in the first passage through the lung (Barbash et al. 2003; Fischer et al. 2009). This can readily be changed by placing a micro-catheter in vessels supplying the target parenchyma with blood thereby providing a chance for all cells to perfuse the target parenchyma.

For more discrete functioning cells, an intra-parenchymal injection might be even more attractive for reasons such as shielding the cells from the exposure to the bloodstream and accurate anatomical placement. In difficult to reach organs, minimally invasive direct parenchymal transplantation could be performed by the trans-vessel wall technique described within this thesis. That technique might, however, not be suitable for treating a large ischemic lesion in humans. On the contrary, in discrete lesions where only a niche cell needs to be replaced, such as in type I diabetes, where the cells do not possess properties for diapedesis, the Extroducer could potentially really show its worth. The next natural step is transplantation of insulin producing cells to swine before planning for clinical trials.

The Extroducer is not limited to cell transplantation. Its main design is to provide a working channel by endovascular technique to the parenchyma in various, otherwise, inaccessible organs. Through that working channel, other procedures such as local chemotherapy-, irradiation-, growth factor administration, tissue sampling, electrophysiological diagnostics and thermo-therapy becomes possible. Further, combined with optical spectroscopic analysis, it might even be possible to perform infra-light histological analysis of tissue via the Extroducer.

3.1 Conclusions and future research
We have discussed the rationale for using endovascular methods for cell transplantation and described findings from our group and other groups, showing that selective intra-arterial administration is a safe way, with a short follow up time, to increase engraftment levels compared to intravenous delivery. However, not all cell systems are optimal for intra-luminal transplantation. These factors might be dependent on integrin expression and endothelium interactions. For cells that lack the capacity to perform diapedesis, and especially for more specific niche cell systems in organ systems that are difficult to reach, we have also developed a system for trans-vessel wall parenchymal access. The Extroducer system has been evaluated both for long term effects and feasibility for pancreas access. *Ergo*, endovascular intervention should provide a number of methods for efficient and safe cell transplantation in current and future clinical practice. The transplantation method must be decided on a disease to disease, cell to cell and patient to patient manner. Future research should investigate the possibilities of providing cells meant for intravasal transplantation with the necessary properties for performing diapedesis.

4. References

Adler, P. H., W. Yu, et al. (1990). "On the tensile and torsional properties of pseudoelastic Ni-Ti." *Scripta Metallurgica et Materila* 24: 943-947

Akesson, E., J. H. Piao, et al. (2007). "Long-term culture and neuronal survival after intraspinal transplantation of human spinal cord-derived neurospheres." *Physiol Behav* 92(1-2): 60-6

Amar, A. P., B. V. Zlokovic, et al. (2003). "Endovascular restorative neurosurgery: a novel concept for molecular and cellular therapy of the nervous system." *Neurosurgery* 52(2): 402-12; discussion 412-3

Bajada, S., I. Mazakova, et al. (2008). "Updates on stem cells and their applications in regenerative medicine." *J Tissue Eng Regen Med* 2(4): 169-83

Bale, R. and G. Widmann (2007). "Navigated CT-guided interventions." *Minim Invasive Ther Allied Technol* 16(4): 196-204

Bang, O. Y., J. S. Lee, et al. (2005). "Autologous mesenchymal stem cell transplantation in stroke patients." *Ann Neurol* 57(6): 874-82

Barbash, I. M., P. Chouraqui, et al. (2003). "Systemic delivery of bone marrow-derived mesenchymal stem cells to the infarcted myocardium: feasibility, cell migration, and body distribution." *Circulation* 108(7): 863-8

Ben-Haim, S., W. F. Asaad, et al. (2009). "Risk factors for hemorrhage during microelectrode-guided deep brain stimulation and the introduction of an improved microelectrode design." *Neurosurgery* 64(4): 754-62; discussion 762-3

Bertuzzi, F., S. Marzorati, et al. (2006). "Islet cell transplantation." *Curr Mol Med* 6(4): 369-74

Borlongan, C. V., M. Hadman, et al. (2004). "Central nervous system entry of peripherally injected umbilical cord blood cells is not required for neuroprotection in stroke." *Stroke* 35(10): 2385-9

Bruder, S. P., N. Jaiswal, et al. (1997). "Growth kinetics, self-renewal, and the osteogenic potential of purified human mesenchymal stem cells during extensive subcultivation and following cryopreservation." *J Cell Biochem* 64(2): 278-94

Buckner, C. D., R. A. Clift, et al. (1974). "Marrow transplantation for the treatment of acute leukemia using HL-A-identical siblings." *Transplant Proc* 6(4): 365-6

Butcher, E. C. (1991). "Leukocyte-endothelial cell recognition: three (or more) steps to specificity and diversity." *Cell* 67(6): 1033-6

Castleman, L. S., S. M. Motzkin, et al. (1976). "Biocompatibility of nitinol alloy as an implant material." *J Biomed Mater Res* 10(5): 695-731

Chen, J., Y. Li, et al. (2001). "Therapeutic benefit of intracerebral transplantation of bone marrow stromal cells after cerebral ischemia in rats." *J Neurol Sci* 189(1-2): 49-57

Chien, S., R. G. King, et al. (1975). "Viscoelastic properties of human blood and red cell suspensions." *Biorheology* 12(6): 341-6

Childs, R., A. Chernoff, et al. (2000). "Regression of metastatic renal-cell carcinoma after nonmyeloablative allogeneic peripheral-blood stem-cell transplantation." *N Engl J Med* 343(11): 750-8

Clausen, F., T. Lorant, et al. (2007). "T lymphocyte trafficking: a novel target for neuroprotection in traumatic brain injury." *J Neurotrauma* 24(8): 1295-307

Cognard, C., A. Weill, et al. (1998). "Intracranial berry aneurysms: angiographic and clinical results after endovascular treatment." *Radiology* 206(2): 499-510

Cronqvist, M., R. Wirestam, et al. (2005). "Diffusion and perfusion MRI in patients with ruptured and unruptured intracranial aneurysms treated by endovascular coiling: complications, procedural results, MR findings and clinical outcome." *Neuroradiology* 47(11): 855-73

Daar, A. S. and H. L. Greenwood (2007). "A proposed definition of regenerative medicine." *J Tissue Eng Regen Med* 1(3): 179-84

Danon, D. and E. Skutelsky (1976). "Endothelial surface charge and its possible relationship to thrombogenesis." *Ann N Y Acad Sci* 275: 47-63

Detante, O., A. Moisan, et al. (2009). "Intravenous administration of 99mTc-HMPAO-labeled human mesenchymal stem cells after stroke: in vivo imaging and biodistribution." *Cell Transplant* 18(12): 1369-79

Dustin, M. L., R. Rothlein, et al. (1986). "Induction by IL 1 and interferon-gamma: tissue distribution, biochemistry, and function of a natural adherence molecule (ICAM-1)." *J Immunol* 137(1): 245-54

Elices, M. J., L. Osborn, et al. (1990). "VCAM-1 on activated endothelium interacts with the leukocyte integrin VLA-4 at a site distinct from the VLA-4/fibronectin binding site." *Cell* 60(4): 577-84

Fay, J. A. (1994). Introduction to Fluid Mechanics. Boston, MIT press.

Feeney, D. M., M. G. Boyeson, et al. (1981). "Responses to cortical injury: I. Methodology and local effects of contusions in the rat." *Brain Res* 211(1): 67-77

Fischer, U. M., M. T. Harting, et al. (2009). "Pulmonary passage is a major obstacle for intravenous stem cell delivery: the pulmonary first-pass effect." *Stem Cells Dev* 18(5): 683-92

Freed, C. R., P. E. Greene, et al. (2001). "Transplantation of embryonic dopamine neurons for severe Parkinson's disease." *N Engl J Med* 344(10): 710-9

Fulton, G. P. (1957). "Microcirculatory terminology." *Angiology* 8(1): 102-4

Fulton, G. P. and B. R. Lutz (1957). "The use of the hamster cheek pouch and cinephotomicrography for research on the microcirculation and tumor growth, and for teaching purposes." *Bmq* 8(1): 13-9

Furlani, D., M. Ugurlucan, et al. (2009). "Is the intravascular administration of mesenchymal stem cells safe? Mesenchymal stem cells and intravital microscopy." *Microvasc Res* 77(3): 370-6

Gavina, M., M. Belicchi, et al. (2006). "VCAM-1 expression on dystrophic muscle vessels has a critical role in the recruitment of human blood-derived CD133+ stem cells after intra-arterial transplantation." *Blood* 108(8): 2857-66

Ghio, M., P. Contini, et al. (1999). "Soluble HLA class I, HLA class II, and Fas ligand in blood components: a possible key to explain the immunomodulatory effects of allogeneic blood transfusions." *Blood* 93(5): 1770-7

Gibbons, G. H. and V. J. Dzau (1994). "The emerging concept of vascular remodeling." *N Engl J Med* 330(20): 1431-8

Glagov, S., R. Vito, et al. (1992). "Micro-architecture and composition of artery walls: relationship to location, diameter and the distribution of mechanical stress." *J Hypertens Suppl* 10(6): S101-4

Gonzalez, N., Y. Murayama, et al. (2004). "Treatment of unruptured aneurysms with GDCs: clinical experience with 247 aneurysms." *AJNR Am J Neuroradiol* 25(4): 577-83

Gordon, P. H., Q. Yu, et al. (2004). "Reaction time and movement time after embryonic cell implantation in Parkinson disease." *Arch Neurol* 61(6): 858-61

Guglielmi, G., F. Vinuela, et al. (1991). "Electrothrombosis of saccular aneurysms via endovascular approach. Part 1: Electrochemical basis, technique, and experimental results." *J Neurosurg* 75(1): 1-7

Gussoni, E., H. M. Blau, et al. (1997). "The fate of individual myoblasts after transplantation into muscles of DMD patients." *Nat Med* 3(9): 970-7

Guzman, R., A. De Los Angeles, et al. (2008). "Intracarotid injection of fluorescence activated cell-sorted CD49d-positive neural stem cells improves targeted cell delivery and behavior after stroke in a mouse stroke model." *Stroke* 39(4): 1300-6

Hagell, P., P. Piccini, et al. (2002). "Dyskinesias following neural transplantation in Parkinson's disease." *Nat Neurosci* 5(7): 627-8

Haider, H., S. Jiang, et al. (2008). "IGF-1-overexpressing mesenchymal stem cells accelerate bone marrow stem cell mobilization via paracrine activation of SDF-1alpha/CXCR4 signaling to promote myocardial repair." *Circ Res* 103(11): 1300-8

Hirshberg, B., S. Montgomery, et al. (2002). "Pancreatic islet transplantation using the nonhuman primate (rhesus) model predicts that the portal vein is superior to the celiac artery as the islet infusion site." *Diabetes* 51(7): 2135-40

Humar, A., R. Kandaswamy, et al. (2000). "Decreased surgical risks of pancreas transplantation in the modern era." *Ann Surg* 231(2): 269-75

Jin, K., Y. Sun, et al. (2005). "Comparison of ischemia-directed migration of neural precursor cells after intrastriatal, intraventricular, or intravenous transplantation in the rat." *Neurobiol Dis* 18(2): 366-74

Johansson, C. B., M. Svensson, et al. (1999). "Neural stem cells in the adult human brain." *Exp Cell Res* 253(2): 733-6

Justicia, C., A. Martin, et al. (2006). "Anti-VCAM-1 antibodies did not protect against ischemic damage either in rats or in mice." *J Cereb Blood Flow Metab* 26(3): 421-32

Kandaswamy, R., A. Humar, et al. (1999). "Vascular graft thrombosis after pancreas transplantation: comparison of the FK 506 and cyclosporine eras." *Transplant Proc* 31(1-2): 602-3

Kondziolka, D., L. Wechsler, et al. (2000). "Transplantation of cultured human neuronal cells for patients with stroke." *Neurology* 55(4): 565-9

Korsgren, O., T. Lundgren, et al. (2008). "Optimising islet engraftment is critical for successful clinical islet transplantation." *Diabetologia* 51(2): 227-32

Le Blanc, K., I. Rasmusson, et al. (2004). "Treatment of severe acute graft-versus-host disease with third party haploidentical mesenchymal stem cells." *Lancet* 363(9419): 1439-41

Lee, S. T., K. Chu, et al. (2008). "Anti-inflammatory mechanism of intravascular neural stem cell transplantation in haemorrhagic stroke." *Brain* 131(Pt 3): 616-29

Lehmann, R., R. A. Zuellig, et al. (2007). "Superiority of small islets in human islet transplantation." *Diabetes* 56(3): 594-603

Lindvall, O. and Z. Kokaia "Stem cells in human neurodegenerative disorders--time for clinical translation?" *J Clin Invest* 120(1): 29-40

Lindvall, O. and Z. Kokaia (2006). "Stem cells for the treatment of neurological disorders." *Nature* 441(7097): 1094-6

Lundberg, J., S. Jonsson, et al. (2010). "New endovascular method for transvascular exit of arteries and veins: developed in simulator, in rat and in rabbit with full clinical integration." *PLoS One* 5(5): e10449

Lundberg, J., S. Jonsson, et al. (2011). "Long Term Follow-up of the Endovascular Trans-Vessel Wall Technique for Parenchymal Access in Rabbit with Full Clinical Integration." *PLoS One In press*

Lundberg, J., K. Le Blanc, et al. (2009). "Endovascular transplantation of stem cells to the injured rat CNS." *Neuroradiology*

Lundberg, J., E. Sodersten, et al. (2011). "Targeted Intra-arterial Transplantation of Stem Cells to the Injured CNS is More Effective than Intravenous Administration - Engraftment is Dependent on Cell Type and Adhesion Molecule Expression." *Cell Transplant*

Ma, B., K. D. Hankenson, et al. (2005). "A simple method for stem cell labeling with fluorine 18." *Nucl Med Biol* 32(7): 701-5

Mayne, R. (1986). "Collagenous proteins of blood vessels." *Arteriosclerosis* 6(6): 585-93

Meaney, T. F., M. A. Weinstein, et al. (1980). "Digital subtraction angiography of the human cardiovascular system." *AJR Am J Roentgenol* 135(6): 1153-60

Meerschaert, J. and M. B. Furie (1995). "The adhesion molecules used by monocytes for migration across endothelium include CD11a/CD18, CD11b/CD18, and VLA-4 on monocytes and ICAM-1, VCAM-1, and other ligands on endothelium." *J Immunol* 154(8): 4099-112

Merani, S., C. Toso, et al. (2008). "Optimal implantation site for pancreatic islet transplantation." *Br J Surg* 95(12): 1449-61

Merli, M., F. Salerno, et al. (1998). "Transjugular intrahepatic portosystemic shunt versus endoscopic sclerotherapy for the prevention of variceal bleeding in cirrhosis: a randomized multicenter trial. Gruppo Italiano Studio TIPS (G.I.S.T.)." *Hepatology* 27(1): 48-53

Miller, R. G., K. R. Sharma, et al. (1997). "Myoblast implantation in Duchenne muscular dystrophy: the San Francisco study." *Muscle Nerve* 20(4): 469-78

Muller, W. A. (2003). "Leukocyte-endothelial-cell interactions in leukocyte transmigration and the inflammatory response." *Trends Immunol* 24(6): 327-34

Murayama, Y., Y. L. Nien, et al. (2003). "Guglielmi detachable coil embolization of cerebral aneurysms: 11 years' experience." *J Neurosurg* 98(5): 959-66

Nagata, S. (1999). "Fas ligand-induced apoptosis." *Annu Rev Genet* 33: 29-55

Ng, P., M. S. Khangure, et al. (2002). "Endovascular treatment of intracranial aneurysms with Guglielmi detachable coils: analysis of midterm angiographic and clinical outcomes." *Stroke* 33(1): 210-7

Nikolic, B., S. Faintuch, et al. (2009). "Stem cell therapy: a primer for interventionalists and imagers." *J Vasc Interv Radiol* 20(8): 999-1012

Pannier, J. L. and I. Leusen (1973). "Circulation to the brain of the rat during acute and prolonged respiratory changes in the acid-base balance." *Pflugers Arch* 338(4): 347-59

Petri, B. and M. G. Bixel (2006). "Molecular events during leukocyte diapedesis." *Febs J* 273(19): 4399-407

Pittenger, M. F., A. M. Mackay, et al. (1999). "Multilineage potential of adult human mesenchymal stem cells." *Science* 284(5411): 143-7

Potten, C. S. and M. Loeffler (1990). "Stem cells: attributes, cycles, spirals, pitfalls and uncertainties. Lessons for and from the crypt." *Development* 110(4): 1001-20

Pulido, R., M. J. Elices, et al. (1991). "Functional evidence for three distinct and independently inhibitable adhesion activities mediated by the human integrin VLA-4. Correlation with distinct alpha 4 epitopes." *J Biol Chem* 266(16): 10241-5

Raymond, J. and D. Roy (1997). "Safety and efficacy of endovascular treatment of acutely ruptured aneurysms." *Neurosurgery* 41(6): 1235-45; discussion 1245-6

Richter, G. M., G. Noeldge, et al. (1990). "Transjugular intrahepatic portacaval stent shunt: preliminary clinical results." *Radiology* 174(3 Pt 2): 1027-30

Ringden, O., M. Uzunel, et al. (2006). "Mesenchymal stem cells for treatment of therapy-resistant graft-versus-host disease." *Transplantation* 81(10): 1390-7

Rothlein, R., M. L. Dustin, et al. (1986). "A human intercellular adhesion molecule (ICAM-1) distinct from LFA-1." *J Immunol* 137(4): 1270-4

Ryan, E. A., J. R. Lakey, et al. (2001). "Clinical outcomes and insulin secretion after islet transplantation with the Edmonton protocol." *Diabetes* 50(4): 710-9

Scharp, D. W., P. E. Lacy, et al. (1991). "Results of our first nine intraportal islet allografts in type 1, insulin-dependent diabetic patients." *Transplantation* 51(1): 76-85

Seldinger, S. I. (1953). "Catheter replacement of the needle in percutaneous arteriography; a new technique." *Acta radiol* 39(5): 368-76

Shapiro, A. M., J. R. Lakey, et al. (1995). "Portal vein thrombosis after transplantation of partially purified pancreatic islets in a combined human liver/islet allograft." *Transplantation* 59(7): 1060-3

Shapiro, A. M., J. R. Lakey, et al. (2000). "Islet transplantation in seven patients with type 1 diabetes mellitus using a glucocorticoid-free immunosuppressive regimen." *N Engl J Med* 343(4): 230-8

Siminiak, T., D. Fiszer, et al. (2005). "Percutaneous trans-coronary-venous transplantation of autologous skeletal myoblasts in the treatment of post-infarction myocardial contractility impairment: the POZNAN trial." *Eur Heart J* 26(12): 1188-95

Slavin, S., A. Nagler, et al. (1998). "Nonmyeloablative stem cell transplantation and cell therapy as an alternative to conventional bone marrow transplantation with lethal cytoreduction for the treatment of malignant and nonmalignant hematologic diseases." *Blood* 91(3): 756-63

Soderman, M., D. Babic, et al. (2008). "Brain imaging with a flat detector C-arm : Technique and clinical interest of XperCT." *Neuroradiology* 50(10): 863-8

Soderman, M., D. Babic, et al. (2005). "3D roadmap in neuroangiography: technique and clinical interest." *Neuroradiology* 47(10): 735-40

Springer, T. A. (1994). "Traffic signals for lymphocyte recirculation and leukocyte emigration: the multistep paradigm." *Cell* 76(2): 301-14

Stamm, C., B. Westphal, et al. (2003). "Autologous bone-marrow stem-cell transplantation for myocardial regeneration." *Lancet* 361(9351): 45-6

Stoeckel, D., A. Pelton, et al. (2004). "Self-expanding nitinol stents: material and design considerations." *Eur Radiol* 14(2): 292-301

Stuve, O., R. Gold, et al. (2008). "alpha4-Integrin antagonism with natalizumab: effects and adverse effects." *J Neurol* 255 Suppl 6: 58-65

Sykova, E., A. Homola, et al. (2006). "Autologous bone marrow transplantation in patients with subacute and chronic spinal cord injury." *Cell Transplant* 15(8-9): 675-87

Thomas, E., R. Storb, et al. (1975). "Bone-marrow transplantation (first of two parts)." *N Engl J Med* 292(16): 832-43

Thomas, E. D., R. Storb, et al. (1975). "Bone-marrow transplantation (second of two parts)." *N Engl J Med* 292(17): 895-902

Thompson, C. A., B. A. Nasseri, et al. (2003). "Percutaneous transvenous cellular cardiomyoplasty. A novel nonsurgical approach for myocardial cell transplantation." *J Am Coll Cardiol* 41(11): 1964-71

Thomson, J. A., J. Itskovitz-Eldor, et al. (1998). "Embryonic stem cell lines derived from human blastocysts." *Science* 282(5391): 1145-7

Tuma, R. F. (2008). Microcirculation. Amsterdam, Academic Press.

Vacanti, J. P. and R. Langer (1999). "Tissue engineering: the design and fabrication of living replacement devices for surgical reconstruction and transplantation." *Lancet* 354 Suppl 1: SI32-4

Wennersten, A., X. Meier, et al. (2004). "Proliferation, migration, and differentiation of human neural stem/progenitor cells after transplantation into a rat model of traumatic brain injury." *J Neurosurg* 100(1): 88-96

Vestweber, D. and J. E. Blanks (1999). "Mechanisms that regulate the function of the selectins and their ligands." *Physiol Rev* 79(1): 181-213

White, S. A., R. F. James, et al. (2001). "Human islet cell transplantation--future prospects." *Diabet Med* 18(2): 78-103

Villiger, P., E. A. Ryan, et al. (2005). "Prevention of bleeding after islet transplantation: lessons learned from a multivariate analysis of 132 cases at a single institution." *Am J Transplant* 5(12): 2992-8

Vulliet, P. R., M. Greeley, et al. (2004). "Intra-coronary arterial injection of mesenchymal stromal cells and microinfarction in dogs." *Lancet* 363(9411): 783-4

Zuk, P. A., M. Zhu, et al. (2001). "Multilineage cells from human adipose tissue: implications for cell-based therapies." *Tissue Eng* 7(2): 211-28

10

Dynamic Relationships of Collagen Extracellular Matrices on Cardiac Differentiation of Human Mesenchymal Stem Cells

Pearly Yong, Ling Qian,
YingYing Chung and Winston Shim
Research and Development Unit, National Heart Centre
Singapore

1. Introduction

Myocardial infarction (MI) results in necrosis, inflammation and scar formation in the myocardium. Such pathological insults place increasing mechanical demands on surviving cardiomyocytes (Boudoulas & Hatzopoulos, 2009). As cardiomyocytes have limited regenerative potential, loss of functional healthy tissue and subsequent left ventricular (LV) remodelling, eventually leads to pathological hypertrophic cardiomyopathy. Hypertrophy of the LV has been documented as a chronic response to MI and invariably progresses to heart failure (Hannigan et al., 2007). Chronic heart failure is a major health problem with patients experiencing a debilitating quality of life.

Cardiac remodelling after MI is characterised by progressive and pathological interstitial fibrosis. During acute phase of cardiac repair, degradation of myocardial extracellular matrix (ECM) coupled with an influx of inflammatory cells and cytokines permits deposition of granulation tissue in the infarct region. At the site of tissue injury, granulation tissue composes of macrophages, myofibroblasts and neovascularisation. Activated myofibroblasts synthesise collagen and other ECM proteins to form dense scar tissue in the infarct in response to inflammatory mediators such as angiotensin II (Ang II) and transforming growth factor-β1 (TGF-β1). Macrophages drive the production of TGF-β1, an essential growth factor for fibroblast production, collagen synthesis and inhibition of collagen degradation (O'Kane & Ferguson, 1997; Sun & Weber, 2000). At the site of MI, increased expression of adhesion molecules (inter-cellular adhesion molecule-1, ICAM-1) and chemoattractant cytokines (monocyte chemotactic protein-1, MCP-1) facilitate migration of inflammatory cells (e.g. macrophages) enabling scavenging of necrotic tissues (Lu et al., 2004). This couples with elevated expression of matrix metalloproteinase-1 (MMP-1) results in remodelling of myocardial ECM by degradation of existing collagen I and III in the injured myocardium (Lu et al., 2004). Furthermore, MMP-9 has been implicated in tissue remodelling by cleaving collagen V at the amino-terminus (Niyibizi et al., 1994). Consequently, this process compromises structural integrity of the ventricles, resulting in myocyte slippage, wall thinning and rupture

(Cleutjens et al., 1995b). Derangements in cardiomyocyte-ECM interactions cause the loss of cellular tensegrity and initiates anoikis in neighbouring healthy tissue (Michel, 2003). It is now well recognised that structural changes in the myocardial ECM can alter collagen-integrin-cytoskeletal-myofibril relations, thus affecting overall geometry and function of the heart (Spinale, 2007).

In non-cartilaginous tissues like the heart, collagen I, III and V are the predominant subtypes of the ECM (Breuls et al., 2009; Linehan et al., 2001). Collagen I is primarily a structural element of the myocardial ECM while collagen V represents a minor, but important component sequestered within collagen I fibres. However, collagen V levels increase in inflammation and scar tissue. The relative resistance of collagen V to mammalian collagenases makes it transiently available during tissue remodelling. The temporal availability of collagen V during active extracellular remodelling implies that it may play an important role in ECM remodelling and tissue stiffness (Breuls et al., 2009; Ruggiero et al., 1994). In fact, collagen V plays a deterministic role in collagenous fibril structure, matrix organisation and stiffness (Fichard et al., 1995).

Binding of ECM to integrins provides a linkage between the ECM and cellular cytoskeleton. Integrins are heterodimeric receptors composed of non-covalently bound α and β subunits. (Brancaccio et al., 2006). Dynamic integrin-ECM interactions result in bidirectional signalling and determines cell morphology, gene expression, migration, proliferation, differentiation and death. Perkins et al. (2010) showed that integrin-mediated adhesion is mandatory for maintenance of the sarcomeric architecture. They proposed that disintegration of the Z-line and progressive muscle degeneration can occur once the adhesion complex comprising of integrins, talin or integrin linked kinase (ILK) is not replenished. In the myocardium, integrins can function as mechanotransducers that transmit mechanical ECM cues to the myocyte, resulting in changes to myocyte biology and function (Ross & Borg, 2001). Integrins $\alpha_2\beta_1$, $\alpha_1\beta_1$, $\alpha_3\beta_1$, $\alpha_v\beta_3$, $\alpha_{IIb}\beta_3$ are collagen binding heterodimers and adhesion to collagen V has been reported to be primarily mediated by integrin $\alpha_2\beta_1$ and $\alpha_1\beta_1$ (Ruggiero et al., 1994). Integrins $\alpha_2\beta_1$ and $\alpha_1\beta_1$ may play a significant role in remodelling of the heart where there is increased collagen synthesis and collagen V expression, although we have previously shown $\alpha_v\beta_3$, but not $\alpha_2\beta_1$, in a collagen V associated cardiac differentiation of human mesenchymal stem cells (hMSCs) (Tan et al., 2010).

Increased ejection fraction (EF) and fractional shortening (FS) parameters, coupled with a reduction in the amount of fibrotic scar tissue have been highlighted following cellular therapy (Chacko et al., 2009). Our previous study showed that cardiomyocyte-like cells (CLCs) that were differentiated from MSCs, improved systolic performance without compromising end-diastolic pressure of the infarcted myocardium when compared to MSCs. CLCs may facilitate hemodynamic recovery by preserving tissue elasticity in the collagen V-expressing peri-infarct borders. This unique cell/matrix relationship may be more conducive to a functionally adaptive remodelling response in maintaining contractile efficiency of post-infarcted myocardium (Tan et al., 2010).

Experimental data show that MSC transplantation inhibits LV remodelling and improves heart function in animals with MI (Xu et al., 2005). Despite the ability of angiogenic mechanisms to reduce infarct mass, only partial restoration of ventricular contraction occurs as myocytes are not regenerated (Gaudette & Cohen, 2006). In addition, cardiac differentiation and retention of surviving transplanted MSCs in-vivo is limited (Feygin et al.,

2007). Influence of ECM proteins and integrin interactions on MSC differentiation have been widely investigated for chrondrogenic and osteogenic differentiation (Djouad et al., 2007; Gronthos et al., 2001). Conversely, studies investigating ECM role in cardiac differentiation of MSCs is limited. Unravelling of integrin roles in cardiac differentiation of MSCs would aid in understanding of mechanisms leading to retention and integration of stem cells in myocardium.

We have previously reported in-vitro differentiation of human MSCs towards CLCs and shown that collagen V promoted adhesion and cardiac gene expression in CLCs (Shim et al., 2004; Tan et al., 2010). In the present study, we further examine the role of individual integrins in cardiac differentiation of CLCs.

2. Materials and methods

2.1 Isolation and culture of bone marrow derived MSCs

Bone marrow was isolated from the sternum of patients undergoing open-heart surgery. They were collected in 17 IU/ml heparin using a 23-gauge needle. Bone marrow aspirates were topped up to 15 ml with Dulbecco's modified Eagle's medium-low glucose (DMEM-LG, GIBCO) supplemented with 10% fetal bovine serum (FBS, Hyclone) and 1% penicillin-streptomycin (Gibco, Invitrogen). To deplete bone marrow asiprates of mature blood lineages, 15 ml of bone marrow blood mixture was overlaid onto 15 ml of Histopaque®-1077 (Sigma-Aldrich) and centrifuged for 1500 rpm (Kubota Centrifuge) for 30 minutes at 4°C. The enriched cell fraction was collected from the interphase, washed once with 5 ml of media and centrifuged at 1200 rpm (Kubota Centrifuge) for 10 minutes. Resuspended cells were then transferred into tissue culture flasks with basal normal growth medium (NGM) comprising DMEM-LG supplemented with 10% FBS for 9 - 11 days to yield plastic adherent MSCs. Subconfluent cells were harvested using 1X Trypsin-EDTA solution for endothelial cell culture (Sigma-Aldrich), 14 – 21 days after initial plating and maintained as MSCs in basal NMG or differentiated towards CLCs in a myogenic differentiation medium (MDM) as previously described (Shim et al., 2004).

Type V collagen (Sigma-Aldrich) and Type I collagen (BD™) were coated on 6-well plates or tissue culture flasks at $10\mu g/cm^2$ for 3 hours at room temperature. Plates and flasks were washed twice with phosphate buffered saline (PBS) and kept at 4°C until required.

2.2 Fluorescence microscopy

Frozen tissue sections of the explanted ventricular rat hearts were fixed in 4% paraformaldehyde (PFA), permeabilised with 0.1% Triton X-100, and further blocked in 5% bovine serum albumin (BSA). This was followed by overnight incubation at 4°C with primary antibodies, including collagen I (Southern Biotech), collagen III (Affinity Bioregent) collagen V (Biotrend) and anti-α-sarcomeric actinin (Sigma-Aldrich) diluted in 1% BSA. Sections were incubated with Alexa Fluor® 488/555/660 - conjugated secondary antibodies (Molecular Probes) in 0.1% BSA at room temperature for 3 hours before staining the nuclei with DAPI. Immunofluorescence microscopy was performed with Zeiss Axiovert 200 M fluorescence microscope, using the Metamorph software (version 6.2, Molecular Devices) or Leica MZ 16 FA Fluorescence Steromicroscope, using the Leica Application Suite software (Version 3.3.0, Leica).

2.3 Flow cytometry

Sternum-derived bone marrow MSCs were differentiated into CLCs and characterised by flow cytometry after 14 days in a MDM. CLCs cultured on uncoated, collagen I or V coated tissue culture flasks were stained with antibodies directed towards integrin subunits α_1 (Abcam), α_2 (Santa Cruz), α_v (Fitzgerald), β_1 (Chemicon) and β_3 (Cell Signaling). Cells were treated with Fix & Perm® Cell Permeabilisation Kit (Invitrogen) and subsequently blocked in PBS containing 5% BSA, 1% FBS and 5 mM ethylenediaminetetracetic acid (EDTA) for 30 minutes at 4°C on a roller. CLCs were then incubated with directly conjugated antibodies for 30 minutes at 4°C. Indirectly conjugated antibodies were incubated for 2 hours at 4°C and subsequently stained with their respective Alexa Fluor® 555 conjugated secondary antibodies (Invitrogen) for 2 hours at 4°C. Isotype controls were stained in parallel with the test samples. Samples were washed in PBS containing 2% BSA, 2% FBS and 5 mM EDTA after each antibody staining and fixation step. All samples were fixed in PBS containing 4% PFA/PBS, washed and resuspended in PBS containing 2% FBS and 0.09% sodium azide (NaZ). Data analysis was performed using FACSDiva software (version 6.1.2, BD™), FlowJo software (version 6.4, Tree Star, Inc.). Histogram overlays were performed and the change in median fluorescence intensity and overton subtraction percentages were computed.

2.4 Integrin neutralisation assays

Integrin neutralisation assays were performed on CLCs using neutralising antibodies against the integrin α_1 (Millipore) subunit and $\alpha_v\beta_3$ (Millipore) heterodimer, at 1μg/ml and 10 μg/ml respectively. CLCs treated with 1μg/ml or 10 μg/ml isotype IgG (Abcam/Dako) antibodies and untreated CLCs served as controls. After trypsin digestion, CLCs were incubated with neutralising and isotype control antibodies for 2 hours at 4°C. 50,000 untreated and treated CLCs were seeded on collagen V pre-coated 6-well plates. Plated CLCs were harvested after 72 hours of culture at 37°C, 5% CO_2. Total RNA was extracted using the RNeasy Mini Kit (Qiagen) and treated with RNAse free DNase solution (Qiagen). DNAse treated RNA samples were stored at -80°C until required.

2.5 Real-time reverse transcriptase polymerase chain reaction for quantitation of cardiac gene expression

First strand cDNA was synthesised from total RNA using the SuperScript™ III First-Strand Synthesis System (Invitrogen) and equal concentrations of cDNA were loaded into tubes containing QuantiFast SYBR Green PCR mastermix (Qiagen). Real-time reverse transcriptase polymerase chain reaction (RT-PCR) was performed on the Rotor-Gene Q thermocycler (Qiagen) using standard cycling parameters and relative gene expression of the following cardiac transcripts was quantitated using the $\Delta\Delta C_T$ method. These transcripts include β actin (BA), cardiac α-actin (CAA), skeletal muscle α-actin (SKAA), troponin T (Trop T), troponin C (Trop C), Nkx2.5 and GATA4 (Sigma-Aldrich). Target gene expression values were normalised relative to the untreated CLCs. BA served as a housekeeping gene for the real time RT-PCR experiments. No template controls were concurrently processed with test samples to rule out the presence of contaminated reagents and nucleic acids.

Gene	Acession Number	Primer Sequence	Product Size (bp)
CAA	NM_005159	5'-CTTCTAAGATGCCTTCTCTCTCCA-3'	147
		5'-TAT TAG AAG CAC AAA CAA ATT GCA-3'	
SKAA	NM_001100.3	5'-CGAGACCACCTACAACAGCA-3'	132
		5'-GCGGTGATCTCTTTCTGCAT-3'	
Trop C	NM_003280.2	5'-CTACAAGGCTGCGGTAGAGC-3'	76
		5'-CAGCACGAAGATGTCGAAGG-3'	
Trop T	NM_000364.2	5'-ATCCCCGATGGAGAGAGAGT-3'	128
		5'-ACGAGCTCCTCCTCCTCTTT-3'	
Nkx2.5	NM_004387	5'-GATTCCGCAGAGCAACTCG-3'	105
		5'-GGAGCTGTTGAGGTGGGATCG-3'	
GATA4	NM_002052.3	5'-TCCAAACCAGAAAACGGAAG-3'	77
		5'-AAGGCTCTCACTGCCTGAAG-3'	
BA	NM_001101	5'-TCCCTGGAGAAGAGCTACGA-3'	194
		5'-AGCACTGTGTTGGCGTACAG-3'	

Table 1. Primer sequences for real time reverse transcriptase polymerase chain reaction (RT-PCR). Transcripts obtained from RT-PCR assays were all less than 200 bp. CAA, cardiac α-actin; SKAA, skeletal muscle α-actin; Trop T, troponin T; Trop C, troponin C; BA, β actin.

2.6 Cell labelling

CLCs were labelled with 1 mmol/L Vybrant CellTracker chloromethyldialkylcarbocyanie (CM-Dil; Molecular Probes) overnight at 37°C and rinsed 3 times before trypsin disgestion and transplantation. MSCs were labelled with 10mmol/L Vybrant carboxy fluorescein diacetate succinimidyl ester (CFDA-SE; Molecular Probes). Cells were resuspended in a final concentration of $1 \times 10^6/0.1$ ml to $5 \times 10^6/0.2$ ml.

2.7 Rat myocardial infarction model

MI was created in n=20 female Wistar rats per group. Each rat weighed approximately 350 - 400g in body weight. The animals were subjected to left thoracotomy and the left anterior descending artery (LAD) was exposed and ligated. After which rats were allowed a week for recovery before given treatment of either injection with labelled cells or placebo to the area of infarction. Cyclosporin A was administered at a dose of 5mg/kg body weight at 3 days before and daily following treatment for 6 weeks until end point.

2.8 Echocardiography

Baseline echocardiography was performed on each rat before MI and 6 weeks after treatment. Echocardiography images were acquired using Vivid 7 ultrasound machine (General Electric VingMed) equipped with i13L linear probe operated at 14MHz. Rats were anaesthetised using 1% - 2% isofluorane with 1L/hr oxygen and then fixed in the supine position on a heated platform. Rats were then shaved at the chest and abdominal areas before electrocardiography (ECG) electrodes were placed onto the left and right leg as well as the left upper extremity. All analysis was performed offline with EchoPAC workstation (General Electric Healthcare).

2.9 Statistical analysis

One-way analysis of variance (ANOVA) was used to determine statistical significance between different treatment groups. Tukey Honestly Significant Difference (HSD) post-hoc analyses were used to determine statistical significance between treatment groups using SPSS 13 software (SPSS Inc.). $p < 0.05$ was considered statistically significant. All data are presented as mean ± standard deviation (SD).

3. Results

3.1 Integrin expression and cardiac differentiation

Flow cytometric analysis showed that α_v and β_1 were the predominant subunits of integrins in CLCs, independent of substrate surface (Table 2). In comparison to collagen V matrix, CLCs cultured on collagen I showed a higher expression of integrin α_1 (59.4 ± 13.7% vs. 78.0 ± 0.9%) and β_3 (44.7 ± 10.6% vs. 56.0 ± 21.8%) subunits. Furthermore, with the exception of α_1 subunit, α_2, α_v, β_1 and β_3 integrins in CLCs cultured on either collagen matrices showed a reduction of expression in comparison to CLCs cultured on polystyrene tissue culture surface.

	CLC		
Integrin Subunit	Uncoated	Collagen I	Collagen V
α1	58.5 ± 1.8	78.0 ± 0.9	59.4 ± 13.7
α2	59.4 ± 6.1	39.9 ± 11.5	44.3 ± 12.8
αv	91.6 ± 0.5	83.8 ± 5.7	81.8 ± 4.6
β1	93.4 ± 0.8	78.5 ± 8.6	79.1 ± 8.6
β3	57.6 ± 2.4	56.0 ± 21.8	44.7 ± 10.6

Table 2. Flow cytometric analysis showed that integrin α_v and β_1 were the predominant subunits in CLCs. CLCs cultured on collagen I showed increased levels of α_1 and β_3. Data were derived from 3 independent experiments and the overton percentage positive results are expressed as mean ± SD. MSCs, Mesenchymal stem cells; CLCs, Cardiomyocyte-like cells.

3.2 CLCs enhance cardiac gene expression via integrin α_1 and $\alpha_v\beta_3$ on collagen V matrices

We previously reported that collagen V matrix enhanced cardiac gene expression when compared to CLCs seeded on collagen I matrix. Collagen V selectively upregulated expression of cardiac transcription factors (GATA4, Nkx2.5), calcium handling transporter (RyR2) and sarcomeric myofilament proteins (Trop T, Trop C, SKAA) in CLCs (Tan et al., 2010). Neutralisation of $\alpha_v\beta_3$ integrin or α_1 subunit in this study did not affect CAA and SKAA gene expression in CLCs that were cultured on collagen V matrix. Furthermore, no significant changes in Nkx2.5 or GATA4 expression was observed in α_1 subunit neutralised CLCs. However, Nkx2.5 down regulation was observed in CLCs neutralised with $\alpha_v\beta_3$, although similar down regulation was also evident in the isotype control experiment. Gene expression of Trop C reduced significantly after $\alpha_v\beta_3$ integrin neutralisation. In contrary, α_1

subunit neutralisation upregulated Trop C expression. Furthermore, there was a concomitant upregulation of Trop T following α_1 integrin neutralisation.

Integrin Neutralisation Antibody	CAA		SKAA		Trop C		Nkx2.5		Trop T		GATA4	
	Isotype	Test	Isotype	Test	Isotype	Test	Isotype	Test	Isotype	Test	Isotype	Test
$\alpha_v \beta_3$	0.87 ± 0.00	1.00 ± 0.10	1.32 ± 0.13	1.15 ± 0.00	0.94 ± 0.10	0.12 ± 0.02	0.23 ± 0.21	0.22 ± 0.16	N.D.	N.D.	N.D.	N.D.
α_1	0.52 ± 0.05	0.91 ± 0.02	0.99 ± 0.12	1.02 ± 0.10	1.17 ± 0.11	1.45 ± 0.40	1.02 ± 0.22	0.90 ± 0.22	1.04 ± 0.05	1.63 ± 0.16	0.87 ± 0.00	0.63 ± 0.45

Table 3. CLCs cultured on collagen V were treated with integrin α_1 (1 µg/ml) neutralising antibodies. Untreated and isotype IgG (1 µg/ml) treated CLCs served as controls for this experiment. Optimal concentrations of test and control antibodies were predetermined in a series of titration experiments. CLCs cultured on collagen V were treated with integrin $\alpha_v \beta_3$ (10 µg/ml) neutralising antibodies. Untreated and isotype IgG (10 µg/ml) treated CLCs served as controls for this experiment. Results are expressed as mean ± SD. CAA, cardiac α-actin; SKAA, skeletal muscle α-actin; Trop T, troponin T; Trop C, troponin C, N.D., not done; MSCs, Mesenchymal stem cells; CLCs, Cardiomyocyte-like cells.

3.3 CLCs integrate into collagen V-rich cardiac syncytium

Consistent with our previous report (Tan et al., 2010), collagen I as the main constituent of cardiac ECM in intact rat myocardium, was found to co-localise with collagen III matrix in the epicardium and perimysial space between major muscle bundles dispersed throughout the myocardium (Fig. 1A). On the other hand, collagen V was predominantly observed in the endomysial space surrounding healthy cardiomyocytes and in the perivascular structures within the myocardium. Following MI by ligating the LAD artery, significant wall thinning was observed in the anterior wall of the LV (Fig.1B). Accumulation of collagen matrices was evident in the infarcted and non-infarcted zones 7 weeks post infarction. Spatial remodelling and redistribution of collagen matrices were observed whereby perimysial collagen I diminished significantly and upregulation of collagen I and III were observed in the pericardium and epicardium of infarcted as well as non-infarcted zones. Furthermore, fibrosis consisted mainly of collagen I matrix was prominently found in the endocardium of infarcted zone while it co-localised with collagen III matrix in the pericardium/epicardium of the non-infarcted and infarcted zones (Fig. 1Bii & 1Biii). In contrast, collagen V fibrils were sparsely detected in the epicardium of infarct, but were prominently found in the peri-vascular structures within the infarct (Fig. 1Biii). In contrast to redistribution of collagen I matrix, collagen V remained in the endomysial matrix of individual muscle fibres in the non-infarcted borders (Fig.1Bii) and also surrounding isolated, but viable cardiac fibres in the infarct.

Myocardial transplanted CLCs were closely associated with collagen V matrix in the endomysial space in the peri-infarct border of the myocardium (Fig. 2A). In contrast, similarly transplanted MSCs were only found in collagen I-rich infarct despite the presence of isolated, collagen V-expressing, myofibres at the infarct borders (Fig. 2B). Furthermore, CLCs were often intimately engrafted among α-actinin stained native cardiomyocytes that were surrounded by collagen V, but not collagen I, matrices (Fig. 2C and 2D). On the contrary, transplanted MSCs were sequestered in the infarct that was dominated with collagen I matrix and isolated from viable and α-actinin stained myocardium that expressed collagen V matrix (Fig. 2E).

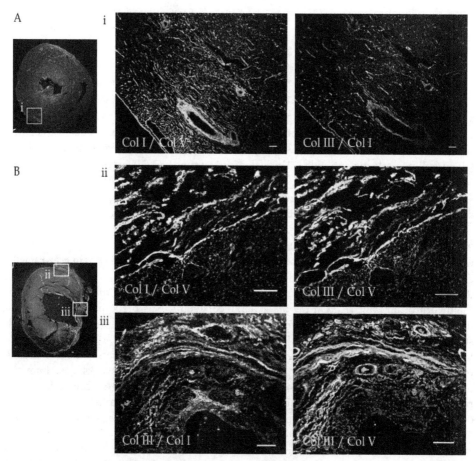

Fig. 1. (A) Collagen distribution in an intact myocardium. (Ai) Higher magnification of the boxed area showing collagen I and III distribution in the perimysium while collagen V was expressed in the endomysial space. (B) Collagen distribution in an infarcted myocardium. (Bii) Higher magnification of the myocardium, epicardium and pericardium at the boxed area. Collagen V was predominantly expressed at the peri-infarct border surrounding viable myocytes and vasculature structures in the infarct region. Collagen I and III were positively stained in the infarcted epicardium and pericardium. (Biii) Higher magnification demonstrating severe thinning of the LV anterior wall. Co-localisation of collagen I and III extended from the pericardium into the infarcted myocardium whereas collagen I was primarily localised in the endocardium. Collagen V was expressed in the vessels and sparsely in the infarct. Scale bar: 200μm.

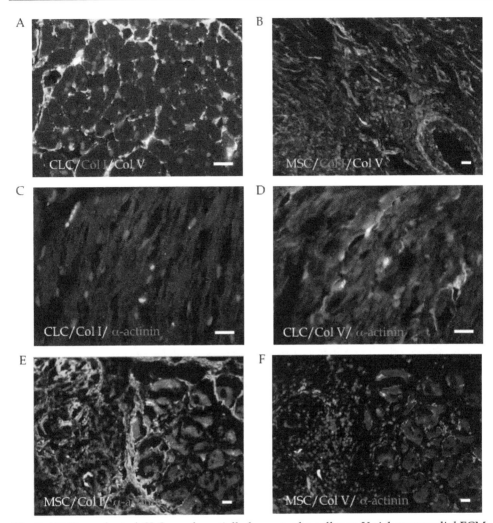

Fig. 2. (A) Transplanted CLCs preferentially home to the collagen V-rich myocardial ECM.
(B) Transplanted MSCs localised in the collagen I enriched infarct zone away from the
collagen V peri-infarct region. (C) Engraftment of CLCs in the α-actinin stained
myocardium (D) showing an affinity towards collagen V matrix in the absence of collagen
I staining. (E) MSCs were embedded in the collagen I-rich infarct zone and were isolated
from α-actinin expressing cardiomyocytes. (F) Collagen V was sparsely distributed in the
infarcted region, but mainly surrounded viable myocytes at the peri-infarct border. Scale
bar: 20μm. MSCs: Mesenchymal stem cells; CLCs: Cardiomyocyte-like cells; Col I:
Collagen I; Col V: Collagen V.

3.4 CLC therapy at high doses improve cardiac hemodynamics

Consistent with their muscular engraftment, LV echocardiography confirmed a better
cardiac performance of transplanted CLCs, 6 weeks post cell transplant (Table 4).

Transplanted CLCs (2.2 ± 0.3 mm, p<0.05), but not MSCs (2.1 ± 0.3 mm), improved LV anterior wall thickness as compared to control infarcted animal (1.8 ± 0.4 mm). Nevertheless, other cardiac parameters indicated that CLCs and MSCs contributed comparably to functional improvements by reducing chamber dilatation and moderating negative LV remodelling.

M-Mode	SF (n=15)	MSC (n=19)	CLC (n=17)	Statistical Significance
LVIDed (mm)	7.7 ± 0.9	7.3 ± 0.6	7.1 ± 0.7	NS
LVIDes (mm)	5.0 ± 1.1	4.2 ± 0.6+	4.1 ± 0.9*	+p<0.05 vs. SF *p<0.01 vs. SF
IVSed (mm)	1.3 ± 0.2	1.3 ± 0.1	1.4 ± 0.1	NS
IVSes (mm)	1.8 ± 0.4	2.1 ± 0.3	2.2 ± 0.3*	*p<0.05 vs. SF
AWT (%)	49.8 ± 16.3	53.6 ± 14.7+	54.0 ± 15.6*	+p<0.05 vs. SF *p<0.05 vs. SF
FS (%)	35.0 ± 5.6	42.4 ± 5.3+	43.1 ± 6.6*	+p<0.05 vs. SF *p<0.005 vs. SF
EF (%)	60.4 ± 7.9	68.7 ± 6.3+	69.8 ± 9.5*	+p<0.05 vs. SF *p<0.005 vs. SF

Table 4. Ultrasound echocardiography assessment of post cellular therapy treated rats. 2D ultrasound echocardiography assessments showed significant improvements in cell transplanted animals. SF: Serum free control; CLC: Cardiomyocyte-like-cells; MSCs: Mesenchymal stem cells; LVIDed: Left ventricular internal dimension at end diastolic; LVID: Left ventricular internal dimension at end systolic; IVSed: Interventricular septum at end diastolic, IVSes: Interventricular septum at end systolic; AWT: Anterior wall thickening; FS: Fractional shortening; EF: Ejection fraction.

4. Discussion

Integrins and ECM are important modulators of stem cell behaviours. To date, cardiac cell therapy supported only modest benefits, likely due to low engraftment of transplanted cells in the infarcted myocardium. Exploration of specific integrin/ECM interaction may improve engraftment and survival of transplanted cells and ultimately, mechanical function of the heart. Our current study examines integrin/ECM interactions on cardiac gene expression of CLCs and distribution of transplanted CLCs in infarcted myocardium.

The distribution and quantity of type I and III collagens in the heart play an important role in maintaining cardiac function. Alterations of collagen population and distribution in the myocardium affect size and shape of the heart chambers as well as myocardial diastolic and systolic function (Cleutjens et al., 1995a; Janicki & Brower, 2002). However, it is unclear if such alterations could affect stem cell migration and differentiation in the myocardium.

We have previously demonstrated that CLCs showed preferential adhesion to collagen V over collagen I matrix by interacting with subsets of integrins (Shim et al., 2004; Tan et al., 2010). van Laake et al. (2010) reported that pre and post transplanted human embryonic cardiomyocytes (hESC-CM) express integrins matching ECM types they encountered in their environment. Therefore, the integrin modulating role of collagen V may aid in the observed retention of the myocardial transplanted CLCs. Furthermore, intimate engraftment of the transplanted CLCs with collagen V-expressing, α-actinin positive, native cardiomyocytes supports an unique role of collagen V in the myocardium. Moreover, differential expression of α_1 and β_3 integrin between collagen I and V cultured CLCs coupled with the preferential homing demonstrated between transplanted MSCs and CLCs suggested a key role of collagen V matrix, not only in cellular retention, but cardiac differentiation of the transplanted stem cells. This is consistent with modulation of cardiac gene expression of CLCs demonstrated in relation to α_1 and $\alpha_v\beta_3$ neutralisation in vitro, although such relationship was not examined in vivo. Nevertheless, the comparable cardiac outcomes achieved in spite of selective homing of the transplanted cells, indicate that different reparative mechanisms may be initiated by MSCs and CLCs. Despite a positive trend of systolic improvement by CLCs, further mechanistic studies are warranted to discern their specific contribution to systolic and diastolic components of cardiac performance.

Integrin α_1 is known to transduce ECM signals to the cytoskeleton that activate downstream mitogen activated protein kinase (MAPK) and extracellular signal-regulated kinase 1 (ERK1) signalling pathways that phosphorylate and activate GATA4 (Akazawa & Komuro, 2003). However, GATA4 expression was unaffected by integrin α_1 neutralisation despite the upregulated Trop C and Trop T belonging to downstream genes known to be activated by GATA4 (Liang et al., 2001; Tidyman et al., 2003). Similarly, neutralisation of $\alpha_v\beta_3$ integrin attenuated Trop C expression despite GATA4 was previously shown to be unaffected by neutralisation of $\alpha_v\beta_3$ (Tan et al., 2010). It is unclear if the modulation of myofilamental gene expression demonstrated was secondary to other nuclear transcription factors. However, integrins are known to mechanotransduce signals to activate Raf-MEK-ERK-1/2 cascade that has been shown to elicit cardiomyocyte growth, increased fetal-gene expression and cytoskeletal reorganisation in neonatal cardiomyocytes (Lorenz et al., 2009). Nevertheless, it is unclear if reduced expression of integrin demonstrated on either collagen surface as compared to CLCs cultured on uncoated polystrene surface was associated with enhanced proliferation of CLCs as previously reported (Tan et al 2010). However, contrary to our previous data, SKAA was not down regulated by integrin $\alpha_v\beta_3$ neutralisation in the current study. This could be due to donor variations. Indeed, donor variation in integrin expression has been documented from different bone marrow isolates and passage numbers, resulting in different growth and proliferation potential (ter Brugge et al., 2002).

Despite beneficial effects of collagen V on cardiac gene expression and stem cell distribution, it should be noted that collagen distribution in the infarcted rat hearts may be different from humans during MI. Furthermore, a 3D structure like the heart may transmit different environmental cues to integrins as compared to 2D environments provided in tissue culture experiments. It remains to be determined whether inhibitory antibodies may transactivate other integrin receptors during epitope occupancy. In addition, the promiscuity of integrins renders it technically challenging to identify whether a single integrin or interplay of synergistic interactions between a few integrins is required for regulation of cardiac gene expression. Future studies employing siRNA techniques that selectively silence α_1 or $\alpha_v\beta_3$ integrin may provide additional information regarding the regulation of cardiac gene expression of CLCs on collagen V matrix ex vivo or in the transplanted milieu of infarcted myocardium.

5. Conclusion

In conclusion, our study indicates that α_1 and $\alpha_v\beta_3$ integrins drive cardiac gene expression of CLCs. Integrin families and ECM are important regulators of cardiac differentiation and myocardial distribution of adult MSCs and CLCs. Specific modulation of interaction between subclasses of collagen and integrin subunits in the post-infarct myocardial ECM could potentially offer a unique opportunity in cardiac regenerative medicine.

6. Acknowledgements

This study was supported by grants from National Medical Research Council, Biomedical Research Council and National Research Foundation of Singapore to W.S.

7. References

Akazawa, H., & Komuro, I. (2003). Roles of cardiac transcription factors in cardiac hypertrophy. *Circ Res, 92*(10), 1079-1088.

Boudoulas, K. D., & Hatzopoulos, A. K. (2009). Cardiac repair and regeneration: The rubik's cube of cell therapy for heart disease. *Dis Model Mech, 2*(7-8), 344-358.

Brancaccio, M., Hirsch, E., Notte, A., Selvetella, G., Lembo, G., & Tarone, G. (2006). Integrin signalling: The tug-of-war in heart hypertrophy. *Cardiovasc Res, 70*(3), 422-433.

Breuls, R. G., Klumpers, D. D., Everts, V., & Smit, T. H. (2009). Collagen type v modulates fibroblast behavior dependent on substrate stiffness. *Biochem Biophys Res Commun, 380*(2), 425-429.

Chacko, S. M., Khan, M., Kuppusamy, M. L., Pandian, R. P., Varadharaj, S., Selvendiran, K., et al. (2009). Myocardial oxygenation and functional recovery in infarct rat hearts transplanted with mesenchymal stem cells. *Am J Physiol Heart Circ Physiol, 296*(5), H1263-1273.

Cleutjens, J. P., Kandala, J. C., Guarda, E., Guntaka, R. V., & Weber, K. T. (1995b). Regulation of collagen degradation in the rat myocardium after infarction. *J Mol Cell Cardiol, 27*(6), 1281-1292.

Cleutjens, J. P., Verluyten, M. J., Smiths, J. F., & Daemen, M. J. (1995a). Collagen remodeling after myocardial infarction in the rat heart. *Am J Pathol, 147*(2), 325-338.

Djouad, F., Delorme, B., Maurice, M., Bony, C., Apparailly, F., Louis-Plence, P., et al. (2007). Microenvironmental changes during differentiation of mesenchymal stem cells towards chondrocytes. *Arthritis Res Ther, 9*(2), R33.

Feygin, J., Mansoor, A., Eckman, P., Swingen, C., & Zhang, J. (2007). Functional and bioenergetic modulations in the infarct border zone following autologous mesenchymal stem cell transplantation. *Am J Physiol Heart Circ Physiol, 293*(3), H1772-1780.

Fichard, A., Kleman, J. P., & Ruggiero, F. (1995). Another look at collagen v and xi molecules. *Matrix Biol, 14*(7), 515-531.

Gaudette, G. R., & Cohen, I. S. (2006). Cardiac regeneration: Materials can improve the passive properties of myocardium, but cell therapy must do more. *Circulation, 114*(24), 2575-2577.

Gronthos, S., Simmons, P. J., Graves, S. E., & Robey, P. G. (2001). Integrin-mediated interactions between human bone marrow stromal precursor cells and the extracellular matrix. *Bone, 28*(2), 174-181.

Hannigan, G. E., Coles, J. G., & Dedhar, S. (2007). Integrin-linked kinase at the heart of cardiac contractility, repair, and disease. *Circ Res, 100*(10), 1408-1414.

Janicki, J. S., & Brower, G. L. (2002). The role of myocardial fibrillar collagen in ventricular remodeling and function. *J Card Fail, 8*(6 Suppl), S319-325.

Liang, Q., De Windt, L. J., Witt, S. A., Kimball, T. R., Markham, B. E., & Molkentin, J. D. (2001). The transcription factors gata4 and gata6 regulate cardiomyocyte hypertrophy in vitro and in vivo. *J Biol Chem, 276*(32), 30245-30253.

Linehan, K. A., Seymour, A. M., & Williams, P. E. (2001). Semiquantitative analysis of collagen types in the hypertrophied left ventricle. *J Anat, 198*(Pt 1), 83-92.

Lorenz, K., Schmitt, J. P., Vidal, M., & Lohse, M. J. (2009). Cardiac hypertrophy: Targeting raf/mek/erk1/2-signaling. *Int J Biochem Cell Biol, 41*(12), 2351-2355.

Lu, L., Zhang, J. Q., Ramires, F. J., & Sun, Y. (2004). Molecular and cellular events at the site of myocardial infarction: From the perspective of rebuilding myocardial tissue. *Biochem Biophys Res Commun, 320*(3), 907-913.

Michel, J. B. (2003). Anoikis in the cardiovascular system: Known and unknown extracellular mediators. *Arterioscler Thromb Vasc Biol, 23*(12), 2146-2154.

Niyibizi, C., Chan, R., Wu, J. J., & Eyre, D. (1994). A 92 kda gelatinase (mmp-9) cleavage site in native type v collagen. *Biochem Biophys Res Commun, 202*(1), 328-333.

O'Kane, S., & Ferguson, M. W. (1997). Transforming growth factor beta s and wound healing. *Int J Biochem Cell Biol, 29*(1), 63-78.

Perkins, A. D., Ellis, S. J., Asghari, P., Shamsian, A., Moore, E. D., & Tanentzapf, G. (2010). Integrin-mediated adhesion maintains sarcomeric integrity. *Dev Biol, 338*(1), 15-27.

Ross, R. S., & Borg, T. K. (2001). Integrins and the myocardium. *Circ Res, 88*(11), 1112-1119.

Ruggiero, F., Champliaud, M. F., Garrone, R., & Aumailley, M. (1994). Interactions between cells and collagen v molecules or single chains involve distinct mechanisms. *Exp Cell Res, 210*(2), 215-223.

Shim, W. S., Jiang, S., Wong, P., Tan, J., Chua, Y. L., Tan, Y. S., et al. (2004). Ex vivo differentiation of human adult bone marrow stem cells into cardiomyocyte-like cells. *Biochem Biophys Res Commun, 324*(2), 481-488.

Spinale, F. G. (2007). Myocardial matrix remodeling and the matrix metalloproteinases: Influence on cardiac form and function. *Physiol Rev, 87*(4), 1285-1342.

Sun, Y., & Weber, K. T. (2000). Infarct scar: A dynamic tissue. *Cardiovasc Res, 46*(2), 250-256.

Tan, G., Shim, W., Gu, Y., Qian, L., Chung, Y. Y., Lim, S. Y., et al. (2010). Differential effect of myocardial matrix and integrins on cardiac differentiation of human mesenchymal stem cells. *Differentiation, 79*(4-5), 260-271.

ter Brugge, P. J., Torensma, R., De Ruijter, J. E., Figdor, C. G., & Jansen, J. A. (2002). Modulation of integrin expression on rat bone marrow cells by substrates with different surface characteristics. *Tissue Eng, 8*(4), 615-626.

Tidyman, W. E., Sehnert, A. J., Huq, A., Agard, J., Deegan, F., Stainier, D. Y., et al. (2003). In vivo regulation of the chicken cardiac troponin t gene promoter in zebrafish embryos. *Dev Dyn, 227*(4), 484-496.

van Laake, L. W., van Donselaar, E. G., Monshouwer-Kloots, J., Schreurs, C., Passier, R.,
    Humbel, B. M., et al. (2010). Extracellular matrix formation after transplantation of
    human embryonic stem cell-derived cardiomyocytes. *Cell Mol Life Sci, 67*(2), 277-
    290.
Xu, X., Xu, Z., Xu, Y., & Cui, G. (2005). Effects of mesenchymal stem cell transplantation on
    extracellular matrix after myocardial infarction in rats. *Coron Artery Dis, 16*(4), 245-
    255.

Permissions

The contributors of this book come from diverse backgrounds, making this book a truly international effort. This book will bring forth new frontiers with its revolutionizing research information and detailed analysis of the nascent developments around the world.

We would like to thank Taner Demirer, MD, FACP, for lending his expertise to make the book truly unique. He has played a crucial role in the development of this book. Without his invaluable contribution this book wouldn't have been possible. He has made vital efforts to compile up to date information on the varied aspects of this subject to make this book a valuable addition to the collection of many professionals and students.

This book was conceptualized with the vision of imparting up-to-date information and advanced data in this field. To ensure the same, a matchless editorial board was set up. Every individual on the board went through rigorous rounds of assessment to prove their worth. After which they invested a large part of their time researching and compiling the most relevant data for our readers. Conferences and sessions were held from time to time between the editorial board and the contributing authors to present the data in the most comprehensible form. The editorial team has worked tirelessly to provide valuable and valid information to help people across the globe.

Every chapter published in this book has been scrutinized by our experts. Their significance has been extensively debated. The topics covered herein carry significant findings which will fuel the growth of the discipline. They may even be implemented as practical applications or may be referred to as a beginning point for another development. Chapters in this book were first published by InTech; hereby published with permission under the Creative Commons Attribution License or equivalent.

The editorial board has been involved in producing this book since its inception. They have spent rigorous hours researching and exploring the diverse topics which have resulted in the successful publishing of this book. They have passed on their knowledge of decades through this book. To expedite this challenging task, the publisher supported the team at every step. A small team of assistant editors was also appointed to further simplify the editing procedure and attain best results for the readers.

Our editorial team has been hand-picked from every corner of the world. Their multi-ethnicity adds dynamic inputs to the discussions which result in innovative outcomes. These outcomes are then further discussed with the researchers and contributors who give their valuable feedback and opinion regarding the same. The feedback is then collaborated with the researches and they are edited in a comprehensive manner to aid the understanding of the subject.

Apart from the editorial board, the designing team has also invested a significant amount of their time in understanding the subject and creating the most relevant covers. They scrutinized every image to scout for the most suitable representation of the subject and create an appropriate cover for the book.

The publishing team has been involved in this book since its early stages. They were actively engaged in every process, be it collecting the data, connecting with the contributors or procuring relevant information. The team has been an ardent support to the editorial, designing and production team. Their endless efforts to recruit the best for this project, has resulted in the accomplishment of this book. They are a veteran in the field of academics and their pool of knowledge is as vast as their experience in printing. Their expertise and guidance has proved useful at every step. Their uncompromising quality standards have made this book an exceptional effort. Their encouragement from time to time has been an inspiration for everyone.

The publisher and the editorial board hope that this book will prove to be a valuable piece of knowledge for researchers, students, practitioners and scholars across the globe.

List of Contributors

Stina Simonsson, Cecilia Borestrom and Julia Asp
Department of Clinical Chemistry and Transfusion Medicine, Institute of Biomedicine, University of Gothenburg, Gothenburg, Sweden

Britta Eiz-Vesper and Rainer Blasczyk
Institute for Transfusion Medicine, Hannover Medical School, Hannover, Germany

Jeane Visentainer and Ana Sell
Maringa State University, Brazil

Adriana Gutiérrez-Hoya, Rubén López-Santiago, Octavio Rodríguez-Cortes and Martha Moreno-Lafont
Departamento de Inmunología, Escuela Nacional de Ciencias Biológicas – Instituto Politécnico Nacional, México

Jorge Vela-Ojeda and Laura Montiel-Cervantes
Unidad Médica de Alta Especialidad, Centro Médico Nacional La Raza, Instituto Mexicano del Seguro Social, México

Helga Maria Schmetzer
Department of Medicine III, José Carreras Unit for Hematopoietic Stem Cell Transplantation, Ludwig Maximilian University of Munich, Germany

Christoph Schmid
Stem Cell Transplantation Unit, Klinikum Augsburg, Ludwig Maximilian University of Munich, Germany

Diana N. Eissens, Arnold van der Meer and Irma Joosten
Radboud University Nijmegen Medical Centre, The Netherlands

Nadia Zghoul and Said Dermime
Immunology & Innovative Cell Therapy Unit, Department of Biomedical Research, Dasman Diabetes Institute, Kuwait

Mahmoud Aljurf
Adult Haematology/Oncology, King Faisal Specialist Hospital and Research Centre, Kingdom of Saudi Arabia

Yannick Willemen, Zwi Berneman, Viggo Van Tendeloo and Evelien Smits
Laboratory of Experimental Hematology, Vaccine and Infectious Disease Institute, Belgium

Khadija Guerti
Laboratory of Experimental Hematology, Vaccine and Infectious Disease Institute, Belgium
Laboratory of Medical Microbiology, Vaccine and Infectious Disease Institute, Belgium
Laboratory of Immunology, Antwerp University Hospital, University of Antwerp, Belgium

Herman Goossens
Laboratory of Medical Microbiology, Vaccine and Infectious Disease Institute, Belgium

Johan Lundberg and Staffan Holmin
Department of Clinical Neuroscience, Karolinska Institutet and Department of Neuroradiology, Karolinska University Hospital, Stockholm, Sweden

Pearly Yong, Ling Qian, YingYing Chung and Winston Shim
Research and Development Unit, National Heart Centre, Singapore